Advances in MRI of the Knee for
Osteoarthritis

Advances in MRI of the Knee for
Osteoarthritis

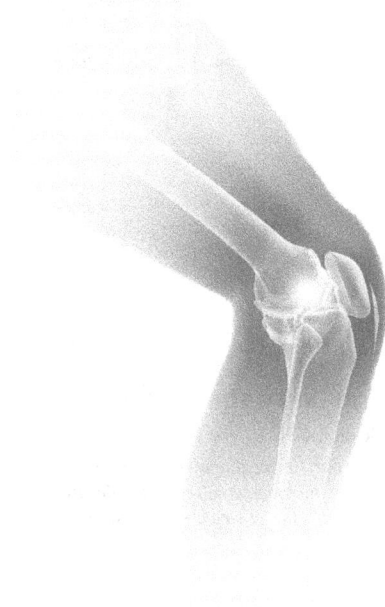

edited by

Sharmila Majumdar
University of California, San Francisco, USA

W🌐 World Scientific

NEW JERSEY · LONDON · SINGAPORE · BEIJING · SHANGHAI · HONG KONG · TAIPEI · CHENNAI

Published by

World Scientific Publishing Co. Pte. Ltd.

5 Toh Tuck Link, Singapore 596224

USA office: 27 Warren Street, Suite 401-402, Hackensack, NJ 07601

UK office: 57 Shelton Street, Covent Garden, London WC2H 9HE

British Library Cataloguing-in-Publication Data
A catalogue record for this book is available from the British Library.

ADVANCES IN MRI OF THE KNEE FOR OSTEOARTHRITIS

ISBN-13 978-981-4271-70-7
ISBN-10 981-4271-70-5

Typeset by Stallion Press
Email: enquiries@stallionpress.com

Contents

8. Bone and Osteoarthritis 235

*by Janet Goldenstein, Gabrielle Blumenkrantz,
Radu I. Bolbos and Xiaojuan Li*

Contributors

Gabrielle Blumenkrantz, PhD
University of California
San Francisco
Department of Radiology and Biomedical Imaging
Joint Bioengineering Graduate Group
University of California San Francisco and
University of California
Berkeley, CA

Radu I. Bolbos, PhD
University of California
San Francisco
Department of Radiology and Biomedical Imaging

Julio Carballido-Gamio, PhD
University of California
San Francisco
Department of Radiology and Biomedical Imaging
Grupo Tecnológica Santa Fe, S. A. de C.V.
Mexico City, Mexico

Ryan Doan
Cleveland Clinic
Lerner College of Medicine
Cleveland OH

Felix Eckstein, MD, PhD
Paracelsus Private Medical University Salzburg
Institute of Anatomy and Musculoskeletal Research
Salzburg, Austria
Chondrometrics GmbH, Ainring
Germany

Janet Goldenstein, PhD
University of California
San Francisco
Department of Radiology and Biomedical Imaging
Joint Bioengineering Graduate Group
University of California San Francisco and
University of California
Berkeley, CA

Brian Hargreaves, PhD
Stanford University
Radiological Sciences Laboratory

Tobias D. Henning, MD
University of California
San Francisco
Department of Radiology and Biomedical Imaging
Technical University of Munich
Germany
Department of Radiology

Alexej Jerschow, PhD
New York University
Chemistry Department
New York, NY

Roland Krug, PhD
University of California
San Francisco
Department of Radiology and Biomedical Imaging

Xiaojuan Li, PhD
University of California
San Francisco
Department of Radiology and Biomedical Imaging
Joint Bioengineering Graduate Group
University of California San Francisco and
University of California
Berkeley, CA

Thomas M. Link, MD
University of California
San Francisco
Department of Radiology and Biomedical Imaging

C. Benjamin Ma, MD
University of California
San Francisco
Department of Orthopaedic Surgery

Sharmila Majumdar, PhD
University of California
San Francisco
Department of Radiology and Biomedical Imaging
Joint Bioengineering Graduate Group
University of California San Francisco and
University of California
Berkeley, CA

Reinhard Meier, MD
University of California
San Francisco
Department of Radiology and Biomedical Imaging
Technical University of Munich
Germany
Department of Radiology

Ravinder R. Regatte, PhD
New York University Langone Medical Center
Center for Biomedical Imaging
Department of Radiology
New York, NY

Michael D. Ries, MD
University of California
San Francisco
Department of Orthopaedic Surgery

Ehsan Saadat
University of California
San Francisco, School of Medicine

Richard B. Souza, PhD, PT
University of California
San Francisco
Department of Radiology and Biomedical Imaging
Department of Physical Therapy and Rehabilitation Science

Preface

In the last decade there has been a focused need for developing non-invasive biomarkers for disease diagnosis, monitoring response to therapy and for designing therapeutics. In the field of musculoskeletal diseases with the aging population, increased activity and sports-related injuries, there has been an increased focus on osteoarthritis. The public-private partnership or the Osteoarthritis Initiative sponsored through the National Institute of Arthritis and Musculoskeletal and Skin Diseases underlines the overwhelming need and keen interest amongst scientists, clinicians, pharmaceutical companies and the government to develop biomarkers for assessing osteoarthritis.

Radiography has been the established tool for assessing osteoarthritis presence, and severity of disease. However, in osteoarthritis, in addition to the bony changes depicted by the X-ray images, cartilage, bone, bone marrow and other tissues are involved. It is within this context that magnetic resonance imaging has been proposed as a non-invasive imaging technique, with potential for quantitative evaluation of the whole joint, including cartilage, bone, meniscus and ligaments.

This book arose from a multi-disciplinary collaboration between radiologists, orthopedic surgeons, engineers and physicists and a recognition within the team that a concise reference guide was needed to introduce the field to a diverse group. It covers the basics of anatomy, etiology of osteoarthritis, methodologies for morphological and functional imaging of cartilage and bone. It is expected that this book will serve as a reference and guide to a wide range of individuals, who are delving into the area of osteoarthritis imaging for the first time, as well as those who are already in the field but in need of a quick refresher.

Sharmila Majumdar, PhD
University of California
San Francisco
Department of Radiology and Biomedical Imaging

1

Anatomy and Physiology of the Knee

by Richard B. Souza and Ryan Doan

Preview

This chapter details the normal anatomy and physiology of the knee. The focus of this chapter centers on those anatomical structures that are involved in osteoarthritis (OA). The chapter begins with MRI images of the healthy knee in all three cardinal planes (Figs. 1 to 3). These images will serve as a source of healthy tissue that can be referred back to in later chapters when discussing pathology within the knee joint.

The knee joint, once described as a simple hinge joint, is in fact a much more complex structure. There are three articulations: one between each femoral condyle and its associated tibial condyle, and one between the patella and the femur. This joint is a common location for pathology, with OA being one of the most common conditions affecting the knee. The three bones that form the knee joint (femur, tibia, and patella) are covered in thick articular cartilage and supported by several ligaments both inside and outside the joint capsule. Furthermore, the knee joint is supported by muscles on the anterior, medial and posterior aspects of the joint. The lateral joint is supported by dense connective tissue. Inside the joint, two fibrocartilagenous crescent-shaped menisci provide cushioning and improve joint congruity. Additional supportive anatomy includes several bursae and fat pads located throughout the knee joint. From the architecture and physiology of bone to the integrity of the menisci, the knee requires an orchestra of events to protect the articular cartilage from the degenerative process of OA.

1

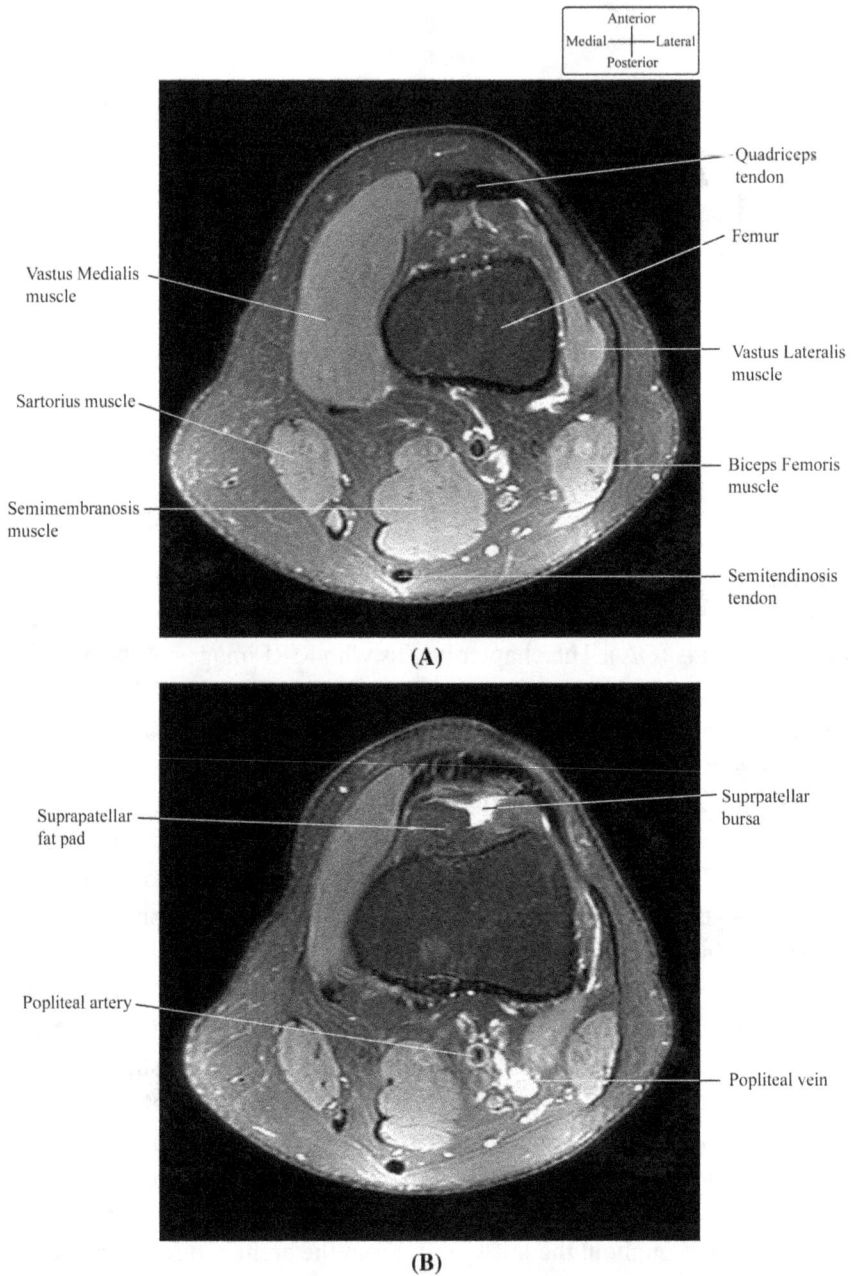

Fig. 1. Axial T_2-weighted magnetic resonance images of the knee and surrounding structures.

(C)

(D)

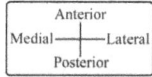

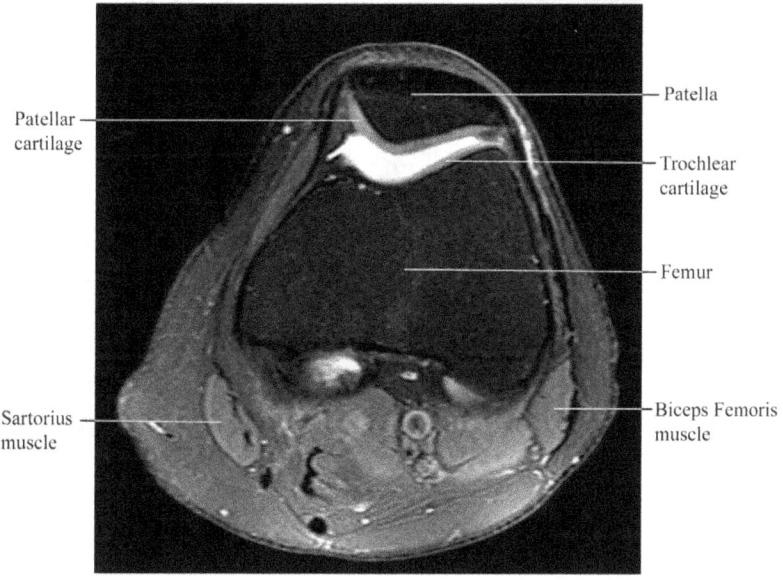

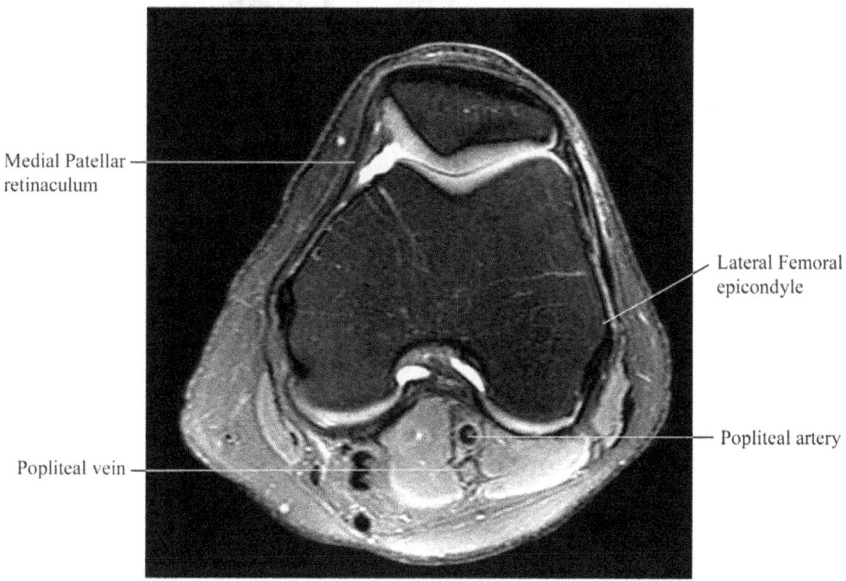

Fig. 1. (*Continued*)

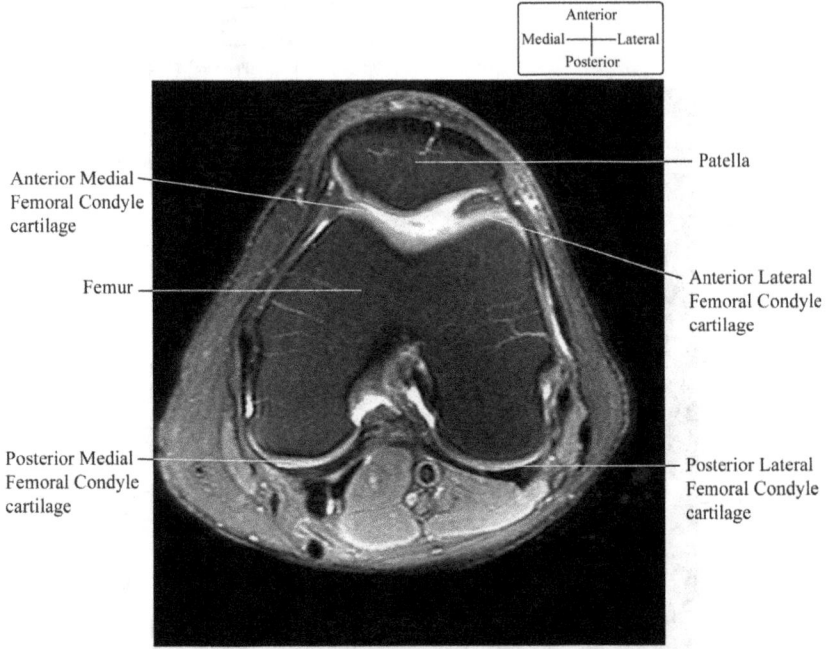

(E)

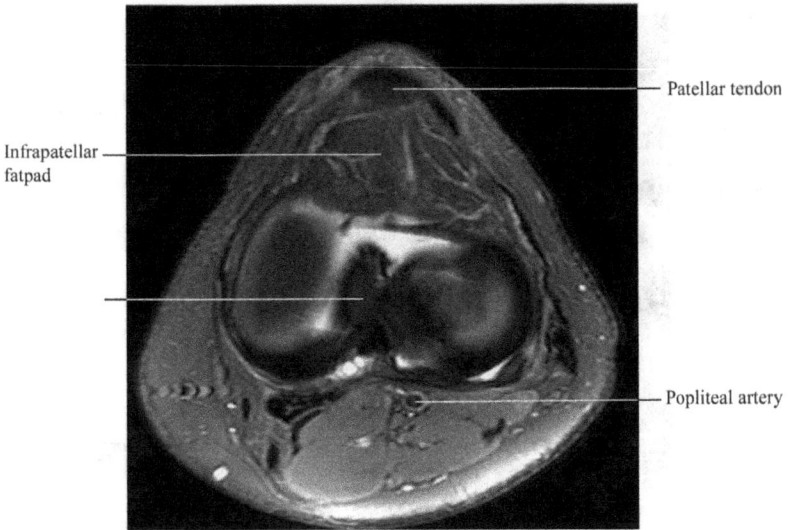

(F)

Fig. 1. (*Continued*)

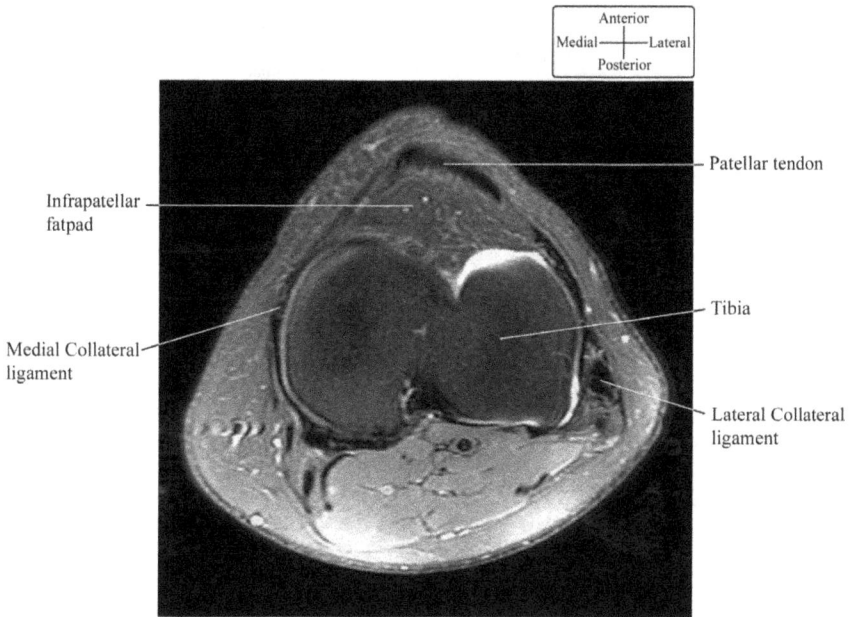

Anterior
Medial——Lateral
Posterior

Patellar tendon

Infrapatellar fatpad

Tibia

Medial Collateral ligament

Lateral Collateral ligament

(G)

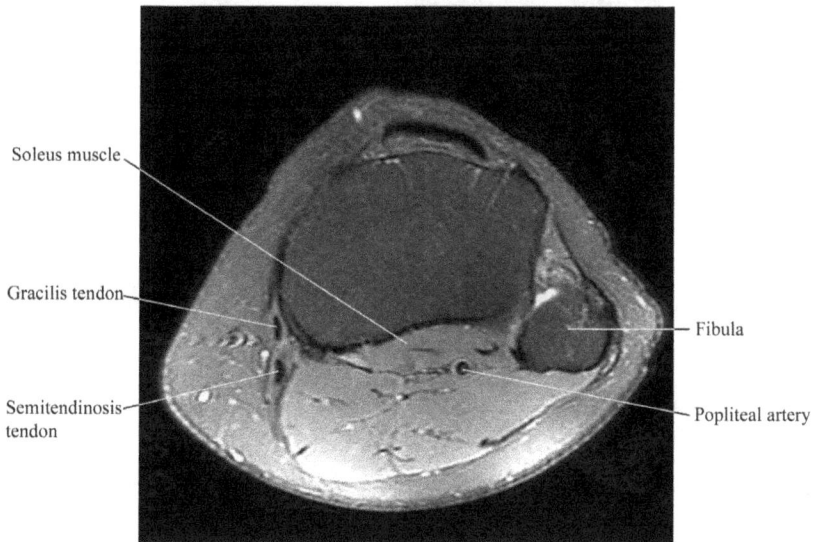

Soleus muscle

Gracilis tendon

Fibula

Semitendinosis tendon

Popliteal artery

(H)

Fig. 1. *(Continued)*

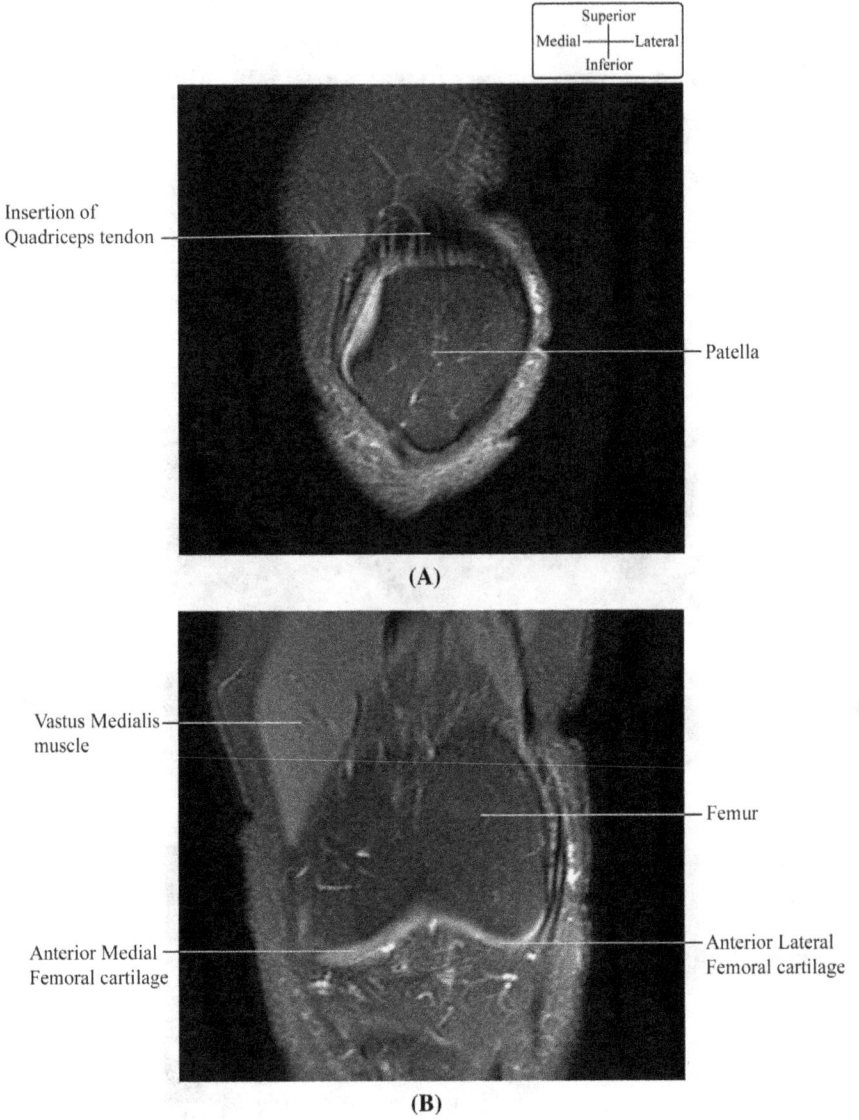

Fig. 2. Coronal T$_2$-weighted magnetic resonance images of the knee and surrounding structures.

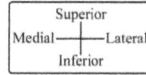

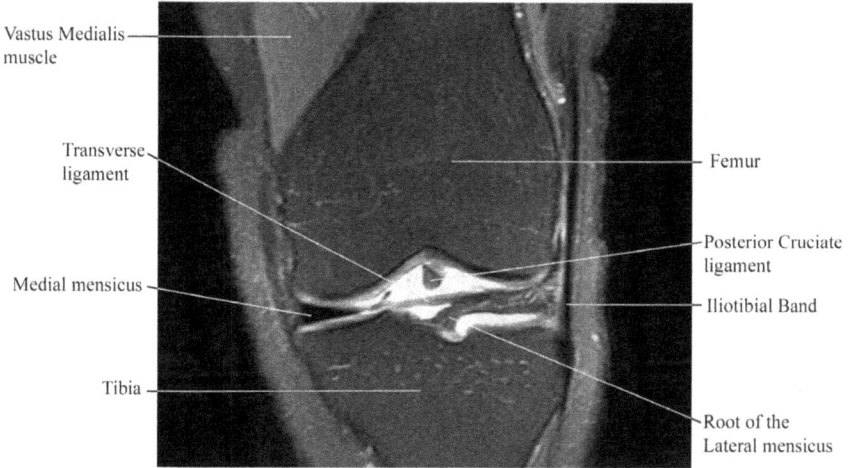

(C)

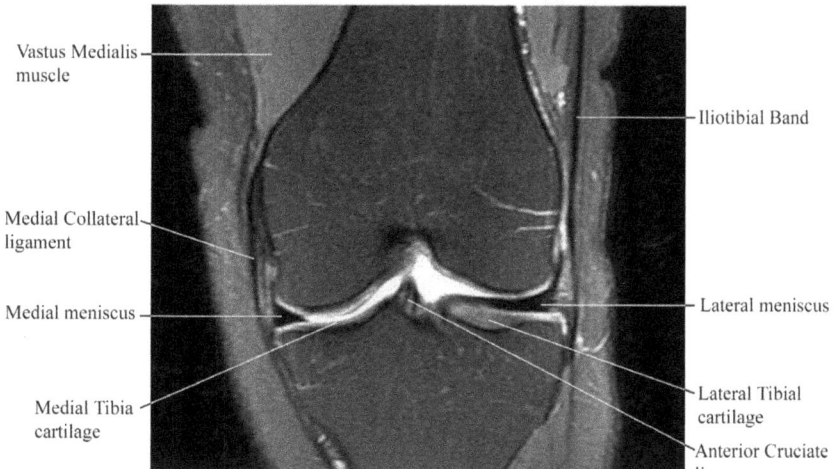

(D)

Fig. 2. (*Continued*)

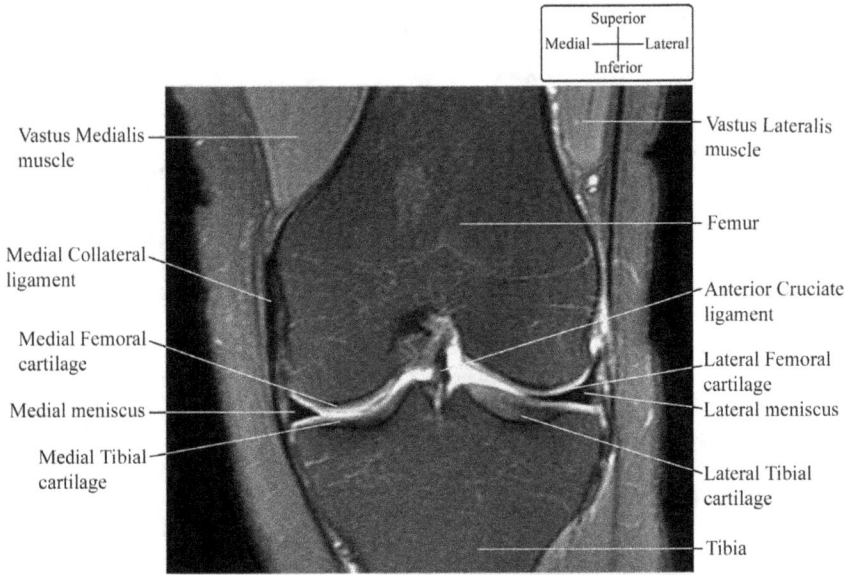

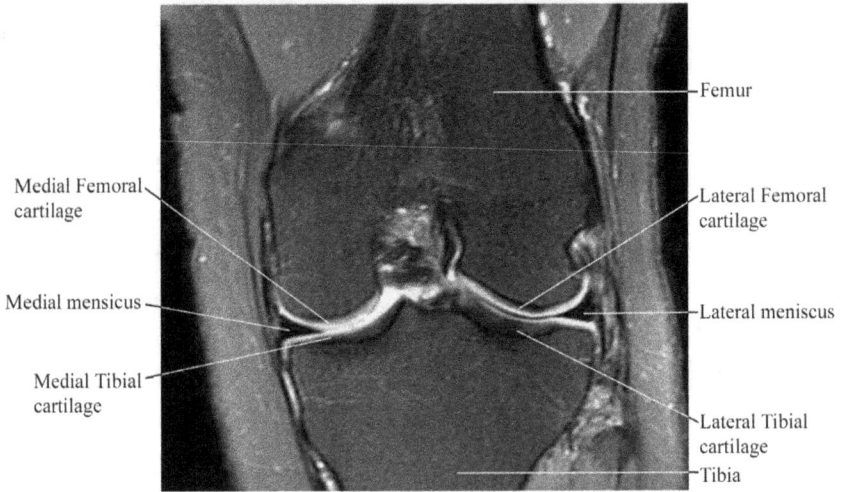

Fig. 2. (*Continued*)

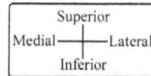

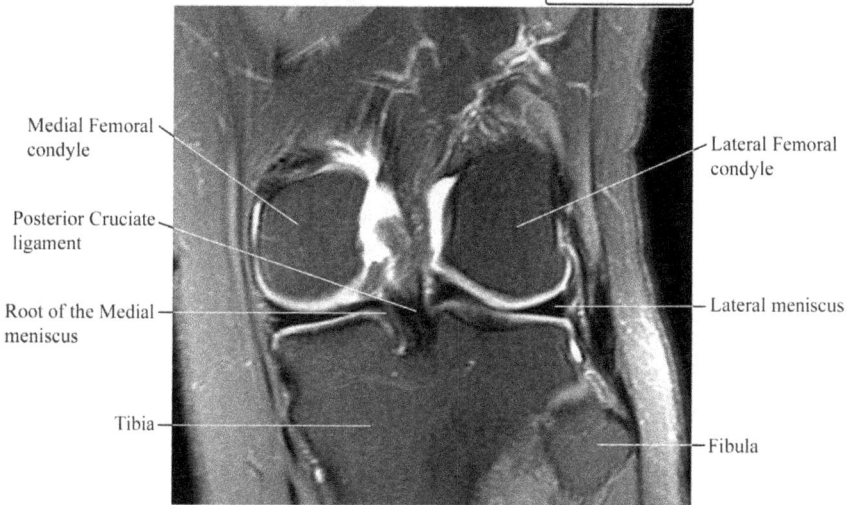

(G)

Medial Femoral condyle

Posterior Cruciate ligament

Root of the Medial meniscus

Tibia

Lateral Femoral condyle

Lateral meniscus

Fibula

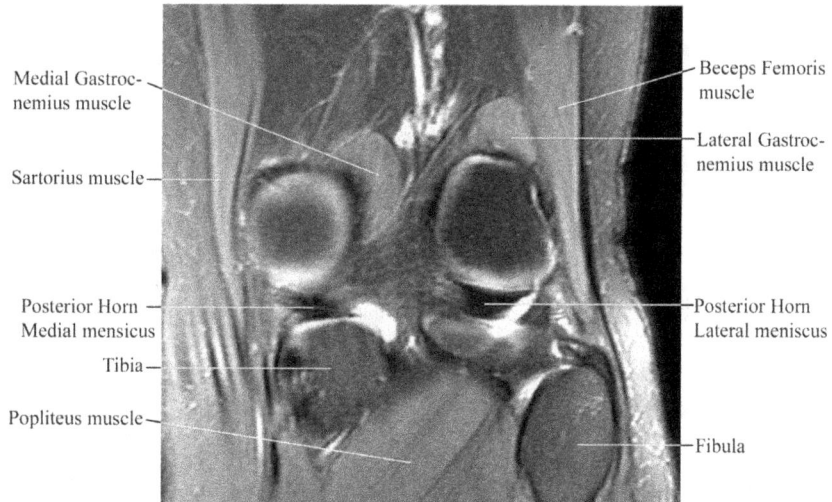

(H)

Medial Gastroc-nemius muscle

Sartorius muscle

Posterior Horn Medial menscius

Tibia

Popliteus muscle

Beceps Femoris muscle

Lateral Gastroc-nemius muscle

Posterior Horn Lateral meniscus

Fibula

Fig. 2. (*Continued*)

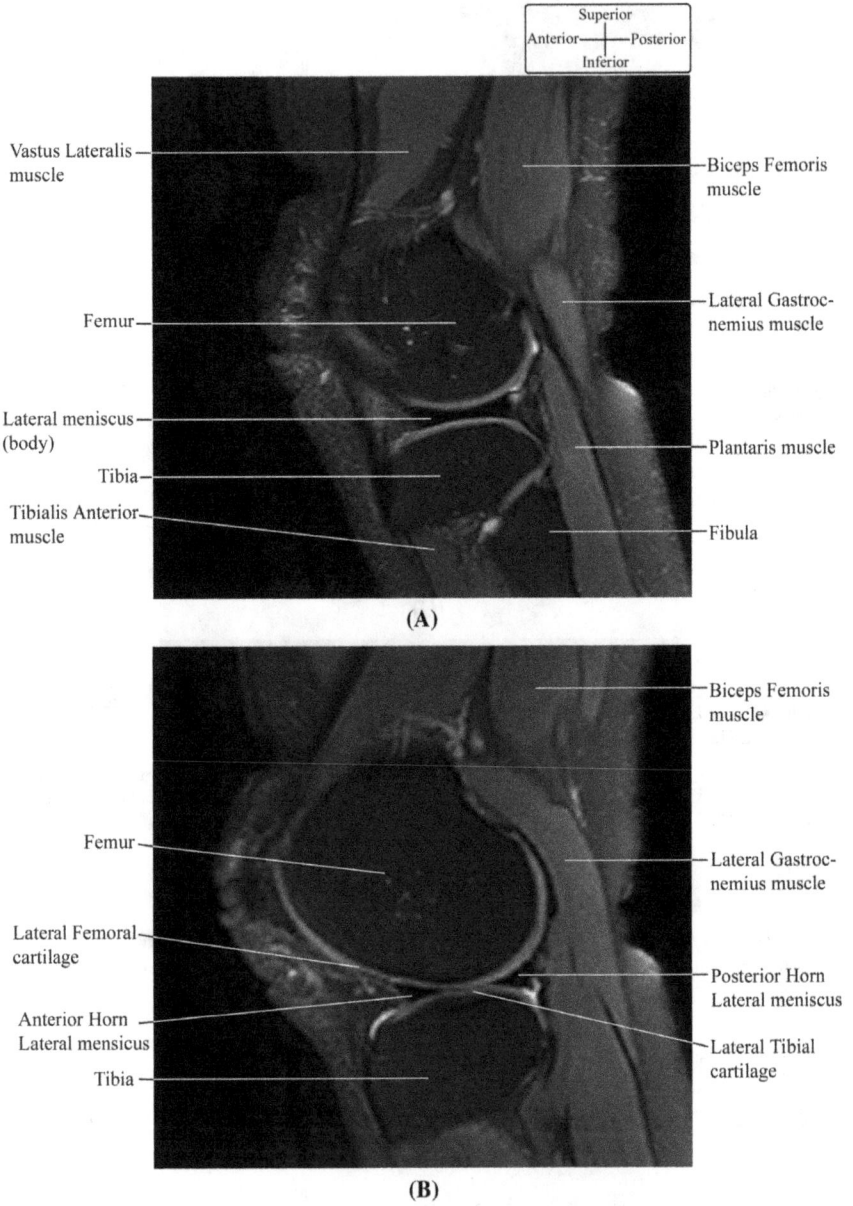

Fig. 3. Sagittal T_2-weighted magnetic resonance images of the knee and surrounding structures.

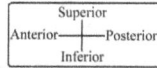

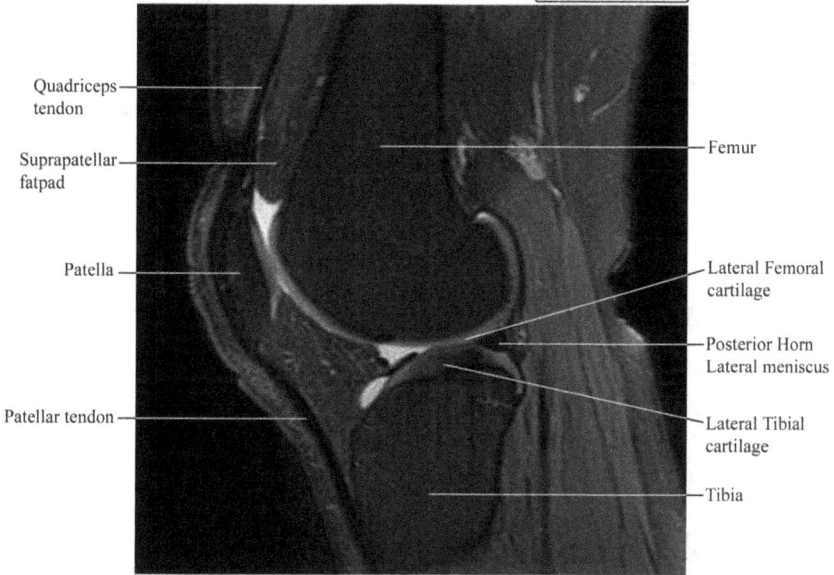

(C)

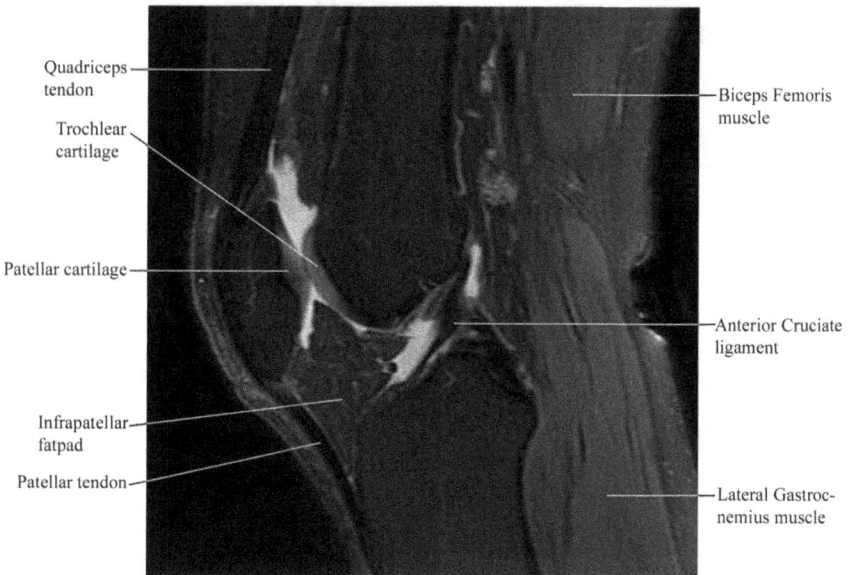

(D)

Fig. 3. (*Continued*)

	Superior	
Anterior	┼	Posterior
	Inferior	

Quadriceps tendon

Femur

Transverse ligament

Tibia

Semi-membranosis muscle

Medial Gastroc-nemius muscle

Posterior Cruciate ligament

Popliteus muscle

(E)

Vastus Medialis muscle

Medial Femoral cartilage

Medial meniscus

Medial Tibial cartilage

Addcutor Magnus muscle

Posterior Horn Medial meniscus

Medial Gastroc-nemius muscle

(F)

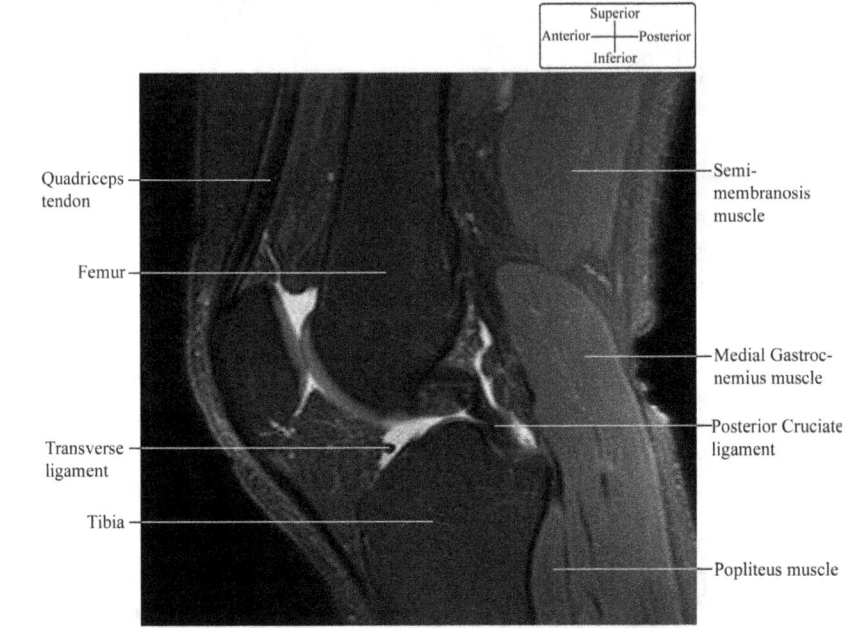

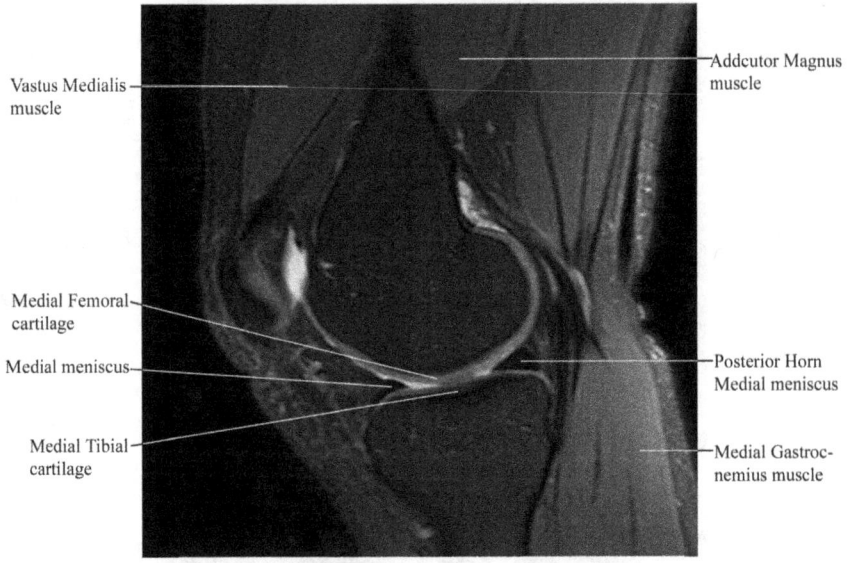

Fig. 3. (*Continued*)

(G)

(H)

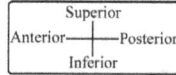

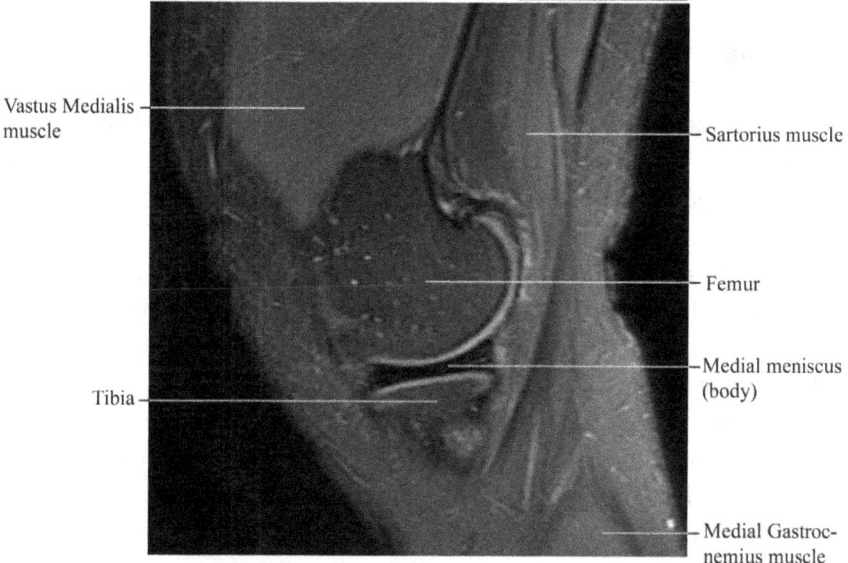

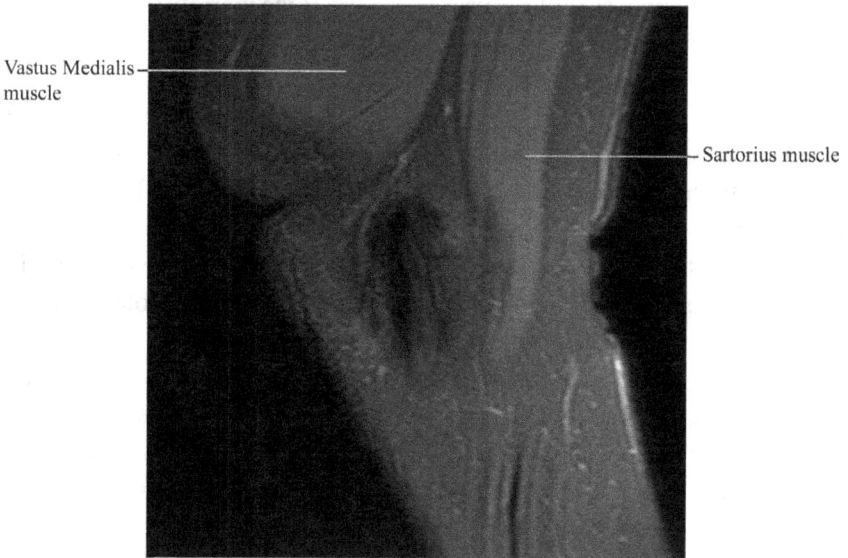

Fig. 3. (*Continued*)

Bone

Bone Structure

Bone is organized into compact bone and cancellous or trabecular bone. The cortex, or compact bone, consists of dense bone tissue. It forms the outer shell of the bone as well as much of the diaphysis, the shaft-like portion of long bones. In contrast, cancellous bone is relatively porous with bony spicules called trabeculae spanning pores. Cancellous bone is found within the epiphysis, the area at the ends of the long bones.

Other tissues found in close proximity to bone include periosteum, endosteum, blood vessels, nerves, and bone marrow. Periosteum is a fibrous layer that surrounds the outer surface of the bone. It includes fibroblasts, collagen, nerves and a pool of osteoprogenitor cells. These osteoprogenitor cells can differentiate into osteoblasts and play important roles in fracture healing. Endosteum is also a fibrous layer and it lines the inner surfaces of bones, which include the inner surface of cortical bone and the surface of the trabeculae. The composition of endosteum is similar to that of periosteum, but it is usually thinner. Osteoprogenitor cells in the endosteum contribute to bone remodeling, as will be discussed later. Bone marrow tissue fills the pores in trabecular bone. It is composed of adipocytes, hematopoetic stem cells, and mesenchymal stem cells. Hematopoeitic stem cells are precursor cells that can differentiate to form leukocytes, erythrocytes, platelets, and osteoclasts. Mesenchymal stem cells are also found in the bone marrow, adherent to the surface of the trabeculae. These cells can differentiate to form chondrocytes, myocytes, adipocytes, and osteoblasts.

Bone tissue itself consists of two major components: bone matrix and cells. Bone matrix is made up of type 1 collagen, proteoglycans, glycoproteins, hydroxyapatite ($Ca_{10}(PO_4)_6(OH)_2$), and various growth and regulatory factors. The matrix provides the actual structure for bone, provides much of the mechanical properties for bone, and supports the growth of bone cells . The cellular component of bone includes osteoblasts, osteoclasts, and osteocytes. These cells are responsible for formation, resorption, and maintenance of the bone matrix.

Bone matrix is structured as a series of lamellae. Each lamella is a layer of mineralized extracellular matrix that contains collagen fibers oriented parallel to each other, in a helical course. Furthermore, in cortical bone, adjacent lamellae have collagen fiber orientations that are approximately perpendicular to each other. In trabeculae, the collagen fibers in the lamellae are oriented parallel to the long axis of the bony spicule. This anisotropy is responsible for the unique mechanical properties of bone. Osteocytes are housed in lacunae between lamellae. These cells extend processes into the lamellae through canaliculi, giving osteocytes the ability to communicate with each other and receive signals from the extracellular matrix. Blood vessels penetrate bone in canals called Volkmann's canals, providing the tissue with important nutrients.

Bone Remodeling

Bone is constantly undergoing remodeling in response to mechanical stresses as well as metabolic factors. During remodeling, old bone is broken down and replaced with new bone. The first step of this process is resorption of old bone by osteoclasts, phagocytic cells derived from hematopoetic stem cells. Ostoeoclasts bind to the surface of the bone through adhesion molecules in the bone matrix, then form a seal around the area that will be resorbed. They will then release acid and metalloproteinases to break down the bone matrix. During this breakdown, growth factors and collagenases impregnated in the matrix are released, providing further stimulus for bone remodeling. Following resorption, osteoblasts lay down new unmineralized bone matrix in the lamellar arrangement described earlier. Osteoblasts that become trapped in the matrix during this process will eventually become osteocytes. Mineralization of bone matrix follows within 12 to 15 days as calcium and phosphate diffuse into the area and crystallize.

Osteoblasts and osteoclasts work together in a system called the basic multicellular unit. Osteoblasts have receptors for vitamin D, parathyroid hormone, and estrogen. Presence of these hormones stimulates osteoblasts through these receptors, enabling osteoblasts to produce a hormone called Receptor Activator of NF-kappaB Ligand(RANKL). RANKL binds Receptor Activator of NF-kappaB (RANK) receptors on osteoclasts, stimulating bone resorption. As bone resorption progresses, growth factors released from the matrix such as Transforming Growth Factor-Beta (TGF-β), Bone Morphogenic Protein (BMP), and Platelet Derived Growth Factor (PDGF) stimulate the differentiation and activation of osteoblasts to matrix-producing cells.

Fracture Healing

Upon injury, mesenchymal stem cells will be recruited to the site of fracture. These pluripotent stem cells will initially condense, forming cellular aggregates joined by adhesion molecules such as Neural Cell Adhesion Molecule (NCAM) and N-cadherin. After aggregation, these mesenchymal stem cells will begin to differentiate into chondrocytes. These proliferating chondrocytes express collagen-2 and Indian hedgehog protein (Ihh). Collagen 2 is incorporated into the extracellular matrix. Ihh expression may stimulate the proliferation of prehypertrophic chondrocytes through production of Parathyroid Hormone Related Protein (PTH-RP). Bone morphogenic protein-7 (BMP7) also stimulates proliferation of these chondrocytes while Fibroblast Growth Factor-3 (FGF3) inhibits proliferation. Runx2 stimulates these proliferative chondrocytes to become hypertrophic. The chondrocytes separate, enlarge in size and begin secretion of type X collagen and Vascular Endothelial Growth Factor (VEGF). VEGF stimulates angiogenesis; osteoprogenitors derived from mesenchymal stem cells arrive with the invasion of new blood vessels. Osteoprogenitors differentiate into osteoblasts under the control of Runx2, Ihh and BMPs. Differentiated osteoblasts secrete osteoid over the cartilage matrix. Hypertrophic chondrocytes die as the surrounding matrix is calcified. Osteoblasts trapped in the matrix differentiate into osteocytes. Invading osteoclasts, differentiated from a monocyte lineage, initiate remodeling. These break down matrix using cathepsin K, metalloproteinases and hydrochloric acid. These osteoclasts are followed by differentiated osteoblasts, which will fill in bone. The combined action of osteoblasts and osteoclasts help the bone achieve its final form.

Anatomical Structures of Knee

The knee includes the distal end of the femur, the proximal end of the tibia, and the patella. The distal end of the femur is composed of two condyles, which articulate with the proximal tibia. The anterior portion of the condyle is relatively flat compared with the posterior portion. This flattened area serves as the weight-bearing portion of the condyle. The anterior condyles are separated by a groove called the trochlea or patellofemoral groove. The posterior aspect of the condyles are rounded and separated by the intercondylar notch. The posterior intercondylar region provides attachment points for the anterior and posterior cruciate ligaments.

The proximal end of the tibia is also composed of two condyles, also called plateaus, that articulate with the femoral condyles. The medial plateau is slightly larger and flatter than the lateral plateau. The plateaus are separated by the intercondylar region, which provides attachment sites for the medial meniscus, lateral meniscus, anterior cruciate ligament, and posterior cruciate ligament. The tibial tuberosity is also located between the plateaus, on the anterior surface of the tibia. It serves as the attachment point for the patellar tendon.

The patella is a sesamoid bone that is roughly triangular in shape. Its proximal edge is wider than the distal edge, providing a broad attachment for the quadriceps femoris tendon. The narrow distal edge provides an attachment for the patellar ligament, which connects the patella to the tibial tuberosity. The posterior aspect of the patella has a medial and lateral facet, which articulate with the medial and lateral condyles of the femur, respectively. The lateral facet is larger than the medial facet.

Cartilage

Cartilage Structure

Cartilage is found in the human body in one of three different forms: hyaline cartilage, elastic cartilage, and fibrocartilage. Hyaline cartilage is the most common form, found in joint (articular) surfaces, nose, larynx, trachea, and bronchi. Fibrocartilage, a type of cartilage that is more dense, fibrous and resistant to tensile loading, serves as a key component in intervertebral discs, menisci of the knee, tendon insertions, sternoclavicular joints, mandibular joints, and the pubic symphysis. Elastic cartilage, as its name suggests, is the most flexible form of cartilage and helps form the external ear, the epiglottis, and part of the larynx.

The three types of cartilage all share a basic structure composed of chondrocytes and extracellular matrix, but differ in the components of their extracellular matrix. Chondrocytes, the cellular component of cartilage, are responsible for production and maintenance of the extracellular matrix. Hyaline cartilage contains an extracellular matrix (ECM) primarily made up of hyaluronic acid, proteoglycans, type II collagen, and water. The ECM of fibrocartilage is more fibrous and dense because of the abundance of type I collagen and the relative scarcity of water and proteoglycans. Elastic cartilage ECM has all of the same components of the hyaline cartilage ECM, with the addition of elastic fibers that provide it with its unique flexibility.

Interactions between the components of the ECM in articular cartilage form the basis for much of the mechanical properties of cartilage. Proteoglycans are molecules that consist of glycosaminoglycans attached to a protein. In articular cartilage, the most abundant proteoglycan is aggrecan. The aggrecan molecule is composed of chains of two types of glycosaminoglycans, chondroiton sulfate and keratin sulfate, attached to a central protein core. The structure has often been compared to a "bottle brush," with the protein representing the metal core and the glycosaminoglycan chains representing the brush bristles. Hundreds of aggrecan molecules may noncovalently bind to a hyaluronate molecule, resulting in fixation of aggrecan. Thus, these aggrecan molecules are unable to move within the cartilage matrix. These fixed aggrecan molecules attract water with the negative charges on their glycosaminoglycan chains and trap water between molecules, resulting in swelling of the extracellular matrix. This hydrostatic swelling is balanced by tension in type II collagen fibers. The negative charges on these glycosaminoglycans also repel each other when the cartilage matrix is compressed, providing cartilage with resiliency.

When viewed in cross-section, articular cartilage is organized into four zones based on depth from the surface. The most superficial layer of articular cartilage, zone 1 or tangential zone, primarily consists of collagen fibers that are parallel to the joint surface. This layer is under tension and resists swelling from the deeper layers. The layer deep to the superficial zone is zone 2, or the transitional zone. In zone 2, collagen fibers are arranged in random orientations. Zone 3 is characterized by collagen fibers that are oriented radially from the deepest layer of the cartilage to the surface. Lastly, zone 4 mainly consists of calcified cartilage and serves as the attachment of cartilage to underlying subchondral bone.

In the knee joint, hyaline cartilage covers the articulating surfaces of the femur, tibia, and patella. Hyaline cartilage, also known as articular cartilage, facilitates the sliding motion of the joint. Fibrocartilage can also be found in the knee joint, especially following injury. A mixture of fibrocartilage-like cartilage and hyaline-like cartilage makes up the meniscus.

Histology of Cartilage

A variety of histological techniques have been employed to stain articular cartilage. Hematoxylin and eosin is a commonly used staining combination that has been applied to all tissues of the body. It is a nonspecific stain that colors nuclei blue and cytoplasm pink. It can be used to evaluate general morphological features of articular cartilage tissue. However, in the study of articular cartilage, it is often helpful to employ stains that are specifically directed against proteoglycans and collagen. Proteoglycan staining can be achieved by the use of safranin O or toluidine blue. The intensity of staining has been correlated with proteoglycan content for both of these stains. However, safranin O provides a superior correlation. For this reason, safranin O is the most widely used cartilage staining technique. It is often used in combination with fast green FCF and hematoxylin, which stain protein and nuclei, respectively. The safranin O/fast green FCF/hematoxylin combination stains the extracellular matrix red, the subchondral bone gray, and nuclei blue. Alcian blue is another stain for proteoglycans that has been used in the past. However, the intensity of staining is not correlated to proteoglycan content. Thus, it is not often used in histological analysis because it provides no information on proteoglycan changes that are often seen in osteoarthritis. Lastly, sirius red F3BA is a stain for collagen that has been used in the past. However, it is difficult to obtain quantitative correlation of staining intensity to collagen content, so this method is not a popular method of histological cartilage characterization.

Joint Capsule and Ligaments

Capsule

A strong fibrous capsule surrounds the knee joint. It attaches proximally at the femur just superior to the femoral condyles. Distally, it attaches to the articular margin of the tibia. Laterally the articular capsule is deficient, allowing the popliteus tendon to exit the knee joint before attaching on the tibia. However, the capsule is reinforced extracapsularly by the iliotibial tract that originates at the proximal femur and inserts at the lateral tibial condyle (Gerde's tubercle). In addition, the lateral capsule is supported by the lateral collateral ligament (LCL) and the medial capsule by the medial collateral ligament (MCL). The oblique popliteal ligament arises from the semimembranosus tendon and supports the posterior joint capsule as is passes from the medial tibial condyle to the posterior femur. Additionally, the posterior capsule is supported by the arcuate popliteal ligament.

Ligaments

The LCL is round and cord-like, extending from the lateral epicondyle of the femur to the head of the fibula. The MCL is a broad, flat ligament that attaches from the medial epicondyle of the femur to the proximal medial tibia. The deep fibers of the MCL penetrate the joint capsule and attach firmly to the medial meniscus. The LCL prevents tibial adduction (varus) and the MCL prevents tibial abduction (valgus). The MCL is weaker than the LCL and more susceptible to injury. Its direct attachment to the medial meniscus often results in the concomitant injury of the MCL and medial meniscus together. Intracapsularly, the knee joint is supported by the anterior cruciate ligament (ACL) and the posterior cruciate ligament (PCL). The ACL is a two-bundle ligament consisting of an anteromedial and posterolateral band. Together these bands prevent anterior tibial translation and knee joint hyperextension. The PCL is the stronger of the two cruciate ligaments and attaches from the central aspect of the tibia posteriorly and passes anteriorly to the lateral aspect of the medial femoral condyle. The PCL prevents anterior femur translation.

Menisci

The crescent-shaped menisci of the knee consist of fibrocartilage arranged in concentric plates in the medial and lateral knee joint. They function to deepen the joint surface, increasing the congruity at the tibiofemoral joint, as well as serve as shock absorbers. The circumference of each crescent is thick, convex and attached to the joint capsule as well as the tibial plateaus via coronary ligaments. Conversely, the inner borders of the menisci are thin, concave and free, making them prone to tears. Superiorly, they are concave to provide congruent articulation for the round femoral condyles.

The roots of the menisci attach mesially near the tibial spines. Just as the lateral root is becoming anchored to the tibial plateau, a meniscofemoral ligament arises and attachs to the lateral femoral condyle. Anteriorly, the transverse ligament connects the medial and lateral menisci.

The blood supply to the menisci is often described by dividing each meniscus into thirds: the outer third, the middle third and the inner third. The outer third, sometimes referred to as the "red zone" has a rich blood supply and capable of healing in cases of injury. The inner third, called the "white zone" is devoid of circulating blood and incapable of healing when torn. The middle third, the "pink zone" is a transition between the inner and outer thirds with limited capacity to heal. It is becoming increasingly apparent that injuries to the meniscus are highly detrimental to articular cartilage health.

Molecularly, the medial and lateral menisci consist primarily of type I collagen. The matrix of the meniscus is not unlike articular cartilage discussed previously; however, the concentration of chondrocytes and proteoglycan molecules is much lower.

Muscles

The knee joint is supported by several muscle groups that surround the knee joint. The quadriceps is the primary muscle group located anterior to the knee joint. It functions to generate knee extensor torque and attaches to the tibial tuberosity via the patellar tendon. The four muscles that comprise the quadriceps group are the vastus medialis, vastus intermedius, vastus lateralis and the rectus femoris. The vastus medialis is located on the medial aspect of the anterior thigh and originates from the medial border of the linea aspera on the posterior femur. Its fibers wrap around medially and anteriorly, inserting into the superior medial patella via the broad quadriceps tendon. The vastus intermedius lies on the anterior aspect of the femur, deep to the rectus femoris. It originates from the anterior and lateral aspects of the femoral shaft and inserts into the superior margin of the patella via the quadriceps tendon. The vastus lateralis is the largest of the quadriceps muscles and originates from the lateral border of the linea aspera. Its fibers wrap around the femur laterally and anteriorly, inserting into the superior lateral patella via the quadriceps tendon. The rectus femoris, the only of the four quadriceps muscles to cross the hip joint, lies on the anterior aspect of the femur, superficial to the vastus intermedius. It originates from the anterior inferior iliac spine and inserts into the superior margin of the patella via the quadriceps tendon. The strong fibrous quadriceps tendon envelopes the patella and continues inferiorly via the patellar tendon before inserting on the tibial tuberosity.

Posteriorly, the hamstrings are the primary knee flexor group. Four muscle heads comprise the hamstrings; two laterally and two medially. The biceps femoris is the two-headed lateral hamstring. This long head of the bicep femoris originates from the ischial tuberosity while the short head originates along the linea aspera. The two heads join at the distal femur and attach to the head of the fibula and lateral tibia. While the long head crosses the hip joint to provide hip extension torque, both heads act together to generate knee flexion torque. The two medial hamstrings are the semimembranosus and semitendinosus. Both muscles originate from the ischial tuberosity along with the long head of the biceps. They extend distally and medially together and insert on the posterior medial tibia. After inserting on the tibia, the tendon of the semimembranosus reflects superiorly and laterally to form the oblique popliteal ligament which helps support the posterior joint capsule.

Additional knee flexors include the gastrocnemius, the plantaris and the popliteus muscles. The gastrocnemius forms part of the calf muscle and originates at the femoral condyles. The medial and lateral heads of the gastrocnemius extend distally from each of the femoral condyles, respectively. They fuse together to insert on the Achilles tendon which ultimately is attached to the posterior calcaneus. The gastrocnemius helps support the posterior knee joint and provides flexion torque upon contraction. The small belly of the plantaris muscle originates from the posterior femur above the lateral condyle and has a long slender tendon that inserts along with the Achilles tendon to the posterior calcaneus. The thin triangular-shaped popliteus originates from the lateral femoral condyle and inserts along the proximal medial tibia. While it assists with knee flexion, its primary function is to internally rotate the tibia, a movement necessary to unlock the knee joint in extension.

The medial aspect of the knee joint is supported by the pes anserine muscle group. This group consists of the sartorius muscle, the gracilis muscle, and the aforementioned semitendinosus muscle. The sartorius muscle originates from the anterior superior iliac spine of the pelvis and courses obliquely across the anterior thigh before inserting at the medial surface of the tibia. While a knee flexor, it also generates hip flexion, and hip external rotation torque. The gracilis is a long strap-like muscle that is part of the hip adductors group as well. It originates from the inferior ramus of the pubis and ischium and inserts along with the sartorius and semitendinosus into the medial aspect of the proximal tibia.

Bursae and Fat Pads

Bursae

Structures of the knee joint may become inflamed in the absence or in combination with osteoarthritis. One such structure that is a common site for inflammation is the bursae of the knee joint. Several bursae are found around the knee joint. These are the suprapatellar (quadriceps) bursa, popliteal bursa, anserine bursa, gastrocnemius bursa, semimembranosus bursa, prepatellar bursa, and subcutaneus and deep infrapatellar bursae. The bursae are typically located between tendons and bones and function to decrease friction. They consist of a pouch of synovial membrane with small amounts of synovial fluid that acts as a lubricant. However, with excessive loads, the bursa can become inflamed and the synovial walls can become thickened and swell. This typically presents as a large focal deformity at the sight of the bursa.

The suprapatellar bursa is located between the femur and the quadriceps tendon and is a direct extension from the superior joint capsule of the knee. The popliteal bursa lies between the tendon of the popliteus and the lateral condyle of the tibia and travels into the joint capsule under the lateral meniscus. The anserine bursa in located between the tendons of the pes anserine (sartorius, gracilis, semitendinosus) and the medial tibial condyle. The gastrocnemius bursa is found deep in the medial head of the gastrocnemius, over the posterior medial femoral and tibial condyles. The semimembranosus bursa is located between the medial head of the gastrocnemius and the tendon of the semimembranosus. The prepatellar bursa lies superior to the anterior patella, just beneath the skin overlying the patella. It allows for the skin to move freely over the anterior patellar surface during knee flexion and extension. The two infrapatellar bursae are located just superficial and deep to the patellar tendon, and function to withstand pressures during kneeling.

Fat Pads

Three fat pads occupy the anterior knee: the quadriceps, prefemoral, and infrapatellar fat pads. The largest fat pad of the knee joint is the infrapatellar fat pad or Hoffa's fat pad. It has been extensively studied due to its proposed role in various pathologies. Located just inferior to the inferior patellar pole, the infrapatellar fat pad occupies much of the space between the patella and the tibia. It extends inferiorly to the deep infrapatellar bursa located at the insertion of the patellar ligament into the tibial tuberosity. The infrapatellar fat pad attaches to several structures including the intercondylar notch via the ligamentum mucosum, the patellar tendon, the inferior pole of the patella and the anterior horns of the menisci.

The two smaller fat pads are the quadriceps and the prefemoral fat pads. The quadriceps fat pad, also known as the anterior suprapatellar fat pad, lies superior to the suprapatellar pole between the distal quadriceps tendon anteriorly, and the suprapatellar recess posteriorly. Just deep (posterior) to the suprapatellar recess and the suprapatellar bursa is the prefemoral fat pad, which lies on the anterior femoral shaft, superior to the trochlear groove.

Fat pads of the knee are highly vascularized and highly innervated. Terminal extensions of the genicular arteries anastomose in the fat pads richly supplying them and their synovial coverings. Substance P immunore-active pain fibers have been found to be widespread and equally distributed throughout the fat pads, retinaculum, and synovium.

Several functions of the fat pads have been proposed including synovial fluid secretion, dead space occupiers, and joint stability. Current research concludes that the infrapatellar fat pad appears to play a role in biomechanical support and neurovascular supply to the adjacent structures.

Nociceptors

Histochemical and anatomical studies have investigated the prevalence of substance P in the structures surrounding the knee. Substance P is a neurotransmitter found in afferent nerve fibers. It is believed that this neurotransmitter is associated with the cascade of events that result in the perception of pain. These events include activation of afferent nerve fibers that enter the dorsal horn of the spinal cord at the appropriate segmental level. The impulses are propagated to the contralateral side at that level and ascend the spinal cord in the spinothatlamic tract, entering the brainstem as the spinal lemniscus, before arriving to the thalamus and continuing to the primary sensory cortex on the post central gyrus. It is there where pain is perceived and then further understood through secondary sensory processing. These substance P fibers have been found in tissues surrounding the knee joint including the medial and lateral retinaculum, the infrapatellar and suprapatellar fat pads, the synovial lining, periosteum and subchondral plate of the patella, femur and tibia.

Conclusion

This chapter has detailed the normal anatomy and physiology of the knee joint. Particular detail was provided for cartilage and bone anatomy. However, many of the supportive structures of knee, such as the menisci and the ligaments are also believed to be involved in OA. As you read later chapters and learn about the details of OA, refer back to this chapter for the normal anatomy and physiology of the knee.

References and Suggested Readings

Drake RL, Vogl W, Mitchell A. *Gray's Anatomy for Students*. Philadelphia: Churchill Livingstone, 2004.

Gray H, Carter HV, Pick TP, Howden R. *Gray's Anatomy*, 15th edn. Iselin: Barnes & Noble, 1995.

Hodges PW, Mellor R, Crossley K, Bennell K. Pain induced by injection of hypertonic saline into the infrapatellar fat pad and effect on coordination of the quadriceps muscles. *Arthritis Rheum* 2009;15:70–77.

Hyllested JL, Veje K, Ostergaard K. Histochemical studies of the extracellular matrix of human articular cartilage — a review. *Osteoarthr Cartil* 2002;10:333–343.

Jacobson JA, Lenchik L, Ruhoy MK, Schweitzer ME, Resnick D. MR imaging of the infrapatellar fat pad of Hoffa. *Radiographics* 1997;17:675–691.

Junqueira LC, Carneiro J. *Basic Histology: Text and Atlas*, 11th edn. Columbus: McGraw Hill Companies, 2005.

Kandel ER, Schwartz JH, Jessell TM. *Principles of Neural Science*, 4th edn. Columbus: McGraw-Hill Professional, 2000.

Kierszenbaum AL. *Histology and Cell Biology*. St. Louis: Mosby, 2002.

Maralcan G, Kuru I, Issi S, Esmer AF, Tekdemir I, Evcik D. The innervation of patella: anatomical and clinical study. *Surg Radiol Anat* 2005;27:331–335.

Marieb EM, Hoehn K. *Human Anatomy and Physiology*, 7th edn. San Francisco: Pearson Benjamin Cummings, 2007.

Moore K, Dalley AF. *Clinically Oriented Anatomy*, 4th edn. Philadelphia: Lippincott Williams & Wilkins, 2006.

Netter F. *Atlas of Human Anatomy*, 3rd edn. Los Angeles: Icon Learning Systems, 2003.

Stoller DW. *Stoller's Atlas of Orthopaedics and Sports Medicine*. Philadelphia: Lippincott Williams & Wilkins, 2007.

Stoller DW, Tirman P, Bredella MA. *Diagnostic Imaging*. Salt Lake City: Amirsys, 2003.

Tortura GJ. *Principles of Human Anatomy*, 7th edn. New York: HarperCollins College, 1995.

Witoński D, Wagrowska-Danielewicz M. Distribution of substance-P nerve fibers in the knee joint in patients with anterior knee pain syndrome. A preliminary report. *Knee Surg Sports Traumatol Arthrosc* 1999;7:177–183.

Wojtys EM, Beaman DN, Glover RA, Janda D. Innervation of the human knee joint by substance-P fibers. *Arthroscopy* 1990;6:254–263.

2

Clinical Presentation and Natural History of Osteoarthritis

by Ehsan Saadat, Radu I. Bolbos and Michael D. Ries

Introduction

Osteoarthritis (OA) is the most common form of arthritis and a leading cause of chronic disability in the United States. OA has a pervasive presence. For example, in a prospective population-based cohort study of determinants and prognosis of chronic diseases in the elderly (the Rotterdam study), only 135 of 1040 individuals aged 55 to 65 years were free of radiographic signs of OA in the hands, knees, hips or the spine.[1,2] The pervasive presence of osteoarthritis, and its debilitating toll on the level of physical activity of patients is a key factor in the large societal burden of OA. OA currently affects at least 20 million Americans[3] and the World Health Organization (WHO) estimates OA to be a leading cause of chronic disability in at least 10% of population aged 60 and older.[4] Knee OA alone has been associated with chronic disability as often as heart or chronic lung disease.[5] It is estimated that over $33 billion are spent annually in the US for its treatment and for lost days of work.

The incidence of osteoarthritis in the US is expected to increase from 15% of the population (40 million) in 1995 to 18% of the population (59 million) by 2020.[3] For knee osteoarthritis, a study investigating the rate of progression of preexisting radiographic OA (the Framingham study) found that in a population with the mean age of 70.8 years, the incidence of radiographic knee OA in women was 2% per year, and 1% per year developed symptomatic, radiographic knee OA, versus 1.4% and 0.7% of men, respectively.[6] The prevalence of radiographic knee OA rises in women from 1%–4% in those 24 to 45 years of age to 53%–55% in those of age 80 years and older. In men, the prevalence rises from 1%–6% in those 45 years and younger to 22%–33% in those 80 years and older.[7–10]

Despite the pervasive presence of OA and its debilitating burden on the society, no disease-modifying or preventative treatment is available which has proven to be effective in modifying the natural history of OA. This contributes to the impact of this disease in the modern society. In recent years, the frequency of this articular disorder has increased as advances in medicine have lead to a prolonged life expectancy for humans.

Epidemiologic studies, as well as basic science research, have elucidated much of what is known about predisposing and protective factors for OA and the natural history of the disease. Imaging technology has had a particularly significant impact in our recent understanding of OA etiopathogenesis as more advanced Magnetic Resonance Imaging (MRI) techniques have been able to demonstrate degenerative changes of the joint earlier, allowing for long-term study in human subjects.[11–15]

The following chapter will provide an overview of OA pathophysiology and clinical diagnosis. Special attention will be paid to pathogenesis of OA as this will lay the groundwork for discussion of advanced MRI methods to detect such changes in following chapters.

Definition of Osteoarthritis

No single terminology or classification system of degenerative joint disease is universally accepted. "Arthrosis" refers to mechanical loss of articular cartilage while "arthritis" refers to joint inflammation in association with arthrosis. Originally, the term "arthritis deformans" was used as a descriptive term for both degenerative arthritis and rheumatoid arthritis. However, since joint deformities can accompany many articular processes, this term is not acceptable. Presently, "degenerative arthritis," "degenerative joint disease" and "osteoarthritis" are used frequently, though "degenerative joint disease" is the best general phrase to describe degenerative processes in any type of articulation, with "osteoarthritis" reserved for degenerative disease of synovial joints.[16]

The term "osteoarthritis" implies an inflammatory disease. However, although inflammatory cells may be present, osteoarthritis is considered to be an intrinsic disease of articular cartilage in which biochemical and metabolic alterations result in its breakdown. OA is joint failure, a disease in which all structures of the joint have undergone pathologic change, often in concert. The pathologic *sine qua non* of OA is hyaline articular cartilage loss, present in a focal and, initially, nonuniform manner. This is accompanied by increasing thickness and sclerosis of the subchondral bony plate, by outgrowth of osteophytes at the joint margin, by stretching of the articular capsule, by mild synovitis in many affected joints, and by weakness of muscles bridging the joint. In the knees, meniscal degeneration is part of the disease. There are numerous pathways that lead to joint failure, but the initial step is often joint injury in the setting of a failure of protective mechanisms.

It must be noted that even though cartilage thinning is discussed as the main characteristic of osteoarthritis, thickening, not thinning, of articular cartilage may occur after injury, a finding repeatedly documented in animal models in which the knee has been rendered unstable with surgical techniques.[17,18] Cartilage, like other connective tissues, swells when injured; however, the cause of post-traumatic cartilage thickening is not well-established; an increase in proteoglycan content, water, or both, may be important in the pathogenesis of cartilage thickening.[17,19] Long-term studies in such knees have indicated that cartilage breakdown and loss may follow the stage of cartilage thickening.[20] Similarly, thickening of articular cartilage may represent an early manifestation of osteoarthritis in humans, and progressive loss of articular cartilage may indicate more advanced disease.

The most recent consensus definition of OA is as follows: "OA diseases are a result of both mechanical and biologic events that destabilize the normal coupling of degeneration and synthesis of articular cartilage chondrocytes and extracellular matrix, and subchondral bone. Although they may be initiated by multiple factors, including genetic, developmental, metabolic, mechanical, and traumatic, OA diseases involve all of the tissues of the diarthroidal joint. Ultimately, OA diseases are manifested by morphologic, biochemical, molecular, and biomechanical changes of both cells and matrix which lead to a softening, fibrillation, ulceration, loss of articular cartilage, sclerosis and eburnation of subchondral bone, osteophytes, and subchondral cysts. When clinically evident, OA diseases are characterized by joint pain, tenderness, limitation of movement, crepitus, occasional effusion, and variable degrees of inflammation without systemic effects."[21] This definition captures several key factors in our recent understanding of OA etiopathogenesis. As elaborated by Mitchell and Cruess,[22] articular degeneration may result from either an abnormal concentration of force across a joint with normal cartilage matrix or a normal concentration of force across an abnormal joint with underlying cartilaginous or subchondral osseous anomalies. Eventually, of course, abnormalities of force and articular structure will appear together, leading to the clinical picture of OA as will be discussed in more detail in this chapter.

Primary and Secondary Osteoarthritis

Traditionally, degenerative joint disease has been classified further into primary (idiopathic) and secondary types. Primary or idiopathic OA is defined as a process of articular degeneration in the absence of any underlying mechanical abnormalities in the joint. Secondary OA is regarded as a result of a previous underlying factor. This classification is, however, widely regarded as misleading. Careful evaluation of many examples of "idiopathic" OA reveals an underlying cause which was overlooked or misdiagnosed initially. It appears likely that primary degenerative joint disease does not truly exist and this classification stems from our limited understanding of the disease etiopathology and diagnostic capabilities.

Clinical Presentations of Osteoarthritis

The symptomatic osteoarthritic joint presents with a wide spectrum of signs and symptoms including pain, limited range of motion and deformity. Crepitus, crackling or popping sounds and sensations experienced under the joints, may be present with or without pain. Effusions, abnormal collection of fluid in a joint space, may be present, usually without heat or erythema. Symptoms range in intensity from mild to severe and can lead to chronic disability. End-stage osteoarthritis of weight-bearing joints is extremely painful. Symptomatic OA may be associated with depression and sleep disturbance in addition to disability.[23,24] Depression in association with hip or knee OA is more predictive of disability than a radiographic grade. Predictably, antidepressant treatment of a depressed patient suffering from OA has been shown to improve pain, function and quality of life scores.[25]

A description of clinical manifestations of osteoarthritis is presented below. It is important to note that although osteoarthritis is the most common reason for symptomatic joint pain, other causes of joint pain need to be considered in the differential diagnosis of a painful joint, and these will be discussed in the following section. Additionally, osteoarthritis, especially of the knee, can be minimized through weight loss, exercise and injury avoidance. The loss of 11.2 pounds has been associated with a 50% reduction in the risk of developing symptomatic knee OA over a ten-year period.[26]

Symptoms

Pain: Pain associated with weight bearing activity is usually the first and predominant complaint of patients with symptomatic OA and arguably the most debilitating aspect of OA. Joint pain from OA is activity-related. Pain comes on either during or just after joint use and then gradually resolves. Examples include knee or hip pain with going up or down stairs, pain in weight-bearing joints when walking, and, for hand OA, pain after cooking. Early in disease, pain is episodic, triggered often by a day or two of overactive use of a diseased joint, such as a person with knee OA taking a long run and noticing a few days of pain thereafter. As disease progresses, the pain becomes continuous and even begins to be bothersome at night. Stiffness of the affected joint may be prominent, but morning stiffness is usually brief (< 30 minutes).

As cartilage is aneural, the cartilage loss in a joint is not accompanied by pain. Thus, pain in OA likely arises from structures outside the cartilage. Innervated structures in the joint which may be the main pain source include the synovium, ligaments, joint capsule, muscles, and subchondral bone. Most of these are not visualized by X-ray, and the severity of X-ray changes in OA correlates relatively poorly with pain severity.[27]

Based on MRI studies in osteoarthritic knees comparing those with and without pain and on studies mapping tenderness in unanesthetized joints, likely sources of pain include synovial inflammation, joint effusions, and bone marrow edema.[28,29] Modest synovitis develops in many but not all osteoarthritic joints.[30] Some diseased joints have no synovitis, whereas others have synovial inflammation that approaches the severity of joints with rheumatoid arthritis. The presence of synovitis on MRI is correlated with the presence and severity of knee pain.[31,32] Capsular stretching from fluid in the joint stimulates nociceptive fibers there, inducing pain. Increased focal loading as part of the disease not only damages cartilage but also may injure the underlying bone. As a consequence, bone marrow edema appears on the MRI; histologically, this edema may signal the presence of microcracks and scar, which may be the consequences of trauma. These lesions may stimulate bone nociceptive fibers. Also, hemostatic pressure within bone rises in OA, and the increased pressure itself may stimulate nociceptive fibers, causing pain. Lastly, osteophytes themselves may be a source of pain. When osteophytes grow, neurovascular innervation penetrates through the base of the bone into the cartilage and into the developing osteophyte.

Pain may arise from extra-articular sources also, including bursae near the joints, or pain referred from the knee or back. Common extra-articular sources of pain near the knee are anserine bursitis and iliotibial band syndrome.

Stiffness: Morning stiffness may occur with OA. While permanent mechanical loss of motion can gradually occur over time as the disease progresses, stiffness is defined as a temporary sensation that the joint and periarticular musculature are tight and difficult to move. Morning stiffness in OA usually lasts less than 30 minutes; this is in direct contrast to inflammatory arthridities such as rheumatoid arthritis where the morning stiffness can be up to three hours in duration. Also, the morning stiffness in OA is restricted to the region around the affected joints, and is not diffuse, as with rheumatoid arthritis.[33]

Limited joint function: Osteoarthritis will result in decreased function of the joint for recreational, vocational or daily activities. This limitation of function can be due to joint pain, or may also result from a limited range of motion secondary to articular feromity, osteophyte formation, malalignment, muscle weakness or joint instability. Joint proprioception is decreased in OA, though this is associated with minimal clinical impact on the disease.[34]

Physical Examination Signs

Physical examination serves to verify that the symptoms expressed by the patient arise from the joint and are not manifestations of a periarticular process such as bursitis, inflammation of a bursa. In a complete physical examination, each joint is palpated for tenderness, warmth, effusion and crepitus. Observation of a patients gait pattern is important particularly to detect pain on weight bearing and effect of OA on walking ability. Passive and active range of motion, as well as pain associated with both must be evaluated and documented. Depending on the site of involvement, additional findings such as pes anserine bursal tenderness of the knee can be elucidated via the physical examination.

OA may be mono- or poly-articular. The hands, knees, hips and spine are the most frequently affected sites. Involvement of the distal interphalangeal joint (DIP), proximal interphalangeal joint (DIP) and the carpometacarpal joints (CMC), but not metacarpophalangeal (MCP) joints, are very characteristic of OA. MCP, wrist, shoulder and elbow involvement points to an underlying condition (congenital abnormality, trauma) or a systemic disease. Of particular note, unilateral disease of hips or knees often becomes bilateral with time, and this is thought to result from the disruption of joint mechanics in the affected joint that translate to abnormal joint mechanics in the contralateral joint, causing OA with time.[35] Patients who have received total hip arthroplasty are at increased risk for developing contralateral knee OA.[36]

Tenderness: Tenderness is typically present with palpation of the joint margins or with pressure on the joint, except for the hip joint which is too deep to produce tenderness on palpation.

Joint enlargement: Joint effusions, abnormal buildup of joint fluid, are a common cause of joint enlargement. Effusions in OA are generally non-inflammatory; if warmth or erythema is present along with effusion, an inflammatory process such as septic arthritis, rheumatoid arthritis or acute gouty arthritis must be considered.

Bony osteophytes, boney growths, are another cause of joint enlargement in OA. These are characteristically present in the physical examination of distal interphalangeal and proximal interphalangeal joints. Osteophytes are commonly present in the hip and as well as the knee and, are better visualized via imaging.

Crepitus: Crepitus is defined as an audible or palpable sensation of roughness, crunching or crackling over a joint throughout passive or active range of motion. Crepitus is thought to be a result of intra-articular debris or irregularity of joint surfaces. The detection of crepitus in patellofemoral, tibial, or femoral condyles around the knee correlates well with degenerative findings in arthroscopy.[37]

Limitation of range of motion: Range of motion limitations can be caused by pain, loss of cartilage, malalignment of the joint, osteophytes, effusions, flexion contractures or muscle spasms. Flexion contracture (inability to extend the knee) affects standing and walking ability on level surfaces, while limitation of flexion tends to restrict sitting ability and ascending or descending stairs. Subtle losses of range of motion may not be appreciated by the patient but can be elucidated by careful observation of movement during the physical examination (especially for hand OA) or asking the patient to walk a few steps in the examination room.

Malalignment: Varus angulation of the limb due to loss of articular cartilage in the medial compartment of the knee and valgus angulation due to loss of articular cartilage in the lateral compartment of the knee commonly occur in OA. The degree of malalignment can be measured via a goniometer during the physical exam or using a full-length standing X-ray.

Musculature: Muscle bulk and motor weakness of the peripheral joint muscles should be measured and followed. Quadriceps femoris atrophy is not uncommon in the presence of knee OA and is likely related to limp or avoidance of use of the limb during weight bearing activity as a result of arthritic pain. Muscle mass decreases with age, and rebuilding muscle strength is helpful in restoring function.

Acuity and joint distribution of OA: Osteoarthritis is an insidious disease. Most patients are asymptomatic until the sixth decade of life. An acute inflammatory presentation of a joint suggests infection, crystal arthopathy or systemic inflammatory arthritis.

Clinical Differential Diagnosis

OA is the most common cause of chronic knee pain in persons over 45 years of age, but the differential diagnosis is long. An acute monoarticular presence warrants consideration of crystal or infectious arthropathy or a seronegative spondyloarthropathy. Polyarticular disease may need to be distinguished from systemic inflammatory arthritis. Inflammatory arthritis is likely if there is prominent morning stiffness and many other joints are affected. DIP involvement is typical of psoriatic arthritis and may be seen infrequently in rheumatoid arthritis. Symptomatic MCP involvement is uncommon in OA and typical of rheumatoid arthritis. The presence of warmth and edema decreases the likelihood of OA. Evaluation of synovial fluid for total white blood cell count to detect inflammation, and crystal analysis may be indicated. Blood tests are indicated if there is concern about systemic or inflammatory process; these should be normal in OA.

Bursitis, inflammation or irritation or the bursa, occurs commonly around knees and hips. A physical examination should focus on whether tenderness is over the joint line (at the junction of the articular joint surfaces) or is outside of it. Anserine bursitis, medial and distal to the knee, is a common cause of chronic knee pain that may respond to a glucocorticoid injection. However, buritis and OA may also occur together. Prominent nocturnal pain in the absence of end-stage OA merits a distinct workup. For hip pain, OA can be detected by loss of internal rotation on passive movement, and pain isolated to an area lateral to the hip joint usually reflects the presence of trochanteric bursitis.

The most important common alternative diagnoses for OA are presented with a brief description of each:

Rheumatoid arthritis: A chronic systemic inflammatory disorder, rheumatoid arthritis (RA) is a crippling disease affecting approximately 1% of the population in the US. Although similar synovial histopathologic and joint abnormalities are identifiable in most patients, the articular and systemic manifestations, outcomes, and differences in genetic makeup and serologic findings vary widely in individual patients. The cause is unknown, although the disease probably occurs in response to a pathogenic agent in a genetically predisposed host. Possible triggering factors include bacterial, mycoplasmal, or viral infections, as well as endogenous antigens in the form of rheumatoid factor, collagens, and mucopolysaccharides.

Joint involvement is typically symmetric, affecting the wrist, meta-carpal, phalangeal, proximal interphalangeal, elbow, shoulder, cervical spine, hip, knee, and ankle joints. The distal interphalangeal joints are typically spared, in contrast to OA which typically involves such joints in the hand. Extra-articular manifestations include vasculitis, pericarditis, skin nodules, pulmonary fibrosis, pneumonitis, and scleritis. The triad of arthritis, lymphadenopathy, and splenomegaly, known as Felty syndrome, is associated with anemia, thrombocytopenia, and neutropenia.

RA occurs two to four times more often in women than men. The disease occurs in all age groups, but increases in incidence with advancing age, with a peak between the fourth and sixth decades.

Gout: Deposition of monosodium urate crystals in the joints produces gout. Although most patients with gout have hyperuricemia, abnormal uric acid level in the blood, few patients with hyperuricemia develop gout. The causes of hyperuricemia include disorders resulting in over-production or undersecretion of uric acid or a combination of these two abnormalities. Examples of uric acid overproduction include enzy-matic mutations, leukemias, hemoglobinopathies, and excessive purine intake.

The first attack involves sudden onset of painful arthritis, most often in the first metatarsophalangeal joint, but also in the ankle, knee, wrist, finger, and elbow. The intensity of the pain is comparable to that from a septic joint, and differentiation is necessary because the treatment is different. Coexistence of a septic joint is unusual but possible. Chronic gouty arthritis is notable for tophaceous deposits, joint deformity, constant pain, and swelling. Definitive diagnosis is made upon demonstration of intracellular monosodium urate crystals in synovial cell leukocytes.

Primary gout has hereditary features, with a familial incidence of 6%–18%. It is likely that the serum urate concentration is controlled by multiple genes.

The key diagnostic test is detection of monosodium urate crystals in white blood cells in synovial fluid. Negative birefringence of the needle-shaped crystals is seen by their yellow coloration on polarized light microscopy.

Hyperuricemia is usually seen, but up to a fourth of gout patients may have normal uric acid levels. Uric acid levels are elevated when they exceed 7 mg/dL. An elevated white blood cell count and sedimentation rate can be seen in acute gout, and thus these tests cannot be used to differentiate between the two processes. Aspirates should be sent for culture to rule out coexisting infection.

Calcium pyrophasphate deposition disease (pseudogout): Calcium pyrophosphate crystal deposition disease, a goutlike syndrome, is also known as pseudogout or chondrocalcinosis. Crystals of calcium pyrophosphate dihydrate are deposited in a joint, most commonly the knee and not the first metatarsophalangeal joint, as in gout. The diagnosis is made by demonstration of the crystals in tissue or synovial fluid and by the presence of characteristic radiographic findings.

Aging and trauma, as well as conditions such as hyperparathyroidism, gout, hemochromatosis, hypophosphatasia, and hypothyroidism are associated with this disorder.

Hereditary forms of calcium pyrophosphate dihydrate deposition disease are reported, with transmission as an autosomal trait. Idiopathic cases were not rigorously examined for genetic factors or association with other diseases.

Erosive inflammatory OA: Erosive OA is considered a subtype of generalized OA primarily affecting the small joints of the hands with a strong familial predisposition. Women are most commonly affected. Pain, swelling and erythema are prominent findings. Radiographs demonstrate irregular joint spaces loss, osteophytes and bony erosions. Bony ankylosis may occur.

Generalized OA: Generalized OA is similar in presentation to isolated OA, but many more joints are affected, including hands, knees, hips and spine. Similar to erosive inflammatory OA, generalized OA is particularly well defined in women between ages 45 and 65. Genetic predisposition is likely, but unproven, in generalized OA.

Hemochromatosis: Hemochromatosis is a common inherited disorder of iron metabolism in which an inappropriate increase in intestinal iron absorption results in deposition of excessive amounts of iron in parenchymal cells with eventual tissue damage and impaired organ function. Arthropathy develops in 25%–50% of symptomatic patients. It usually occurs after age 50 but may occur as a first manifestation, or long after therapy. The joints of the hands, especially the second and third metacarpophalangeal joints, are usually the first joints involved, a feature that helps to distinguish the chondrocalcinosis associated with hemochromatosis from the idiopathic form. A progressive polyarthritis involving wrists, hips, ankles, and knees may also ensue. Acute brief attacks of synovitis may be associated with deposition of calcium pyrophosphate (pseudogout), mainly in the knees. Radiologic manifestations include cystic changes of the subchondral bones, loss of articular cartilage with narrowing of the joint space, diffuse demineralization, hypertrophic bone proliferation, and calcification of the synovium. The arthropathy tends to progress despite removal of iron by phlebotomy.

Pigmented villonodular synovitis: Pigmented villonodular synovitis (PVNS) is a rare benign neoplasm of the synovium that typically develops in the knee or other large joint during the third or fourth decade of life, but that can occur in any synovial-lined joint at any age. Involvement of the synovium is usually diffuse, producing boggy swelling that can be massive and disproportionate to the degree of discomfort. Rarely PVNS is focal within the joint and presents with locking symptoms. The grossly thickened synovium has friable villi that bleed, leading to diffuse hemosiderin staining of the synovium and bloody or xanthochromic synovial fluid in most, but not all, cases. Plain radiographs do not show specific changes but may reveal erosions and cystic changes in adjacent bone, usually with preserved joint space. Magnetic resonance imaging is the imaging procedure of choice and may point to the correct diagnosis, but definitive diagnosis requires histologic examination of involved tissue. The treatment of choice for most patients is surgical excision.

Hemophilic arthropathy: Hemophilia is a sex-linked recessive genetic disorder characterized by the absence or deficiency of factor VIII (hemophilia A, or classic hemophilia) or factor IX (hemophilia B, or Christmas disease). Hemophilia A is by far the more common type, constituting 85% of cases. Spontaneous hemarthrosis is a common problem with both types of hemophilia and can lead to a chronic deforming arthritis. The frequency and severity of hemarthrosis are related to the degree of clotting factor deficiency. Hemarthrosis is not common in other inherited disorders of coagulation, such as von Willebrand disease or factor V deficiency.

Hemarthrosis becomes evident after one year of age, when the child begins to walk and run. In order of frequency, the joints most commonly affected are the knees, ankles, elbows, shoulders, and hips. Small joints of the hands and feet are occasionally involved.

In the initial stage of arthropathy, hemarthrosis produces a warm, tensely swollen, and painful joint. The patient holds the affected joint in flexion and guards against any movement. Blood in the joint remains liquid because of the absence of intrinsic clotting factors and the absence of tissue thromboplastin in the synovium. The blood in the joint space is resorbed over a period of a week or longer, depending on the size of the hemarthrosis. Joint function usually returns to normal or baseline in about two weeks.

Recurrent hemarthrosis leads to the development of a chronic arthritis. The involved joints remain swollen, and flexion deformities develop. In the later stages of arthropathy, joint motion is restricted and function is severely limited. Joint ankylosis, subluxation, and laxity are features of end-stage disease.

Pathophysiology of Osteoarthritis

General Considerations

As mentioned earlier, articular cartilage is the major target of degenerative changes in osteoarthritis. Normal articular cartilage is strategically located at the ends of bones to perform two functions: (1) bathed in synovial fluid, it ensures virtually friction-free movements within the joint and (2) in weight-bearing joints, it spreads the load across the joint surface in a manner that allows the underlying bones to effectively absorb shock and weight bearing loads. These functions require the cartilage to be elastic (i.e. to regain normal architecture after being compressed, a property referred to as "reversible deformation") and for it to have unusually high tensile strength. These attributes are provided by the two major components of the cartilage: a special type of collagen (type II) and proteoglycans, both produced by chondrocytes. As is the case with adult bones, articular cartilage is not static; it undergoes turnover in which worn out matrix components are degraded and replaced. This balance is maintained by chondrocytes, which not only synthesize the matrix but also secrete matrix-degrading enzymes. Thus, the health of the chondrocytes and their ability to maintain the essential properties of the cartilage matrix determine joint integrity.[38] In osteoarthritis, this process is disturbed by a variety of influences. Other supporting tissues within the joint are also affected by OA: subchondral bone, meniscus, ligaments, periarticular muscle, and synovial membrane (synovium). The roles of these in the pathogenesis of OA will be discussed below as well.

Factors Inducing Susceptibility to OA

Osteoarthritis was previously thought to be a normal consequence of aging, thereby leading to the term "degenerative joint disease." It is now realized that osteoarthritis results from a complex interplay of multiple factors, including joint integrity, genetics, local inflammation, mechanical forces, and cellular biochemical processes.[39] Perhaps the most important of these influences are aging and mechanical effects. Evidence for this includes the increasing frequency of osteoarthritis with advancing age,[9,40] its occurrence in weight-bearing joints, and an increase in the frequency of the disease in conditions that predispose the joints to abnormal mechanical stresses, such as obesity[26,40–49] repetitive loading resulting from occupational exposure, and previous joint deformity.[50–60] Genetic factors also appear to play a role in susceptibility to osteoarthritis, particularly in cases involving the hands and hips. The specific gene or genes responsible for this have not been identified, although linkage to chromosomes 2 and 11 has been suggested in some cases.[61–65] The risk of osteoarthritis of hip and knee is increased in direct proportion to bone density,[66–69] and high levels of estrogens have also been associated with an increased risk of the disease, though conflicting results have been reported.[6,70-77] The overall role played by hormones in the pathogenesis of osteoarthritis remains unclear.

Articular Cartilage in Osteoarthritis

Osteoarthritis is characterized by significant changes in both the composition and the mechanical properties of articular cartilage. Numerous *in vitro* studies have explored the relationship between repetitive, mechanical loading and resultant changes in cellular function and matrix elements. It has been demonstrated that chondrocyte production of the macromolecular extracellular matrix components is dependent upon both the magnitude and frequency of the force applied.[78-80]

Compared with normal cartilage, cartilage from osteoarthritic tissue deforms more readily in response to the same load and more fluid is lost during the application of a given load.[81] The same external load therefore results in different mechanical stimuli in normal and osteoarthritic cartilage.[80] Early in the course of the disease, the degenerating cartilage contains increased water and a decreased concentration of proteoglycans compared with healthy cartilage (Fig. 1). In addition, there appears to be a weakening of the collagen network, presumably caused by decreased local synthesis of type II collagen, and increased breakdown of preexisting collagen. The levels of certain molecular messengers, including Interleukin-1 (IL-1),[82-88] Tumor Necrosis Factor (TNF)[89-92] and nitric oxide,[93-96] are increased in osteoarthritic cartilage and appear to be responsible for some of these changes in the composition of the cartilage.

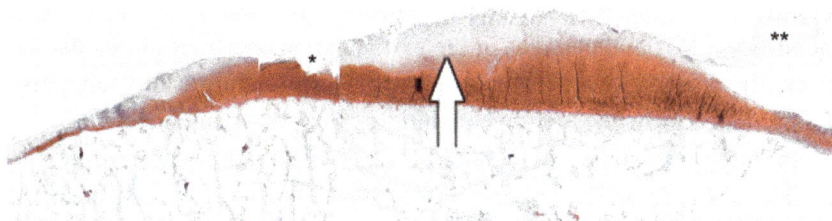

Fig. 1. Sagittal histologic section (Safranin-O stain) of the lateral tibial plateau in a 74-year-old male patient with OA. *indicates a cutting artifact. Cartilage thinning, fibrillation and proteoglycan loss by a 50% reduction in red-staining in the Safranin-O staining is demonstrable at the arrow.[166]

IL-1 is synthesized by chondrocytes and mononuclear cells lining the synovium and acts in multiple ways to suppress synthesis of type 2 (articular cartilage) collagen and promote the formation of type 1 (fibrous cartilage) collagen. Additionally, IL-1 induces catabolic enzymes such as collagenase and suppresses prostaglandin synthesis.[83,84,87] IL-1 caused cartilage damage via proteoglycan loss in an animal model. Not only are levels of IL-1 increased in OA, but the chondrocytes of osteoarthritic joints are more susceptible to the actions of IL-1 than non-arthritic chondrocytes.[88]

TNF is a cytokine with similar but less potent effects as IL-1,[89,91] and plays a role in cartilage damage in rheumatoid arthritis.[91] Competitive inhibition of TNF with anti-TNF antibodies has been found to improve symptoms.[90]

Nitric oxide, a highly reactive gas also known as endothelium-derived relaxing factor, has been implicated as a pathogenic mediator in osteoarthritis. Nitric oxide activates metalloproteinsases in articular cartilage.[93] In a canine model of OA, the inhibition of inducible nitric oxide synthase lessened cartilage deterioration.[94,95] In humans, increased amounts of nitic oxide are measured in diseased versus non-diseased cartilage.[96]

Apoptosis is also increased,[97-99] likely responsible for a decrease in the number of functional chondrocytes. In aggregate, these changes tend to reduce the tensile strength and the resilience of the articular cartilage. In response to these regressive changes, chondrocytes in the deeper layers proliferate and attempt to "repair" the damage by producing new collagen and proteoglycans. Although these reparative changes are initially able to keep pace with the deterioration of cartilage, molecular signals causing chondrocyte loss and changes in the extracellular matrix, as noted earlier, eventually predominate. Factors responsible for this shift from a reparative to a predominantly degenerative picture remain poorly understood.

In the early stages of osteoarthritis, the chondrocytes proliferate, leading to increased numbers of chondrocytes adjacent to areas of chondromalacia and increased affinity of the perilacunar matrix for hematoxylin.[100,101] This process is accompanied by biochemical changes as the water content of the matrix increases and the concentration of proteoglycans decreases. Subsequently, vertical and horizontal fibrillation and cracking of the matrix occur as the superficial layers of the cartilage are degraded. Gross examination at this stage reveals a granular articular surface that is softer than normal. Eventually, full-thickness portions of the cartilage are sloughed, and the exposed subchondral bone plate becomes the new articular surface. Friction smoothes and burnishes the exposed bone, giving it the appearance of polished ivory (bone eburnation).

Histological Appearance and Grading for Cartilage Degeneration

As mentioned earlier, loss of proteoglycan content, cartilage thinning, fissuring and/or delamination, as well as matrix fibrillation and osteophyte formation are all observed in osteoarthritic cartilage, and all these changes are demonstrable via histologic sections (see Figs. 1 to 5). Crucial to any study of osteoarthritis pathogenesis or treatment is the availability of a reliable, reproducible, simple yet comprehensive histologic grading system for articular cartilage abnormalities. Such a system can be utilized to identify specific subsets of patients with varying degrees of disease, provide direct validation for radiographic findings, evaluate animal models of osteoarthritis progression and/or repair and provide an opportunity to advance our understanding of osteoarthritis by allowing for new pathologic findings to be evaluated. The pioneering work of Mankin *et al.* in 1971 resulted in the development of an OA pathology grading system using femoral heads removed during arthroplasty.[102] The Mankin grading system was based on microscopic evaluation of decalcified sections from femoral head articular cartilage removed at surgery. The sections were stained with Safranin O with a light green counter stain. The grading system is based on a combination of cellular changes, biochemical changes as revealed by the intensity of Safranin O staining, and structural changes in the cartilage matrix, including thickness and surface characteristics (Table 1). Since its creation, the Mankin system has been adopted by many investigators and utilized in studies investigating animal models of OA as well as OA spontaneously arising in humans and non-human primates. Despite its widespread use, however, the Mankin system's reproducibility and validity has been questioned.[103,104] The Mankin system is based on cartilage samples from very degenerated hips, and therefore not linear for

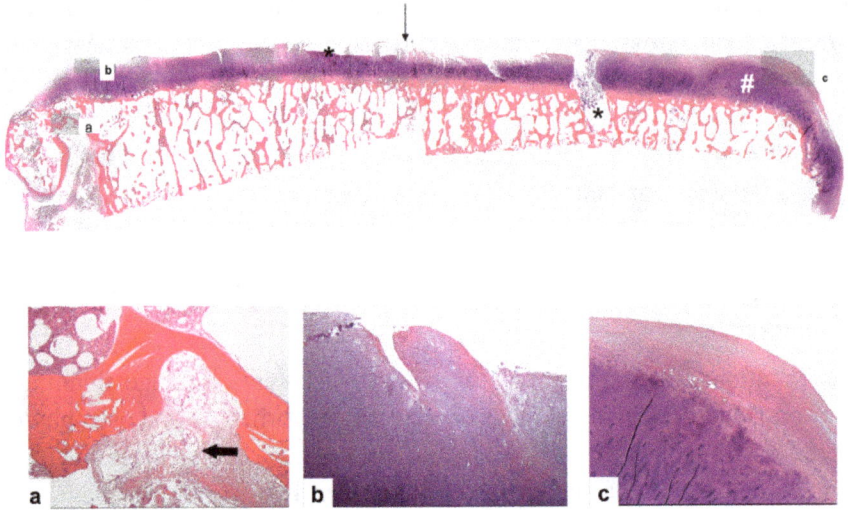

Fig. 2. Tibial histological section (H&E) of a 54-year-old female patient with OA. *indicates sectioning and folding artifacts. Magnified histological areas demonstrate osteophyte **(a)**, fibrocartilage overlying the osteophyte **(b)** and synovial (pannus) tissue overlying normal cartilage. Increased fibrovascular tissue ingrowth (arrow in a) within the bone marrow of the osteophyte leads to increased osteoclast resorption. Black arrow indicates less than 50% thinning and surface fraying of the cartilage in the central tibia.[166]

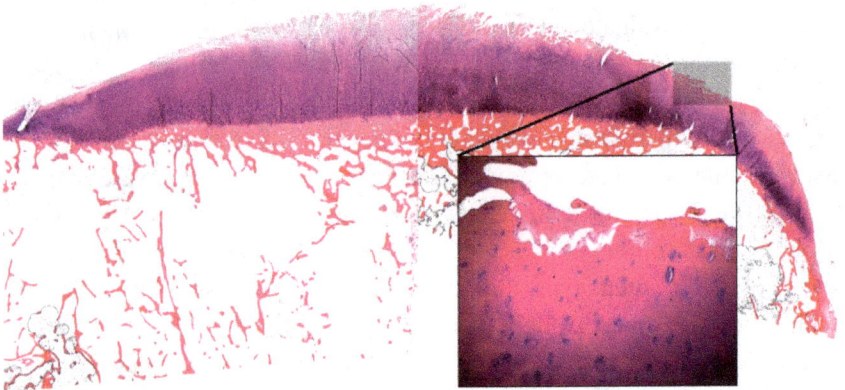

Fig. 3. Histological section (H&E) of the lateral tibial plateau in a 51-year-old male patient with OA. Fraying with fibrillation involving less than 50% of the cartilage surface is observed centrally and posteriorly at the tibia. Magnification shows minor synovial tissue ingrowth in the posterior aspect, degrading the superficial cartilage layer.[166]

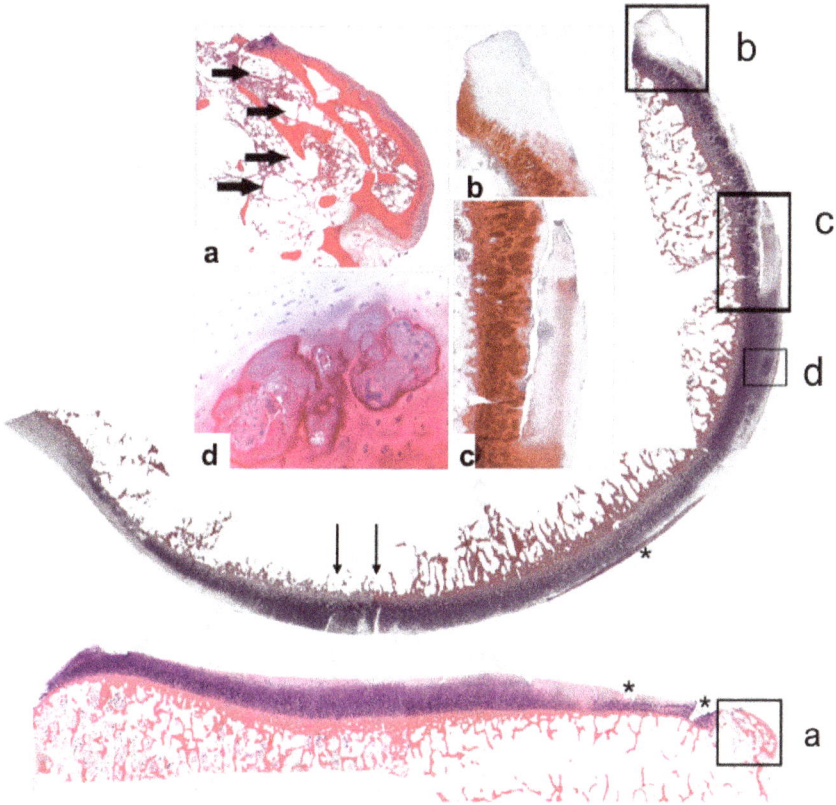

Fig. 4. Complete histological reconstruction of the medial knee compartment (a, d: H&E staining; b, c: Safranin-O staining) in a 68-year-old female osteoarthritic patient. *indicates sectioning and folding artifacts. A number of pathologic processes are depicted in the histological sections: (I) Deep (> 50%) fissures/clefts in the cartilage (two small black arrows). (II) Osteophyte **(a)** with fibrovascular tissue with multiple large vascular sinuses within the marrow, indicating increased vascular flow. (III) In **(b)** a small area of thick fibro-cartilage, with reduced Safranin-O red staining indicating reduced proteoglycan content and increased matrix water content is shown. (IV) In **(d)** necrotic chondrocytes with myxoid degeneration of the surrounding matrix (Weichselbaum's lacunae) are demonstrated in the vicinity of a cartilage lesion **(c)**. (V) In **(c)** horizontal cartilage delamination with reduced proteoglycan content in the separated cartilage layer is shown.[166]

mild or earlier phases of the disease, which is what is most commonly seen in experimental animal models of osteoarthritis.

In 2005, the Osteoarthritis Research Society International (OARSI) introduced the Osteoarthritis Cartilage Histopathology Grading System

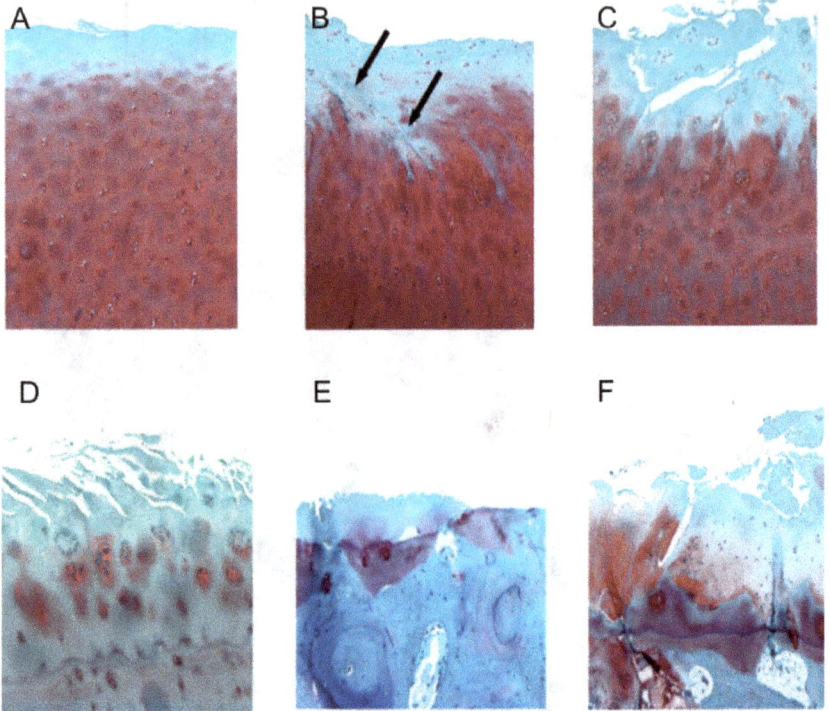

Fig. 5. OA cartilage pathology, OARSI grades 1–6, histologic features, Safranin O stain, original magnification ×5. (**A**) Grade 1: surface intact. The articular surface is uneven and can demonstrate superficial fibrillation. This may be accompanied by cell death or proliferation. The mid zone and deep zone are unaffected. (**B**) Grade 2: surface discontinuity. Focally fibrillation extends through the superficial zone to the superficial zone-mid zone portion ↓. This may be accompanied by cell proliferation, increased or decreased matrix staining and/or cell death in mid zone. (**C**) Grade 3: vertical fissures extending into mid zone. The matrix fibrillation extends vertically downward into the mid zone. As the OA becomes more extensive, the fissures may branch and extend into the deep zone. Cell death and all proliferation may be observed most prominently adjacent to fissures. (**D**) Grade 4: erosion. Cartilage matrix loss is observed which in earliest stage may be only delamination of superficial zone cartilage. More extensive erosion results illustrated in excavation, loss of matrix in fissured domains. (**E**) Grade 5: denudation. The unmineralized hyaline cartilage is completely eroded. The articular surface is mineralized cartilage or bone. Microfracture through the bone plate may result in reparative fibrocartilage occupying gaps in the surface. (**F**) Grade 6: deformation. The processes of microfracture, repair and bone remodelling change the contour of the articular surface. At the earliest phase, illustrated, fibrocartilage has grown along the level of the previously eroded and denuded surface. Fibrocartilaginous articular surfaces, marginal and central osteophytes are processes associated with more extensive articular contour deformation.

Table 1. Mankin scoring system.

I: Structure	
Normal	0
Surface irregularities	1
Pannus and surface irregularities	2
Clefts to transitional zone	3
Clefts to radial zone	4
Clefts to calcified zone	5
Complete disorganization	6
II: Cells	
Normal	0
Diffuse hypercellularity	1
Cloning	2
Hypocellularity	3
III: Safranin-O staining	
Normal	0
Slight reduction	1
Moderate reduction	2
Severe reduction	3
No dye noted	4
IV: Tidemark integrity	
Intact	0
Crossed by blood vessels	1

(OCHGS), to overcome the limitations of the Mankin grading system.[105] This system follows an analogy of the concept widely used in cancer pathology assessment: increasing grade (OA depth progression into articular cartilage) indicates more aggressive disease, whereas increasing stage (horizontal extent of cartilage involvement within one joint compartment irrespective of the severity of underlying disease) indicates greater disease extent. The overall score is a composite of OA grade and stage results, representing a combined assessment of OA severity and extent (Tables 2a and 2b; Fig. 5). In one comparison study[106] between the Mankin grading system and the OCHGS, both were found to have excellent intra- and inter-observer reproducibility and variability and a good positive correlation between the scores. The same study also demonstrated that three inexperienced observers were able to reach excellent intra- and inter-observer variability using the OCHGS, whereas intra-observer variability seemed

Table 2a. OCHGS advanced grading methodology.

Grade (key feature)	Subgrade	Associated criteria (tissue reaction)
Grade 0: Surface and cartilage intact	No subgrade	Intact, uninvolved cartilage
Grade 1: Surface intact	1.0 Cells intact	Matrix: Superficial zone intact, edema and/or fibrillation
	1.5 Cell death	Cells: Proliferation (clusters), hypertrophy Reaction must be more than superficial fibrillation only
Grade 2: Surface discontinuity	2.0 Fibrillation through superficial zone	As above
	2.5 Surface abrasion with matrix loss within superficial zone	+ Discontinuity at superficial zone ± Cationic stain matrix depletion upper 1/3 of cartilage (mid zone) ± Disorientation of chondron columns
Grade 3: Vertical fissures	3.0 Simple fissures	As above
	3.5 Branched/complex fissures	± Cationic stain depletion into lower 2/3 of cartilage (deep zone) ± New collagen formation (polarized light microscopy)
Grade 4: Erosion	4.0 Superficial zone delamination	Cartilage matrix loss, cyst formation within cartilage matrix
	4.5 Mid zone excavation	
Grade 5: Denudation	5.0 Bone surface intact	Surface is sclerotic bone or reparative tissue including fibrocartilage
	5.5 Reparative tissue surface present	
Grade 6: Deformation	6.0 Joint margin osteophytes	Bone remodeling. Deformation of articular surface contour (more than osteophyte formation only)
	6.5 Joint margin and central osteophytes	Includes: Microfracture and repair

Table 2b. OCHGS stage assessment.

Stage	% Involvement (surface, area, and volume)
Stage 0	No OA activity seen
Stage 1	< 10%
Stage 2	10–25%
Stage 3	25–50%
Stage 4	> 50%

more dependent on experience when using the Mankin grading system. There is a lack of data thus far on the correlation of OCHGS to macroscopic and biochemical scores.

Bone Changes in Osteoarthritis

Osteoarthritis (OA) is characterized by progressive alterations in the structural and functional properties of periarticular bone. These skeletal changes are reflective of the factors and processes that control the activities of the bone cell populations that remodel and adapt skeletal tissues to local environmental and systemic factors, as well as to the alterations in articular cartilage and the other tissues comprising the diarthrodial joint. During the course of OA, there are marked changes in the organization and functional properties of the periarticular bone. Importantly, these alterations are not uniform, reflecting the differences in the structural organization of the bone at different periarticular sites including progressive increase in subchondral bone plate thickness, subchondral trabecular bone architecture changes, development of subchondral bone cysts, bone growth at the joint margins (osteophytes), the appearance of bone marrow edema lesions (BMEL), and advancement of the tidemark associated with vascular invasion of the calcified cartilage.[107]

   The architecture and the properties of the periarticular cortical and trabecular bone are modified through the cellular processes of remodeling and modeling. In addition, mechanical factors may directly alter the structural and functional features of the bone tissue via generation of discontinuities (so-called "microcracks") in the absence of direct cellular activity.[108–110] An additional mechanism affecting periarticular bone involves the process of endochondral ossification in which new bone is formed by replacement of a cartilaginous matrix. These cellular processes are reactivated at the joint margins, giving rise to the formation of osteophytes, which represent one of the radiographic characteristics of OA. In addition, a similar cellular process is activated at the site of the tidemark, immediately adjacent to the calcified cartilage. The initial event involves the penetration of the zone of calcified cartilage by vascular elements followed by chondrocyte hypertrophy, deposition of calcified cartilage, and eventual replacement with bone. This results in duplication of the tidemark and advancement of the calcified cartilage into the deep zones of the articular cartilage. Importantly, the replacement of the hyaline cartilage contributes to thinning of the articular cartilage zone and likely adversely affects the integrity and biomechanical properties of the articular surface.[108,109,111–113] All these alterations, especially when accompanied by changes in the shape and contour of the subchondral plate, may adversely affect the capacity of the adjacent articular cartilage to adapt to mechanical loads.[114,115] The role of bone in OA will be discussed in further detail in Chapter 8.

Meniscus in Osteoarthritis

In OA, the meniscus is often torn, macerated, or even totally destroyed, suggesting a strong association between the degenerative disease and the meniscus.[54,116] There are two major categories of meniscal injuries: traumatic lesions and gradual degeneration with aging or other degenerative processes.[117–119]

Traumatic lesions usually occur in younger active individuals caused by a distinct knee trauma when the meniscus is trapped between the femoral condyle and the tibial plateau under excessive forces.[120] The meniscus often splits vertically and parallel to the circumferentially oriented collagen fibers.

Degenerative lesions, described as horizontal cleavages, flap (oblique) or complex tears, or meniscal maceration or destruction, are associated with older age and osteoarthritic disease.[116,118] MRI in patients who had a mean age of 65 years found a meniscal tear in 67% of asymptomatic patients and in 91% of patients who had symptomatic knee OA.[116]

Meniscal lesions may be associated with knee joint symptoms, but most lesions, especially degenerative meniscal lesions, are asymptomatic.[116,121] Still, a meniscal tear may cause severe knee discomfort or even locking of the knee because of a dislocated tear fragment, and surgical treatment often becomes necessary. Englund *et al.*[122] reported that, despite the meniscus preservation during meniscal surgery which may provide some benefits compared with total resection, the reduction in the frequency of knee OA seems to be modest. The reason might be that many of the middle-aged and older surgery patients already have early-stage knee OA at the time of "meniscal" symptoms, and the meniscal tear itself is associated weakly with the development of knee symptoms, but other features of OA may be symptomatic.[123]

The menisci and articular cartilage have many similar components and properties and are subjected to similar stresses. The pathologic processes active in the early-stage OA joint that eventually lead to the cartilage destruction characteristic of OA are not limited only to the joint cartilage but would be expected to affect the integrity of the menisci and ligaments as well.[120] A tear in a meniscus with degenerative changes often is associated with pre-existing structural changes in the articular cartilage that may represent early-stage OA.[118] Shear stress and early proteolytic degradation of the collagenous meniscal matrix may result in decreased tensile strength. A meniscal tear could be the result of the decreased ability of the compromised meniscus to withstand loads and force transmissions during normal knee joint loads.[120]

Meniscal displacement is common, particularly in osteoarthritic knees.[124,125] This feature often is another sign of a degraded or torn meniscus and a possible OA disease process. Meniscal displacement also may contribute to the increased joint space narrowing seen on radiographs, and meniscal tear and displacement are strong determinants of the rate of cartilage loss in knee OA.[50,54,126] Englund emphasized that in middle-aged or elderly people, knees with meniscal damage but without cartilage lesions are at much higher risk of knee OA than knees with intact menisci, suggesting that in many instances the meniscal damage comes before visible cartilage changes.[123]

To date, little is known about the effect of meniscal injury on the risk of disease progression in OA patients. Studies of the meniscectomy suggest the importance of the meniscal function loss as a risk factor for subsequent knee OA.[127] Using semi-quantitative MRI with arthroscopic correlation, Hunter et al.[54] demonstrated a strong association of the meniscal pathology changes with cartilage loss in symptomatic knee OA. In a recent study, Lo and colleagues[128] found a strong association between maceration of the meniscus and BME, suggesting that the meniscus maceration was a prerequisite for a large BME and that BME lesions may be a consequence of impact forces in a knee with an aberrant load distribution or instability resulting from a meniscus damage.

Meniscal tears are commonly present in acute ACL injuries. Both orthopedic and radiology literature have reported a significant association between the meniscus tears and ACL injury, and that these ACL injuries are more commonly associated with the lateral meniscus (LM) tears than medial meniscus (MM) tears.[129] Also, associations between BME and meniscal tears have been demonstrated in studies of the acute ACL injuries reporting that these lesions as predominantly located on the lateral side of the joint.[130–132] Nishimori et al.,[133] reporting clinical findings based on MRI and arthroscopy in patients with acute ACL injuries, emphasized the importance that needs to be attributed to the cartilage damage of the posterior lateral tibial plateau as well as to the posterior horn tears in the LM.

All these findings emphasize the important role of the meniscus in OA development, suggesting that abnormal meniscal function could have potential consequences for cartilage damage. Therefore, identifying risk factors may help to develop preventive interventions targeted toward the osteoarthritic patients.

Ligaments in Osteoarthritis

Cruciate ligaments as well as collateral ligaments have an essential role in maintaining the joint stability. Acute injuries can affect these ligaments, generating abnormal joint functionality that may lead to OA. The anterior cruciate ligament (ACL) is the most frequently injured ligament of the knee joint, but there is little reported about the condition of the posterior cruciate ligament (PCL) in OA.[134,135]

There are relatively few studies that have evaluated the histological changes in both cruciate ligaments in osteoarthritic knees. Young et al.[136]

found abnormal type II collagen deposition in PCL from the spontaneously Dunkin-Hartley osteoarthritic guinea pig model. Stubbs and coworkers[137] suggested that degenerative and traumatic change occurs to the cruciate ligaments in osteoarthritis, and there is indirect evidence that damage to the ACL from osteophyte induced stenosis of the intercondylar notch or previous direct trauma may induce changes in the PCL.

Cushner and colleagues[138] studied the histology of anterior cruciate ligaments (ACLs) in 19 osteoarthritic knees and found evidence of degeneration of ACL, which was not seen in normal control knees. Nelissen and Hoogendorn[134] assessed the posterior cruciate ligaments (PCLs) in 20 arthritic patients and noted marked architectural changes and functional deterioration in those with severe grades of osteoarthritis and rheumatoid arthritis. Allain *et al.*[139] examined the histology as well as the macroscopic appearance of both the cruciate ligaments in osteoarthritic knees and reported that the macroscopic appearance of ACL reflects the histological state of PCL in osteoarthritic knees. Although these studies mention varying degrees of histological changes in the cruciate ligaments, it is not known if the degree of degeneration varies with the radiologic progression of the arthritic process and correlates with the severity of deformity. Reactive bone formation in the intercondylar notch in an osteoarthritic knee causes narrowing and reduction in the height of the notch. This can damage the ACL because of shear forces on the ligament during each movement of flexion and extension.[140] Damage to the PCL has been found to be comparatively less severe in osteoarthritic knees,[139] which might be because of the posterior placement of this ligament as compared with the ACL.

A number of studies have proposed that the articular cartilage sustained irreversible injury during impact after an ACL tear, and thus, cartilage degeneration can continue to occur despite the fact that functional stability of the knee is restored following ACL reconstruction.[141,142] Longitudinal MRI studies reported that there was a high prevalence of radiographic OA, pain, and functional limitations in ACL-injured patients ten to 20 years after injuries.[60,143] ACL-injured patients with post-traumatic OA are also reported to be 15 to 20 years younger than patients with primary OA.[144] Also, a strong association between BME and the progression of structural damage in cartilage and trabecular bone was demonstrated in patients with ACL tears.[145,146]

The medial and lateral collateral ligaments stabilize a joint against valgus and varus stress, respectively. In Hartley Dunkin guinea pigs, a guinea pig strain that "spontaneously" develops osteoarthritis of the knee, it was initially considered that the initial abnormalities arose in the articular cartilage. MRI studies subsequently showed changes in the structure and remodeling of subchondral bone of the Hartley Dunkin guinea pigs, particularly at the insertion sites of the cruciate ligaments, which preceded changes in the articular cartilage by several weeks.[147] In humans, injury to the collateral ligaments of the knee is acknowledged to be a risk factor for knee osteoarthritis.[148] The ligamentous laxity associated with hypermobility syndrome is another well-recognized risk factor for osteoarthritis.[149] Sharma et al.,[150] emphasized the importance of varus or valgus malalignment of the knee as a risk factor for the progression of knee osteoarthritis and the role of collateral ligaments damage as risk factor for incident knee OA.

Periarticular Muscle in Osteoarthritis

The most active shock-absorbing mechanisms for joints involve the use of muscles and joint motion. Knee joint instability as a consequence of periarticular muscle weakness may contribute to OA. Loss of muscle — sarcopenia — in older individuals also may be a contributing factor in the development or progression of OA in weight-bearing joints. The loss of supporting muscle may increase the joint load, which can lead to cartilage damage, especially in the weight-bearing joints. Resistance exercise and muscle strengthening may decrease knee symptoms.[151]

Muscle weakness (which may occur in association with knee OA) and an increase in the latent period of the reflex, which may occur with peripheral neuropathy (nerve damage) resulting from aging or other causes, can reduce the effectiveness of this shock-absorbing mechanism. Although the periarticular muscles serve a primary motor function, Hurley et al.[152] emphasized the importance of the sensory function of muscle and of the proprioceptive impulses that originate in muscle and are transmitted to the central nervous system. Data suggest that muscle weakness caused either by reflex inhibition of muscle contraction or by intra-articular pathology may result in joint degeneration.

It has been shown that the quadriceps muscle is important in providing anteroposterior stability to the knee, and that quadriceps weakness is common in patients who have knee OA.[153] In these patients quadriceps weakness has generally been thought to arise as a consequence of the pain that occurs with loading of the arthritic joint; it was postulated that the pain caused the patient to minimize load bearing, thereby leading to atrophy. Quadriceps weakness also may exist also in subjects who have knee OA but who have no history of joint pain and in whom quadriceps muscle mass is not diminished but is normal or even increased (as a result of obesity).[154] Although weakness in the quadriceps is common in patients with knee osteoarthritis, it has generally been considered to arise as a consequence of the pain that occurs with loading of the affected joint, which leads the patient to minimize load bearing, thereby leading to disuse atrophy of the muscle.[155] Longitudinal studies suggest that, in addition to being the consequence of painful knee osteoarthritis, quadriceps weakness may be a risk factor for incident radiographic knee osteoarthritis.[156,157]

The shock-absorbing function of periarticular muscle in protecting joints other than the knee probably is important also. The expression of OA (e.g. with respect to the frequency and severity of joint pain and the rate of progression of joint damage) may vary at different joint sites, and some of this variability may be influenced by the adequacy of the physiologic shock-absorbing mechanisms that protect the joint.[155]

Synovial Membrane in Osteoarthritis

Synovitis, an inflammation of the synovial membrane, is an important characteristic of chronic inflammatory joint diseases such as rheumatoid arthritis (RA), but can also occur as a secondary inflammatory symptom in OA, when it is primarily induced by biochemical stress on cartilage.[158] The synovial membrane or synovium from patients who have advanced OA commonly exhibits hyperplasia of the lining cell layer and focal infiltration of lymphocytes and monocytes.[159] In advanced OA the intensity of the synovitis may resemble that in rheumatoid arthritis. Synovitis in OA may be caused by phagocytosis of wear particles of cartilage and bone from the abraded joint surface,[160,161] by release from the cartilage of soluble matrix macromolecules[162] (e.g. proteoglycans, collagen, fibronectin fragments), or by the presence of crystals of calcium pyrophosphate dihydrate or calcium hydroxyapatite.[163] Earlier in the course of OA, however, the synovium, even from symptomatic patients who have full-thickness ulceration of the articular cartilage, may be histologically normal, suggesting that the early pain in those cases is not caused by synovitis.[164] Conversely, the severity of articular cartilage damage and of synovitis may be as great in patients who have knee OA but no joint pain as in those who do have knee pain. Hill *et al.*[31] showed in cross-sectional MRI analyses of subjects who had knee OA that synovial thickening was much more common in subjects who had pain than in those who were asymptomatic and, among those who had knee pain, was associated with more severe pain. The same group reported in a 30-month longitudinal study of patients who had symptomatic knee OA, changes in synovitis, as graded by MRI, correlated only modestly with changes in knee pain.[32] The relatively weak correlation suggests that synovitis was not the only or even the major cause of the joint pain. Furthermore, pain was not correlated with the loss of articular cartilage in either the tibiofemoral or patellofemoral compartment, and changes in synovial effusion were not correlated with changes in pain. In contrast, Lo and colleagues[165] found that maximal joint effusion scores on MRI were highly associated with knee pain even after adjustment for bone marrow edema lesion scores, suggesting that effusion (a manifestation of underlying synovitis) was associated independently with knee pain.

Conclusions

Osteoarthritis represents the failure of a whole organ (the synovial joint) and not just of articular cartilage, and results from a complex interaction of anatomy and biochemistry within and outside the joint. While a great deal of information has been gathered about the biochemistry and molecular biology of OA, much is still undetermined about this debilitating and common disease. As Brandt and Radin[155] have elaborated, all the other tissues of the knee joint including bone, menisci, ligaments, periarticular muscles, and synovium, are involved in OA and affect its progression. Clinical and basic science research in OA have broadened their scope from a narrow focus on just the articular cartilage, and are promising to unveil targets for therapeutic intervention.

References

1. Meulenbelt I, Bijkerk C, de Wildt SC, Miedema HS, Valkenburg HA, Breedveld FC, Pols HA, Te Koppele JM, Sloos VF, Hofman A, Slagboom PE, van Duijn CM. Investigation of the association of the CRTM and CRTL1 genes with radiographically evident osteoarthritis in subjects from the Rotterdam study. *Arthritis Rheum* 1997;40(10):1760–1765.

2. Hofman A, Grobbee DE, de Jong PT, van den Ouweland FA. Determinants of disease and disability in the elderly: the Rotterdam Elderly Study. *Eur J Epidemiol* 1991;7(4):403–422.

3. Lawrence RC, Helmick CG, Arnett FC, Deyo RA, Felson DT, Giannini EH, Heyse SP, Hirsch R, Hochberg MC, Hunder GG, Liang MH, Pillemer SR, Steen VD, Wolfe F. Estimates of the prevalence of arthritis and selected musculoskeletal disorders in the United States. *Arthritis Rheum* 1998;41(5):778–799.

4. *Global Economic and Health Care Burden of Musculoskeletal Disease* (World Health Organization, 2001).

5. Guccione AA, Felson DT, Anderson JJ, Anthony JM, Zhang Y, Wilson PW, Kelly-Hayes M, Wolf PA, Kreger BE, Kannel WB. The effects of specific medical conditions on the functional limitations of elders in the Framingham Study. *Am J Public Health* 1994;84(3):351–358.

6. Felson DT, Zhang Y, Hannan MT, Naimark A, Weissman BN, Aliabadi P, Levy D. The incidence and natural history of knee osteoarthritis in the elderly. The Framingham Osteoarthritis Study. *Arthritis Rheum* 1995;38(10):1500–1505.

7. Anderson JJ, Felson DT. Factors associated with osteoarthritis of the knee in the first national Health and Nutrition Examination Survey (HANES I). Evidence for an association with overweight, race, and physical demands of work. *Am J Epidemiol* 1988;128(1):179–189.

8. Felson DT, Naimark A, Anderson J, Kazis L, Castelli W, Meenan RF. The prevalence of knee osteoarthritis in the elderly. The Framingham Osteoarthritis Study. *Arthritis Rheum* 1987;30(8):914–918.

9. Lawrence JS, Bremner JM, Bier F. Osteo-arthrosis. Prevalence in the population and relationship between symptoms and X-ray changes. *Ann Rheum Dis* 1966;25(1): 1–24.

10. van Saase JL, van Romunde LK, Cats A, Vandenbroucke JP, Valkenburg HA. Epidemiology of osteoarthritis: Zoetermeer survey. Comparison of radiological osteoarthritis in a Dutch population with that in 10 other populations. *Ann Rheum Dis* 1989;48(4):271–280.

11. Bolbos RI, Link TM, Ma CB, Majumdar S, Li X. T1rho relaxation time of the meniscus and its relationship with T1rho of adjacent cartilage in knees with acute ACL injuries at 3 T. *Osteoarthr Cartil* 2009;17(1):12–18.

12. Li X, Benjamin Ma C, Link TM, Castillo DD, Blumenkrantz G, Lozano J, Carballido-Gamio J, Ries M, Majumdar S. *In vivo* T(1rho) and T(2) mapping of articular cartilage in osteoarthritis of the knee using 3 T MRI. *Osteoarthr Cartil* 2007;15(7):789–797.

13. Li X, Han ET, Ma CB, Link TM, Newitt DC, Majumdar S. *In vivo* 3T spiral imaging based multi-slice T(1rho) mapping of knee cartilage in osteoarthritis. *Magn Reson Med* 2005;54(4):929–936.

14. Li X, Pai A, Blumenkrantz G, Carballido-Gamio J, Link T, Ma B, Ries M, Majumdar S. Spatial distribution and relationship of T(1rho) and T(2) relaxation times in knee cartilage with osteoarthritis. *Magn Reson Med* 2009;61(6):1310–1318.
15. Rauscher I, Stahl R, Cheng J, Li X, Huber MB, Luke A, Majumdar S, Link TM. Meniscal measurements of T1rho and T2 at MR imaging in healthy subjects and patients with osteoarthritis. *Radiology* 2008;249(2):591–600.
16. Resnick D. Degenerative disease of extraspinal locations. In: Resnick D, editor. *Diagnosis of Bone and Joint Disorders*, Vol. 2. Philadelphia: W. B. Saunders Company, 2002, pp. 1271–1272.
17. Braunstein EM, Brandt KD, Albrecht M. MRI demonstration of hypertrophic articular cartilage repair in osteoarthritis. *Skeletal Radiol* 1990;19(5):335–339.
18. Vignon E, Arlot M, Hartmann D, Moyen B, Ville G. Hypertrophic repair of articular cartilage in experimental osteoarthrosis. *Ann Rheum Dis* 1983;42(1):82–88.
19. Adams ME, Brandt KD. Hypertrophic repair of canine articular cartilage in osteoarthritis after anterior cruciate ligament transection. *J Rheumatol* 1991;18(3): 428–435.
20. Brandt KD, Braunstein EM, Visco DM, O'Connor B, Heck D, Albrecht M. Anterior (cranial) cruciate ligament transection in the dog: a bona fide model of osteoarthritis, not merely of cartilage injury and repair. *J Rheumatol* 1991;18(3):436–446.
21. Kuettner KE, Goldberg VM. Introduction. In: Kuettner KE, Goldberg VM, editors. *Osteoarthritic Disorders*. Rosemont, IL: American Academy of Orthopaedic Surgeons, 1995, pp. xxi–xxv.
22. Mitchell NS, Cruess RL. Classification of degenerative arthritis. *Can Med Assoc J* 1977;117(7):763–765.
23. Davis MA, Ettinger WH, Neuhaus JM, Barclay JD, Segal MR. Correlates of knee pain among US adults with and without radiographic knee osteoarthritis. *J Rheumatol* 1992;19(12):1943–1949.
24. Summers MN, Haley WE, Reveille JD, Alarcon GS. Radiographic assessment and psychologic variables as predictors of pain and functional impairment in osteoarthritis of the knee or hip. *Arthritis Rheum* 1988;31(2):204–209.
25. Lin EH, Katon W, Von Korff M, Tang L, Williams JW Jr, Kroenke K, Hunkeler E, Harpole L, Hegel M, Arean P, Hoffing M, Della Penna R, Langston C, Unutzer J. Effect of improving depression care on pain and functional outcomes among older adults with arthritis: a randomized controlled trial. *JAMA* 2003;290(18):2428–2429.
26. Felson DT, Zhang Y, Anthony JM, Naimark A, Anderson JJ. Weight loss reduces the risk for symptomatic knee osteoarthritis in women. The Framingham Study. *Ann Intern Med* 1992;116(7):535–539.
27. Hannan MT, Felson DT, Pincus T. Analysis of the discordance between radiographic changes and knee pain in osteoarthritis of the knee. *J Rheumatol* 2000;27(6): 1513–1517.
28. Felson DT, Chaisson CE, Hill CL, Totterman SM, Gale ME, Skinner KM, Kazis L, Gale DR. The association of bone marrow lesions with pain in knee osteoarthritis. *Ann Intern Med* 2001;134(7):541–549.
29. Sowers MF, Hayes C, Jamadar D, Capul D, Lachance L, Jannausch M, Welch G. Magnetic resonance-detected subchondral bone marrow and cartilage

defect characteristics associated with pain and X-ray-defined knee osteoarthritis. *Osteoarthr Cartil* 2003;11(6):387–393.

30. Kennedy TD, Plater-Zyberk C, Partridge TA, Woodrow DF, Maini RN. Morphometric comparison of synovium from patients with osteoarthritis and rheumatoid arthritis. *J Clin Pathol* 1988;41(8):847–852.

31. Hill CL, Gale DG, Chaisson CE, Skinner K, Kazis L, Gale ME, Felson DT. Knee effusions, popliteal cysts, and synovial thickening: association with knee pain in osteoarthritis. *J Rheumatol* 2001;28(6):1330–1337.

32. Hill CL, Hunter DJ, Niu J, Clancy M, Guermazi A, Genant H, Gale D, Grainger A, Conaghan P, Felson DT. Synovitis detected on magnetic resonance imaging and its relation to pain and cartilage loss in knee osteoarthritis. *Ann Rheum Dis* 2007;66(12):1599–1603.

33. Altman RD. Classification of disease: osteoarthritis. *Semin Arthritis Rheum* 1991;20(6 Suppl 2):40–47.

34. Bennell KL, Hinman RS, Metcalf BR, Crossley KM, Buchbinder R, Smith M, McColl G. Relationship of knee joint proprioception to pain and disability in individuals with knee osteoarthritis. *J Orthop Res* 2003;21(5):792–797.

35. Mundermann A, Dyrby CO, Andriacchi TP. Secondary gait changes in patients with medial compartment knee osteoarthritis: increased load at the ankle, knee, and hip during walking. *Arthritis Rheum* 2005;52(9):2835–2844.

36. Shakoor N, Block JA, Shott S, Case JP. Nonrandom evolution of end-stage osteoarthritis of the lower limbs. *Arthritis Rheum* 2002;46(12):3185–3189.

37. Ike R, O'Rourke KS. Compartment-directed physical examination of the knee can predict articular cartilage abnormalities disclosed by needle arthroscopy. *Arthritis Rheum* 1995;38(7):917–925.

38. Aigner T, McKenna L. Molecular pathology and pathobiology of osteoarthritic cartilage. *Cell Mol Life Sci* 2002;59(1):5–18.

39. Creamer P, Hochberg MC. Osteoarthritis. *Lancet* 1997;350(9076):503–508.

40. Hartz AJ, Fischer ME, Bril G, Kelber S, Rupley D Jr, Oken B, Rimm AA. The association of obesity with joint pain and osteoarthritis in the HANES data. *J Chronic Dis* 1986;39(4):311–319.

41. Davis MA, Ettinger WH, Neuhaus JM, Hauck WW. Sex differences in osteoarthritis of the knee. The role of obesity. *Am J Epidemiol* 1988;127(5):1019–1030.

42. Felson DT, Anderson JJ, Naimark A, Walker AM, Meenan RF. Obesity and knee osteoarthritis. The Framingham Study. *Ann Intern Med* 1988;109(1):18–24.

43. Hart DJ, Spector TD. The relationship of obesity, fat distribution and osteoarthritis in women in the general population: the Chingford Study. *J Rheumatol* 1993;20(2):331–335.

44. Heliovaara M, Makela M, Impivaara O, Knekt P, Aromaa A, Sievers K. Association of overweight, trauma and workload with coxarthrosis. A health survey of 7,217 persons. *Acta Orthop Scand* 1993;64(5):513–518.

45. Jordan JM, Luta G, Renner JB, Linder GF, Dragomir A, Hochberg MC, Fryer JG. Self-reported functional status in osteoarthritis of the knee in a rural southern community: the role of sociodemographic factors, obesity, and knee pain. *Arthritis Care Res* 1996;9(4):273–278.

46. Kellgren JH. Osteoarthrosis in patients and populations. *Br Med J* 1961; 2(5243):1–6.

47. Kraus JF, D'Ambrosia RD, Smith EG, Van Meter J, Borhani NO, Franti CE, Lipscomb PR. An epidemiological study of severe osteoarthritis. *Orthopedics* 1978;1(1):37–42.

48. Saville PD, Dickson J. Age and weight in osteoarthritis of the hip. *Arthritis Rheum* 1968;11(5):635–644.

49. Spector TD, Hart DJ, Doyle DV. Incidence and progression of osteoarthritis in women with unilateral knee disease in the general population: the effect of obesity. *Ann Rheum Dis* 1994;53(9):565–568.

50. Berthiaume MJ, Raynauld JP, Martel-Pelletier J, Labonte F, Beaudoin G, Bloch DA, Choquette D, Haraoui B, Altman RD, Hochberg M, Meyer JM, Cline GA, Pelletier JP. Meniscal tear and extrusion are strongly associated with progression of symptomatic knee osteoarthritis as assessed by quantitative magnetic resonance imaging. *Ann Rheum Dis* 2005;64(4):556–563.

51. Doherty M, Watt I, Dieppe P. Influence of primary generalised osteoarthritis on development of secondary osteoarthritis. *Lancet* 1983;2(8340):8–11.

52. Englund M, Paradowski PT, Lohmander LS. Association of radiographic hand osteoarthritis with radiographic knee osteoarthritis after meniscectomy. *Arthritis Rheum* 2004;50(2):469–475.

53. Hill CL, Seo GS, Gale D, Totterman S, Gale ME, Felson DT. Cruciate ligament integrity in osteoarthritis of the knee. *Arthritis Rheum* 2005;52(3): 794–799.

54. Hunter DJ, Zhang YQ, Niu JB, Tu X, Amin S, Clancy M, Guermazi A, Grigorian M, Gale D, Felson DT. The association of meniscal pathologic changes with cartilage loss in symptomatic knee osteoarthritis. *Arthritis Rheum* 2006;54(3):795–801.

55. Jacobsen S, Sonne-Holm S. Hip dysplasia: a significant risk factor for the development of hip osteoarthritis. A cross-sectional survey. *Rheumatology (Oxford)* 2005;44(2):211–218.

56. McDermott M, Freyne P. Osteoarthrosis in runners with knee pain. *Br J Sports Med* 1983;17(2):84–87.

57. Murphy SB, Ganz R, Muller ME. The prognosis in untreated dysplasia of the hip. A study of radiographic factors that predict the outcome. *J Bone Joint Surg Am* 1995;77(7):985–989.

58. Neyret P, Donell ST, Dejour H. Osteoarthritis of the knee following meniscectomy. *Br J Rheumatol* 1994;33(3):267–268.

59. Reijman M, Hazes JM, Pols HA, Koes BW, Bierma-Zeinstra SM. Acetabular dysplasia predicts incident osteoarthritis of the hip: the Rotterdam study. *Arthritis Rheum* 2005;52(3):787–793.

60. von Porat A, Roos EM, Roos H. High prevalence of osteoarthritis 14 years after an anterior cruciate ligament tear in male soccer players: a study of radiographic and patient relevant outcomes. *Ann Rheum Dis* 2004;63(3):269–273.

61. Chapman K, Mustafa Z, Dowling B, Southam L, Carr A, Loughlin J. Finer linkage mapping of primary hip osteoarthritis susceptibility on chromosome 11q in a cohort of affected female sibling pairs. *Arthritis Rheum* 2002;46(7):1780–1783.

62. Chapman K, Mustafa Z, Irven C, Carr AJ, Clipsham K, Smith A, Chitnavis J, Sinsheimer JS, Bloomfield VA, McCartney M, Cox O, Cardon LR, Sykes B, Loughlin J. Osteoarthritis-susceptibility locus on chromosome 11q, detected by linkage. *Am J Hum Genet* 1999;65(1):167–174.

63. Holderbaum D, Haqqi TM, Moskowitz RW. Genetics and osteoarthritis: exposing the iceberg. *Arthritis Rheum* 1999;42(3):397–405.

64. Loughlin J, Dowling B, Mustafa Z, Southam L, Chapman K. Refined linkage mapping of a hip osteoarthritis susceptibility locus on chromosome 2q. *Rheumatology (Oxford)* 2002;41(8):955–956.

65. Spector TD, MacGregor AJ. Risk factors for osteoarthritis: genetics. *Osteoarthr Cartil* 2004;12(Suppl A):S39–44.

66. Cooper C, Cook PL, Osmond C, Fisher L, Cawley MI. Osteoarthritis of the hip and osteoporosis of the proximal femur. *Ann Rheum Dis* 1991;50(8):540–542.

67. Hart DJ, Mootoosamy I, Doyle DV, Spector TD. The relationship between osteoarthritis and osteoporosis in the general population: the Chingford Study. *Ann Rheum Dis* 1994;53(3):158–162.

68. Nevitt MC, Lane NE, Scott JC, Hochberg MC, Pressman AR, Genant HK, Cummings SR. Radiographic osteoarthritis of the hip and bone mineral density. The Study of Osteoporotic Fractures Research Group. *Arthritis Rheum* 1995;38(7): 907–916.

69. Zhang Y, Hannan MT, Chaisson CE, McAlindon TE, Evans SR, Aliabadi P, Levy D, Felson DT. Bone mineral density and risk of incident and progressive radiographic knee osteoarthritis in women: the Framingham Study. *J Rheumatol* 2000;27(4):1032–1037.

70. Hannan MT, Felson DT, Anderson JJ, Naimark A, Kannel WB. Estrogen use and radiographic osteoarthritis of the knee in women. The Framingham Osteoarthritis Study. *Arthritis Rheum* 1990;33(4):525–532.

71. Nevitt MC, Cummings SR, Lane NE, Hochberg MC, Scott JC, Pressman AR, Genant HK, Cauley JA. Association of estrogen replacement therapy with the risk of osteoarthritis of the hip in elderly white women. Study of Osteoporotic Fractures Research Group. *Arch Intern Med* 1996;156(18):2073–2080.

72. Nevitt MC, Felson DT, Williams EN, Grady D. The effect of estrogen plus progestin on knee symptoms and related disability in postmenopausal women: The Heart and Estrogen/Progestin Replacement Study, a randomized, double-blind, placebo-controlled trial. *Arthritis Rheum* 2001;44(4):811–818.

73. Oliveria SA, Felson DT, Klein RA, Reed JI, Walker AM. Estrogen replacement therapy and the development of osteoarthritis. *Epidemiology* 1996;7(4): 415–419.

74. Rosner IA, Goldberg VM, Moskowitz RW. Estrogens and osteoarthritis. *Clin Orthop Relat Res* 1986(213):77–83.

75. Samanta A, Jones A, Regan M, Wilson S, Doherty M. Is osteoarthritis in women affected by hormonal changes or smoking? *Br J Rheumatol* 1993;32(5): 366–370.

76. Tsai CL, Liu TK. Estradiol-induced knee osteoarthrosis in ovariectomized rabbits. *Clin Orthop Relat Res* 1993(291):295–302.

77.   Turner AS, Athanasiou KA, Zhu CF, Alvis MR, Bryant HU. Biochemical effects of estrogen on articular cartilage in ovariectomized sheep. *Osteoarthr Cartil* 1997;5(1):63–69.

78.   Korver TH, van de Stadt RJ, Kiljan E, van Kampen GP, van der Korst JK. Effects of loading on the synthesis of proteoglycans in different layers of anatomically intact articular cartilage *in vitro*. *J Rheumatol* 1992;19(6):905–912.

79.   Sah RL, Kim YJ, Doong JY, Grodzinsky AJ, Plaas AH, Sandy JD. Biosynthetic response of cartilage explants to dynamic compression. *J Orthop Res* 1989;7(5): 619–636.

80.   Urban JP. The chondrocyte: a cell under pressure. *Br J Rheumatol* 1994;33(10): 901–908.

81.   Mizrahi J, Maroudas A, Lanir Y, Ziv I, Webber TJ. The "instantaneous" deformation of cartilage: effects of collagen fiber orientation and osmotic stress. *Biorheology* 1986;23(4):311–330.

82.   Agarwal S, Deschner J, Long P, Verma A, Hofman C, Evans CH, Piesco N. Role of NF-kappaB transcription factors in antiinflammatory and proinflammatory actions of mechanical signals. *Arthritis Rheum* 2004;50(11):3541–3548.

83.   Dodge GR, Poole AR. Immunohistochemical detection and immunochemical analysis of type II collagen degradation in human normal, rheumatoid, and osteoarthritic articular cartilages and in explants of bovine articular cartilage cultured with interleukin 1. *J Clin Invest* 1989;83(2):647–661.

84.   Kandel RA, Dinarello CA, Biswas C. The stimulation of collagenase production in rabbit articular chondrocytes by interleukin-1 is increased by collagens. *Biochem Int* 1987;15(5):1021–1031.

85.   Pettipher ER, Higgs GA, Henderson B. Interleukin 1 induces leukocyte infiltration and cartilage proteoglycan degradation in the synovial joint. *Proc Natl Acad Sci USA* 1986;83(22):8749–8753.

86.   Smith MD, Triantafillou S, Parker A, Youssef PP, Coleman M. Synovial membrane inflammation and cytokine production in patients with early osteoarthritis. *J Rheumatol* 1997;24(2):365–371.

87.   Westacott CI, Sharif M. Cytokines in osteoarthritis: mediators or markers of joint destruction? *Semin Arthritis Rheum* 1996;25(4):254–272.

88.   Warnock MG, Sharif M, Elson CJ. IL-1-beta at physiological concentration stimulates degradation of human articular cartilage. *Bone Mineral* 1994;25(Suppl):S36.

89.   Campbell IK, Piccoli DS, Roberts MJ, Muirden KD, Hamilton JA. Effects of tumor necrosis factor alpha and beta on resorption of human articular cartilage and production of plasminogen activator by human articular chondrocytes. *Arthritis Rheum* 1990;33(4):542–552.

90.   Moreland LW, Baumgartner SW, Schiff MH, Tindall EA, Fleischmann RM, Weaver AL, Ettlinger RE, Cohen S, Koopman WJ, Mohler K, Widmer MB, Blosch CM. Treatment of rheumatoid arthritis with a recombinant human tumor necrosis factor receptor (p75)-Fc fusion protein. *N Engl J Med* 1997;337(3):141–147.

91.   Saklatvala J. Tumour necrosis factor alpha stimulates resorption and inhibits synthesis of proteoglycan in cartilage. *Nature* 1986;322(6079):547–549.

92.   Venn G, Nietfeld JJ, Duits AJ, Brennan FM, Arner E, Covington M, Billingham ME, Hardingham TE. Elevated synovial fluid levels of interleukin-6 and tumor

necrosis factor associated with early experimental canine osteoarthritis. *Arthritis Rheum* 1993;36(6):819–826.

93. Murrell GA, Jang D, Williams RJ. Nitric oxide activates metalloprotease enzymes in articular cartilage. *Biochem Biophys Res Commun* 1995;206(1):15–21.

94. Pelletier JP, Jovanovic DV, Lascau-Coman V, Fernandes JC, Manning PT, Connor JR, Currie MG, Martel-Pelletier J. Selective inhibition of inducible nitric oxide synthase reduces progression of experimental osteoarthritis *in vivo*: possible link with the reduction in chondrocyte apoptosis and caspase 3 level. *Arthritis Rheum* 2000;43(6):1290–1299.

95. Pelletier JP, Lascau-Coman V, Jovanovic D, Fernandes JC, Manning P, Connor JR, Currie MG, Martel-Pelletier J. Selective inhibition of inducible nitric oxide synthase in experimental osteoarthritis is associated with reduction in tissue levels of catabolic factors. *J Rheumatol* 1999;26(9):2002–2014.

96. Salvatierra J, Escames G, Hernandez P, Cantero J, Crespo E, Leon J, Salvatierra D, Acuna-Castroviejo D, Vives F. Cartilage and serum levels of nitric oxide in patients with hip osteoarthritis. *J Rheumatol* 1999;26(9):2015–2017.

97. Blanco FJ, Guitian R, Vazquez-Martul E, de Toro FJ, Galdo F. Osteoarthritis chondrocytes die by apoptosis. A possible pathway for osteoarthritis pathology. *Arthritis Rheum* 1998;41(2):284–289.

98. Hashimoto S, Ochs RL, Komiya S, Lotz M. Linkage of chondrocyte apoptosis and cartilage degradation in human osteoarthritis. *Arthritis Rheum* 1998;41(9): 1632–1638.

99. Hashimoto S, Takahashi K, Amiel D, Coutts RD, Lotz M. Chondrocyte apoptosis and nitric oxide production during experimentally induced osteoarthritis. *Arthritis Rheum* 1998;41(7):1266–1274.

100. Miosge N, Hartmann M, Maelicke C, Herken R. Expression of collagen type I and type II in consecutive stages of human osteoarthritis. *Histochem Cell Biol* 2004;122(3):229–236.

101. Walter H, Kawashima A, Nebelung W, Neumann W, Roessner A. Immunohistochemical analysis of several proteolytic enzymes as parameters of cartilage degradation. *Pathol Res Pract* 1998;194(2):73–81.

102. Mankin HJ, Dorfman H, Lippiello L, Zarins A. Biochemical and metabolic abnormalities in articular cartilage from osteo-arthritic human hips. II. Correlation of morphology with biochemical and metabolic data. *J Bone Joint Surg Am* 1971;53(3):523–537.

103. Ostergaard K, Andersen CB, Petersen J, Bendtzen K, Salter DM. Validity of histopathological grading of articular cartilage from osteoarthritic knee joints. *Ann Rheum Dis* 1999;58(4):208–213.

104. Ostergaard K, Petersen J, Andersen CB, Bendtzen K, Salter DM. Histologic/ histochemical grading system for osteoarthritic articular cartilage: reproducibility and validity. *Arthritis Rheum* 1997;40(10):1766–1771.

105. Pritzker KP, Gay S, Jimenez SA, Ostergaard K, Pelletier JP, Revell PA, Salter D, van den Berg WB. Osteoarthritis cartilage histopathology: grading and staging. *Osteoarthr Cartil* 2006;14(1):13–29.

106. Custers RJ, Creemers LB, Verbout AJ, van Rijen MH, Dhert WJ, Saris DB. Reliability, reproducibility and variability of the traditional Histologic/Histochemical

Grading System vs the new OARSI Osteoarthritis Cartilage Histopathology Assessment System. *Osteoarthr Cartil* 2007;15(11):1241–1248.

107.   Goldring SR. The role of bone in osteoarthritis pathogenesis. *Rheum Dis Clin North Am* 2008;34(3):561–571.

108.   Bullough PG. The role of joint architecture in the etiology of arthritis. *Osteoarthr Cartil* 2004;12(Suppl A):S2–9.

109.   Burr DB. Anatomy and physiology of the mineralized tissues: role in the pathogenesis of osteoarthrosis. *Osteoarthr Cartil* 2004;12(Suppl A):S20–30.

110.   Frost HM. Perspective: genetic and hormonal roles in bone disorders: insights of an updated bone physiology. *J Musculoskelet Neuronal Interact* 2003;3(2): 118–135.

111.   Scharstuhl A, Vitters EL, van der Kraan PM, van den Berg WB. Reduction of osteophyte formation and synovial thickening by adenoviral overexpression of transforming growth factor beta/bone morphogenetic protein inhibitors during experimental osteoarthritis. *Arthritis Rheum* 2003;48(12):3442–3451.

112.   van der Kraan PM, van den Berg WB. Osteophytes: relevance and biology. *Osteoarthr Cartil* 2007;15(3):237–244.

113.   Messent EA, Ward RJ, Tonkin CJ, Buckland-Wright C. Differences in trabecular structure between knees with and without osteoarthritis quantified by macro and standard radiography, respectively. *Osteoarthr Cartil* 2006;14(12):1302–1305.

114.   Day JS, Ding M, van der Linden JC, Hvid I, Sumner DR, Weinans H. A decreased subchondral trabecular bone tissue elastic modulus is associated with pre-arthritic cartilage damage. *J Orthop Res* 2001;19(5):914–918.

115.   Day JS, van der Linden JC, Bank RA, Ding M, Hvid I, Sumner DR, Weinans H. Adaptation of subchondral bone in osteoarthritis. *Biorheology* 2004;41(3–4): 359–368.

116.   Bhattacharyya T, Gale D, Dewire P, Totterman S, Gale ME, McLaughlin S, Einhorn TA, Felson DT. The clinical importance of meniscal tears demonstrated by magnetic resonance imaging in osteoarthritis of the knee. J *Bone Joint Surg Am* 2003; 85-A(1):4–9.

117.   Poehling GG, Ruch DS, Chabon SJ. The landscape of meniscal injuries. *Clin Sports Med* 1990;9(3):539–549.

118.   Noble J, Hamblen DL. The pathology of the degenerate meniscus lesion. *J Bone Joint Surg Br* 1975;57(2):180–186.

119.   Smillie IS. The current pattern of internal derangements of the knee joint relative to the menisci. *Clin Orthop Relat Res* 1967;51:117–122.

120.   Englund M. The role of the meniscus in osteoarthritis genesis. *Rheum Dis Clin North Am* 2008;34(3):573–579.

121.   Ding C, Martel-Pelletier J, Pelletier JP, Abram F, Raynauld JP, Cicuttini F, Jones G. Meniscal tear as an osteoarthritis risk factor in a largely non-osteoarthritic cohort: a cross-sectional study. *J Rheumatol* 2007;34(4):776–784.

122.   Englund M, Lohmander LS. Risk factors for symptomatic knee osteoarthritis fifteen to twenty-two years after meniscectomy. *Arthritis Rheum* 2004;50(9): 2811–2819.

123.   Englund M, Niu J, Guermazi A, Roemer FW, Hunter DJ, Lynch JA, Lewis CE, Torner J, Nevitt MC, Zhang YQ, Felson DT. Effect of meniscal damage

on the development of frequent knee pain, aching, or stiffness. *Arthritis Rheum* 2007;56(12):4048–4054.

124. Adams JG, McAlindon T, Dimasi M, Carey J, Eustace S. Contribution of meniscal extrusion and cartilage loss to joint space narrowing in osteoarthritis. *Clin Radiol* 1999;54(8):502–506.

125. Gale DR, Chaisson CE, Totterman SM, Schwartz RK, Gale ME, Felson D. Meniscal subluxation: association with osteoarthritis and joint space narrowing. *Osteoarthr Cartil* 1999;7(6):526–532.

126. Ding C, Martel-Pelletier J, Pelletier JP, Abram F, Raynauld JP, Cicuttini F, Jones G. Knee meniscal extrusion in a largely non-osteoarthritic cohort: association with greater loss of cartilage volume. *Arthritis Res Ther* 2007;9(2):R21.

127. Felson DT, Zhang Y. An update on the epidemiology of knee and hip osteoarthritis with a view to prevention. *Arthritis Rheum* 1998;41(8):1343–1355.

128. Lo GH, Hunter DJ, Nevitt M, Lynch J, McAlindon TE. Strong association of MRI meniscal derangement and bone marrow lesions in knee osteoarthritis: data from the osteoarthritis initiative. *Osteoarthr Cartil* 2009;17(6):743–747.

129. Nikolic DK. Lateral meniscal tears and their evolution in acute injuries of the anterior cruciate ligament of the knee. Arthroscopic analysis. *Knee Surg Sports Traumatol Arthrosc* 1998;6(1):26–30.

130. Tiderius CJ, Olsson LE, Nyquist F, Dahlberg L. Cartilage glycosaminoglycan loss in the acute phase after an anterior cruciate ligament injury: delayed gadolinium-enhanced magnetic resonance imaging of cartilage and synovial fluid analysis. *Arthritis Rheum* 2005;52(1):120–127.

131. Murphy BJ, Smith RL, Uribe JW, Janecki CJ, Hechtman KS, Mangasarian RA. Bone signal abnormalities in the posterolateral tibia and lateral femoral condyle in complete tears of the anterior cruciate ligament: a specific sign? *Radiology* 1992;182(1):221–224.

132. Costa-Paz M, Muscolo DL, Ayerza M, Makino A, Aponte-Tinao L. Magnetic resonance imaging follow-up study of bone bruises associated with anterior cruciate ligament ruptures. *Arthroscopy* 2001;17(5):445–449.

133. Nishimori M, Deie M, Adachi N, Kanaya A, Nakamae A, Motoyama M, Ochi M. Articular cartilage injury of the posterior lateral tibial plateau associated with acute anterior cruciate ligament injury. *Knee Surg Sports Traumatol Arthrosc* 2008;16(3):270–274.

134. Nelissen RG, Hogendoorn PC. Retain or sacrifice the posterior cruciate ligament in total knee arthroplasty? A histopathological study of the cruciate ligament in osteoarthritic and rheumatoid disease. *J Clin Pathol* 2001;54(5):381–384.

135. Hodler J, Haghighi P, Trudell D, Resnick D. The cruciate ligaments of the knee: correlation between MR appearance and gross and histologic findings in cadaveric specimens. *AJR Am J Roentgenol* 1992;159(2):357–360.

136. Young RD, Vaughan-Thomas A, Wardale RJ, Duance VC. Type II collagen deposition in cruciate ligament precedes osteoarthritis in the guinea pig knee. *Osteoarthr Cartil* 2002;10(5):420–428.

137. Stubbs G, Dahlstrom J, Papantoniou P, Cherian M. Correlation between macroscopic changes of arthrosis and the posterior cruciate ligament histology in the osteoarthritic knee. *ANZ J Surg* 2005;75(12):1036–1040.

138. Cushner FD, La Rosa DF, Vigorita VJ, Scuderi GR, Scott WN, Insall JN. A quantitative histologic comparison: ACL degeneration in the osteoarthritic knee. *J Arthroplasty* 2003;18(6):687–692.

139. Allain J, Goutallier D, Voisin MC. Macroscopic and histological assessments of the cruciate ligaments in arthrosis of the knee. *Acta Orthop Scand* 2001;72(3):266–269.

140. Lee GC, Cushner FD, Vigoritta V, Scuderi GR, Insall JN, Scott WN. Evaluation of the anterior cruciate ligament integrity and degenerative arthritic patterns in patients undergoing total knee arthroplasty. *J Arthroplasty* 2005;20(1):59–65.

141. Johnson DL, Urban WP Jr., Caborn DN, Vanarthos WJ, Carlson CS. Articular cartilage changes seen with magnetic resonance imaging-detected bone bruises associated with acute anterior cruciate ligament rupture. *Am J Sports Med* 1998;26(3):409–414.

142. Faber KJ, Dill JR, Amendola A, Thain L, Spouge A, Fowler PJ. Occult osteochondral lesions after anterior cruciate ligament rupture. Six-year magnetic resonance imaging follow-up study. *Am J Sports Med* 1999;27(4):489–494.

143. Lohmander LS, Ostenberg A, Englund M, Roos H. High prevalence of knee osteoarthritis, pain, and functional limitations in female soccer players twelve years after anterior cruciate ligament injury. *Arthritis Rheum* 2004;50(10):3145–3152.

144. Roos H, Adalberth T, Dahlberg L, Lohmander LS. Osteoarthritis of the knee after injury to the anterior cruciate ligament or meniscus: the influence of time and age. *Osteoarthr Cartil* 1995;3(4):261–267.

145. McAlindon TE, Watt I, McCrae F, Goddard P, Dieppe PA. Magnetic resonance imaging in osteoarthritis of the knee: correlation with radiographic and scintigraphic findings. *Ann Rheum Dis* 1991;50(1):14–19.

146. Hunter DJ, Niu J, Zhang Y. Altered perfusion and venous hypertension is present in regions of bone affected by BMLs in knee OA. *Osteoarthr Cartil* 2007(15 Suppl C):C171.

147. Watson PJ, Hall LD, Carpenter TA, Tyler JA. A magnetic resonance imaging study of joint degeneration in the guinea pig knee. *Agents Actions Suppl* 1993;39:261–265.

148. Kannus P. Long-term results of conservatively treated medial collateral ligament injuries of the knee joint. *Clin Orthop Relat Res* 1988(226):103–112.

149. Bird HA, Tribe CR, Bacon PA. Joint hypermobility leading to osteoarthrosis and chondrocalcinosis. *Ann Rheum Dis* 1978;37(3):203–211.

150. Sharma L, Song J, Felson DT, Cahue S, Shamiyeh E, Dunlop DD. The role of knee alignment in disease progression and functional decline in knee osteoarthritis. *JAMA* 2001;286(2):188–195.

151. Kee CC. Osteoarthritis: manageable scourge of aging. *Nurs Clin North Am* 2000;35(1):199–208.

152. Hurley MV. The role of muscle weakness in the pathogenesis of osteoarthritis. *Rheum Dis Clin North Am* 1999;25(2):283–298, vi.

153. Johansson H, Sjolander P, Sojka P. A sensory role for the cruciate ligaments. *Clin Orthop Relat Res* 1991(268):161–178.

154. Slemenda C, Brandt KD, Heilman DK, Mazzuca S, Braunstein EM, Katz BP, Wolinsky FD. Quadriceps weakness and osteoarthritis of the knee. *Ann Intern Med* 1997;127(2):97–104.

155. Brandt KD, Radin EL, Dieppe PA, van de Putte L. Yet more evidence that osteoarthritis is not a cartilage disease. *Ann Rheum Dis* 2006;65(10):1261–1264.

156. Slemenda C, Heilman DK, Brandt KD, Katz BP, Mazzuca SA, Braunstein EM, Byrd D. Reduced quadriceps strength relative to body weight: a risk factor for knee osteoarthritis in women? *Arthritis Rheum* 1998;41(11):1951–1959.

157. Brandt KD, Heilman DK, Slemenda C, Katz BP, Mazzuca SA, Braunstein EM, Byrd D. Quadriceps strength in women with radiographically progressive osteoarthritis of the knee and those with stable radiographic changes. *J Rheumatol* 1999;26(11):2431–2437.

158. Loeuille D, Chary-Valckenaere I, Champigneulle J, Rat AC, Toussaint F, Pinzano-Watrin A, Goebel JC, Mainard D, Blum A, Pourel J, Netter P, Gillet P. Macroscopic and microscopic features of synovial membrane inflammation in the osteoarthritic knee: correlating magnetic resonance imaging findings with disease severity. *Arthritis Rheum* 2005;52(11):3492–3501.

159. Brandt KD, Dieppe P, Radin EL. Etiopathogenesis of osteoarthritis. *Rheum Dis Clin North Am* 2008;34(3):531–559.

160. Myers SL, Flusser D, Brandt KD, Heck DA. Prevalence of cartilage shards in synovium and their association with synovitis in patients with early and endstage osteoarthritis. *J Rheumatol* 1992;19(8):1247–1251.

161. Evans CH. Cellular mechanisms of hydrolytic enzyme release in osteoarthritis. *Arthritis Rheum* 1981;Semin(11 Suppl 1):93–95.

162. Boniface RJ, Cain PR, Evans CH. Articular responses to purified cartilage proteoglycans. *Arthritis Rheum* 1988;31(2):258–266.

163. Brandt KD, Schumacher HR Jr. Osteoarthritis and crystal deposition diseases. *Curr Opin Rheumatol* 1996;8(3):235–237.

164. Myers SL, Brandt KD, Ehlich JW, Braunstein EM, Shelbourne KD, Heck DA, Kalasinski LA. Synovial inflammation in patients with early osteoarthritis of the knee. *J Rheumatol* 1990;17(12):1662–1669.

165. Lo GH, McAlindon T, Niu J. Strong association of bone marrow lesions and effusion with pain in osteoarthritis. *Arthritis Rheum* 2007;56(Suppl):S790.

166. Saadat E, Jobke B, Chu B, Lu Y, Cheng J, Li X, Ries MD, Majumdar S, Link TM. Diagnostic performance of *in vivo* 3-T MRI for articular cartilage abnormalities in human osteoarthritic knees using histology as standard of reference. *Eur Radiol* 2008;18(10):2292–2302.

167. Pritzker KP, Gay S, Jimenez SA, Ostergaard K, Pelletier JP, Revell PA, Salter D, van den Berg WB. Osteoarthritis cartilage histopathology: grading and staging. *Osteoarthr Cartil* 2006;14(1):13–29.

3

Current Radiographic Diagnosis for Osteoarthritis of the Knee

by Ehsan Saadat and Thomas M. Link

Introduction

Plain radiography is to date the primary method for radiologic diagnosis of osteoarthritis (OA). Plain radiography is able to detect the cardinal pathologic processes in OA, such as the appearance of osteophytes, loss of cartilage thickness, as evident by development of joint space narrowing, as well as joint malalignment. However, gross changes such as these appear later in the disease process. Early changes in the cartilage and other articular tissues are not directly visible using radiographs, and plain radiographs are insensitive to focal cartilage loss. Despite its shortcomings, plain radiography is still the primary radiographic method for diagnosis of OA and is the basis for the most widely used epidemiologic grading system for OA, the Kellgren-Lawrence scale, discussed later in this chapter.

This chapter will focus on the clinical utility of plain radiographs in the clinical diagnosis of knee osteoarthritis. Many radiographic techniques are used to obtain images of the knee. Five of the most commonly used views (antero-posterior weight-bearing, lateral, tunnel, merchant and sunrise views) will be presented and the strengths and shortcomings of each will be briefly discussed. Specific radiographic findings for knee osteoarthritis and their correlation to histopathologic findings will be presented. The chapter will conclude with the description of one of the most widely used radiographic grading systems for osteoarthritis, the Kellgren-Lawrence grade.

Radiographic Diagnosis of Knee Osteoarthritis

General Considerations

For radiographic diagnosis of knee osteoarthritis, it is useful to regard the knee joint as consisting of three compartments: medial femorotibial, lateral femorotibial and patellofemoral compartments. Although pathologic changes are evident in all three compartments in OA, radiographic changes are usually present in only one or two of these. Reproducible plain radiographic series are examined in a systematic manner to evaluate the bony and soft tissue anatomy. Subtle radiographic changes are better appreciated by careful comparison of the affected and unaffected knees. In OA, abnormalities in the patellofemoral compartment are commonly observed, usually combined with abnormalities in the femorotibial compartments. Rarely, abnormalities confined to the femorotibial compartments are present.

The ability of the radiograph to allow detection of the pathologic abnormalities depends on the method of examination. Routine techniques (which include antero-posterior weight bearing and lateral radiographs) are limited in their sensitivity to delineate early alterations, though some degree of joint space narrowing, sclerosis, cysts and osteophytes are usually detected in the more involved weight-bearing compartment (medial or lateral femorotibial compartment).[1,2] "Tunnel" projections[3] obtained during knee flexion occasionally may reveal osseous lesions and osteophytes that are not evident on the routine radiographs, particularly those occurring on the posterior portions of the femoral condyles.

Routine non-weight-bearing radiographs of the knee are obtained with the patient lying on the X-ray table. Such radiographs may underestimate the extent of cartilage loss and the degree of angular deformity present and are limited in their sensitivity to delineate early alterations.[4−6] Weight-bearing radiographs should be used to supplement the radiographic examination.[1,2,7−12] This latter technique provides a better assessment of cartilage loss as the joint space width decreases under the body weight. It also allows more accurate delineation of subluxation of femur and tibia and of varus and valgus angulations. Even with the addition of the weight-bearing radiographs to the routine examination, the degree of abnormality in the less involved femorotibial compartment is difficult to determine, and it may be better judged with Magnetic Resonance Imaging. Patellofemoral compartmental analysis requires special radiographic projections, including tangential and oblique views.

Additionally, a radiographic survey of the whole leg in a standing position is used to better evaluate leg length and varus and valgus malalignment. This analysis also provides information about the mechanical condition of the knee, extent of osseous deformity and helps in determining the size of the wedge of the bone that needs to be excised surgically in patients scheduled to undergo tibial osteotomy. Similar weight bearing whole leg radiographs are useful in preoperative assessment of patients undergoing total knee replacement, allowing the assessment of leg alignment and leg length discrepancy.

Antero-Posterior Weight-Bearing Views

The antero-posterior weight-bearing radiograph of the knee is obtained with the beam directed 5° to 7° towards the head with the patient standing (Fig. 1). This view should be used to supplement the radiographic examination.[1,2,7–12] These views should be obtained on vertically-oriented 7 × 17 inch films.[2] Ideally, the weight-bearing radiographs should be obtained with the patient standing on the involved leg alone; some authors suggest that a radiograph exposed with the patient standing and the knees flexed to 30° or 45° (a "standing tunnel projection" or Rosenberg view) is ideal.[13–17] Angulation and subluxation at the knee joint are best

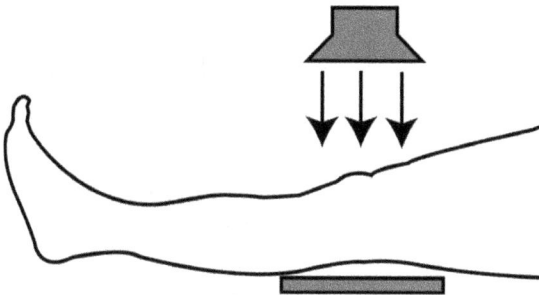

Fig. 1. Anteroposterior radiograph technique: central ray is directed in a cephalad direction with an angle of 5° to 7°. (Courtesy Dana Carpenter PhD, UCSF Department of Radiology and Biomedical Imaging.)

demonstrated on weight-bearing views of the joint. Varus angulation is more frequently observed than valgus angulation. Varus angulation typically results in lateral subluxation of the tibia on the femur, and valgus angulation is associated with medial subluxation of the tibia on the femur and lateral subluxation at the patellofemoral joint. The narrowing of one femorotibial compartment is usually accompanied by narrowing of the contralateral compartment on X-rays.

Lateral Views

A lateral view of the knee is obtained with the knee flexed 20° to 35° (Fig. 2). The lateral view is useful for evaluation of patellar position. Patella alta refers to an abnormally high patella in relation to the femur, which may result in subluxation and dislocation of the patella as the resting position of the patella positions is above the trochlear groove, limiting the bony stability. Patella baja is defined as an abnormally low patella, which most often results from soft tissue contracture and hypotonia of the quadriceps muscle following surgery or trauma to knee. Diagnosis of patella alta and baja are made by comparing the patellar tendon length to the patella height. Normal anatomy includes a 1:1 ratio. A ratio of < 0.8 patellar tendon length: patella height is defined as baja and a ratio > 1.2 is defined as alta.

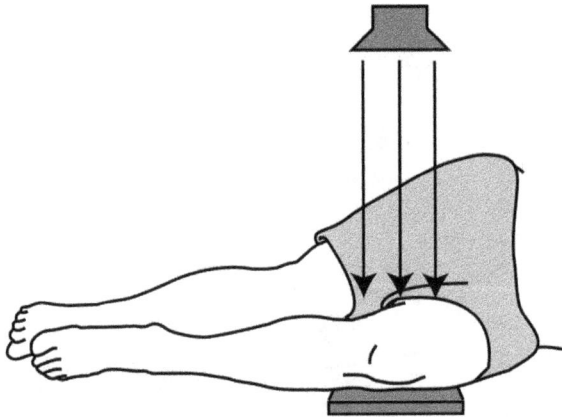

Fig. 2. Lateral radiograph technique: the knee is flexed 20°–35°. (Courtesy Dana Carpenter PhD, UCSF Department of Radiology and Biomedical Imaging.)

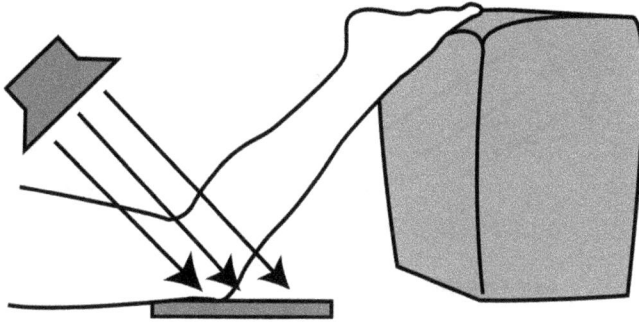

Fig. 3. Tunnel view technique: the knee is flexed 40° to 50° and rests on a sandbag. Central ray is angulated 40° to 50° in a caudal direction. (Courtesy Dana Carpenter PhD, UCSF Department of Radiology and Biomedical Imaging.)

Tunnel Projections

Tunnel projections are angulated frontal views obtained with the knee in 40° to 50° of flexion (Fig. 3). These can be obtained in an antero-posterior or postero-anterior projection. Such images permit improved visualization of the intracondylar notch region and can sometimes reveal abnormalities such as cartilage loss or osteochondral lesions (particularly on the posterior portions of the femoral condyles) that would not be appreciated using antero-posterior weight-bearing films.[3]

Merchant View

The "merchant's view" of the knee is obtained with the patient positioned supine on the table, knee flexed to 45° over the end of the table with the X-ray beam directed supero-inferiorly (30° towards the floor) in the coronal plane (Fig. 4).[18] This view is suitable for evaluation of patellar alignment in the trochlear groove. Unfortunately, this method requires a special film-holding apparatus and patellar magnification is apparent. The direction of the beam can be changed (i.e. from the ankle towards the knee) and radiographs may be acquired with various degrees of knee flexion, which might better assess the patellofemoral joint.[19,20] However patellofemoral malalignment is often greatest at near-full-knee-extension angles which are not possible to view with radiographs. Despite this, the merchant view and

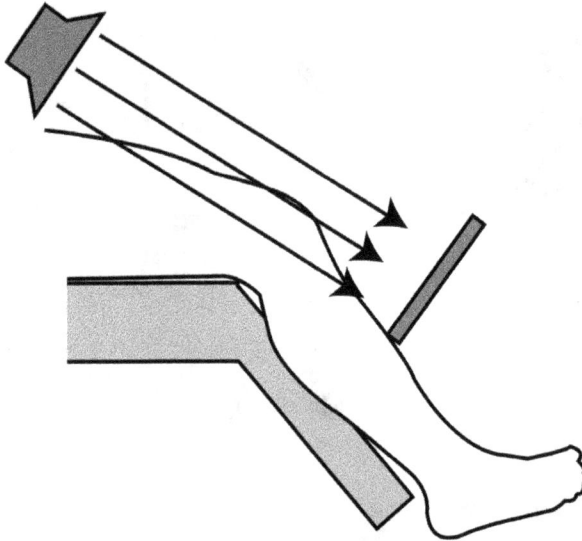

Fig. 4. Merchant view technique: the patient is placed supine on the table and the knees are flexed 45° over the end of the table. The central ray is angled 30° from the horizontal in a caudal direction. (Courtesy Dana Carpenter PhD, UCSF Department of Radiology and Biomedical Imaging.)

a lateral view are usually the first methods used in combination to evaluate patellar alignment.

Sunrise Views

The sunrise view was one of the original methods for evaluation of the patellofemoral joint (Fig. 5). The sunrise view uses the prone position with acute knee flexion. This degree of knee flexion results in the patella's becoming deeply situated within the intercondylar fossa, and renders this technique non-ideal. Furthermore, the sunrise view fails to demonstrate the articular surfaces of the patellofemoral joint and can be painful in the acutely traumatized patient.[21] Hughston[22] suggested that a view obtained with the patient prone and the knee flexed to 50° or 60° was a more suitable technique for visualization of the patellofemoral joint, although in this view distortion is created by severe angulation of the incident beam.

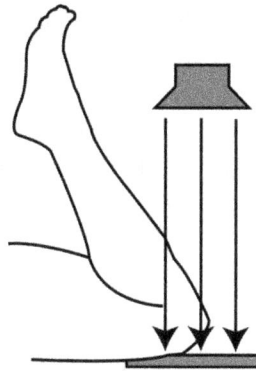

Fig. 5. Sunrise view technique: knee is flexed more than 90°. The patella is situated deep in the intercondylar fossa. (Courtesy Dana Carpenter PhD, UCSF Department of Radiology and Biomedical Imaging.)

Radiographic Findings in Osteoarthritis and Their Correlation to Histopathology

General Remarks

Before a discussion of the specific radiographic findings of knee osteoarthritis, a number of radiographic landmarks about the knee deserve special mention. On routine radiographs, the shallow grooves in the distal articular surface of the femur can be recognized. Blumensaat's line is identified as a condensed linear shadow on a lateral radiograph that represents tangential bone in the intercondylar fossa.[23] The location and appearance of Blumensaat's line is extremely sensitive to changes in knee position and has been used in the past to provide information about the relative position of the patella in lateral projections.[24] Elevation of the distal pole of the patella above this line with the knee flexed 30° has been used as an indicator of patella alta.

The radiographic anatomy of the knee with relation to soft tissues has also been characterized. In the lateral projection of a mildly flexed knee, the collapsed suprapatellar pouch creates a sharp vertical radiodense line between the anterior suprapatellar fat pad and the prefemoral fat pad. This line is usually less than 5 mm in width (but can be as wide as 10 mm). Shadows of increased thickness suggest the presence of intra-articular fluid.[25–27] Intra-articular fluid in the knee may also cause displacement of the ossified fabella.[28] In lateral projections, a thin layer of extrasynovial fat hugs the femoral condyles posteriorly. This fat plane extends from the origin of the femoral condyles to the posterior aspect of the tibial plateau and creates a shape similar to numeral "3". This fat plane becomes distorted in the presence of intra-articular fluid.[29]

Joint Space Narrowing

The progressive cartilage loss in osteoarthritis accounts for the fundamental radiographic change in OA, joint space narrowing. The loss of joint space is usually restricted to the affected compartment. This focal cartilaginous destruction evidenced by focal loss of joint space is what differentiates OA from other causes of joint pain, such as rheumatoid arthritis which involves more diffuse abnormalities in cartilage. Of note, meniscus defects of extrusion of the meniscus, which may be observed in OA, can also cause joint space narrowing detectable by radiography.

Cartilage is not imaged directly using conventional radiographs. Rather, cartilage thickness can be estimated from the width of the joint space, assuming that the opposing joint surfaces are in contact, as is the case in standing. Since articular cartilage itself is not viewed, changes in the internal structure of cartilage such as focal ulceration, are not demonstrated, making this technique rather insensitive to focal pathological changes.

Changes in the thickness and biomechanical properties of articular cartilage in the evolution of osteoarthritis leads to increased transmission of force to the underlying bone. The underlying bone responds initially with increasing local blood flow and bone production; however, this response in later overwhelmed and trabecular microfractures might ensue. These later changes manifest as subchondral sclerosis on radiographs. Sclerotic bone is found consistently in compartments with articular space narrowing,[30] and this feature is striking in areas of the joint denuded of hyaline cartilage. Sclerosis of subchondral bone is more frequent in the tibia or in both the femur and tibia; isolated sclerosis of the femur is unusual.

Osteophytes

Osteophytes are considered by many physicians to be the most characteristic abnormality of degenerative joint disease. Osteophytes develop in areas of joints subjected to low stress; they are considered to be a reparative response of the remaining cartilage, however there is evidence to suggest that osteophytes arise from periosteal or synovial tissues as well.[31] Radiographically, marginal osteophytes appear as variably-sized lips of new bone around the edges of the joints on both femur and tibia. Central, or interior osteophytes simulating intra-articular bodies may also be observed, especially on the femoral condyles. Marginal or central osteophytes contribute to intra-articular surface irregularity as well as sharpening of the tibial spines. It should be noted that although the presence of osteophytes combined with articular space narrowing is usually considered a manifestation of osteoarthritis of the knee, the relationship of osteophytes to the articular disease is subject to debate. It might be that the inclusion of compartments with osteophyte formation and no other finding accounts for a high frequency of tricompartmental involvement in some reported series of patients with osteoarthritis of the knee.

Cyst Formation

Cyst formation is an important and predominant finding in osteo-arthritis.[32–36] The term cyst is commonly used, but is erroneous since these cavities are not lined by epithelium and the term "pseudocyst" should ideally be used. When present, cysts are usually multiple in number and varying in size. However, large cysts (> 2 cm) raise the possibility of an accompanying disorder such as rheumatoid arthritis or a crystal arthropathy; though the union of several small neighboring cysts into large multiloculated lesions is possible.[37] Radiographically, the cysts have a sclerotic margin and are in association with joint space loss and bony eburnation. Cysts are observed within areas of bony sclerosis at sites of increased pressure transmission. The pathogenesis of cystic lesions in degenerative joint disease has received great attention. Although all reports emphasize the importance of concentrated pressure or stress on the articular cartilage and subchondral bone in the development of these lesions, two fundamental theories of cyst pathogenesis have been proposed: synovial fluid intrusion, whereby elevated intra-articular pressure leads to synovial fluid intrusion through cartilage and formation of a subchondral cyst[33,38,39] and bony contusion, whereby the impact of apposing osseous surfaces leads to the fracture and vascular insufficiency of subchondral bone and cyst necrosis.[34,40,41]

Radiographic Grading Systems for Knee Osteoarthritis

The radiographic features currently used to assess osteoarthritis were originally selected to measure various aspects of cartilage loss and subchondral bone reaction. Although several radiographic grading systems have been proposed over the last 20 years, the method developed by Kellgren and Lawrence in 1957 was adopted by the World Health Organization in Rome, in 1961, as the gold standard for cross-sectional and longitudinal epidemiological studies. This system assigns one of five grades (0 to 4) to osteoarthritis at various joint sites. The criteria for increasing severity relate closely to the sequential appearance of osteophytes, joint space loss, subchondral sclerosis and cyst formation. The grading system is outlined in Table 1.

The Kellgren and Lawrence grading system has been criticized for its reliance on the presence of the osteophytes for classification of disease. The time sequence of when bony changes occur and articular cartilage is lost is still controversial. Thus, according to Kellgren and Lawrence, presence of a narrowed, sclerotic joint with deformity cannot be classified as osteoarthritic unless an osteophyte is also present. There also remains the problem of how to classify the individuals with grade 1, doubtful osteophytes.

Table 1. The Kellgren-Lawrence grading system for osteoarthritis.

1. Radiologic features on which grades were based:
  a. Formation of osteophytes on the joint margins or on the tibial spines
  b. Periarticular ossicles (pertaining mostly to proximal and distal interphalangeal joints)
  c. Narrowing of joint cartilage associated with subchondral bone sclerosis
  d. Small pseudocystic areas with sclerotic wall, situated in the subchondral bone
  e. Altered shape of bone ends (pertaining mostly to the head of the femur)

2. Radiographic criteria for assessment of OA

Grade 0	None	No features of OA
Grade 1	Doubtful	Minute osteophyte, doubtful significance
Grade 2	Minimal	Definite osteophyte, unimpaired joint space
Grade 3	Moderate	Moderate diminution of joint space
Grade 4	Severe	Joint space greatly impaired with subchondral bone sclerosis

There is an increasing acceptance that OA may not represent a single disorder but that it is a disease spectrum with a series of subsets that lead to similar clinical and pathological alterations.[42] As a result, many groups have developed specific criteria relating to the differing pathological processes of OA in specific joint sites. For the knee, each of the joint space narrowing, osteophytes and the overall Kellgren-Lawrence grade shows good within-observer reproducibility, but the scoring of the osteophytes was most closely associated with knee pain. Figures 6 to 11 demonstrate representative aspects of Kellgren-Lawrence grades 0 to 4.

Conclusions

Plain radiography is still the primary method for radiologic diagnosis of osteoarthritis. Plain radiography is able to detect the cardinal pathologic processes in OA, such as the appearance of osteophytes, loss of cartilage thickness and joint malalignment, but is insensitive to focal damage to cartilage and its surrounding soft tissues. Further, the demonstrable changes

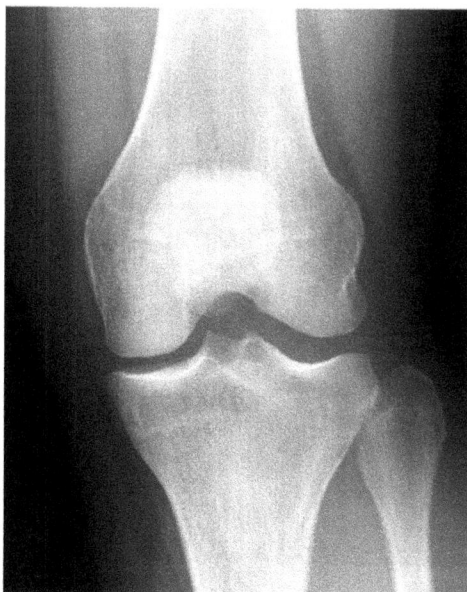

Fig. 6. AP radiograph of normal knee with KL score of 0. No osteophytes or joint space narrowing is observed.

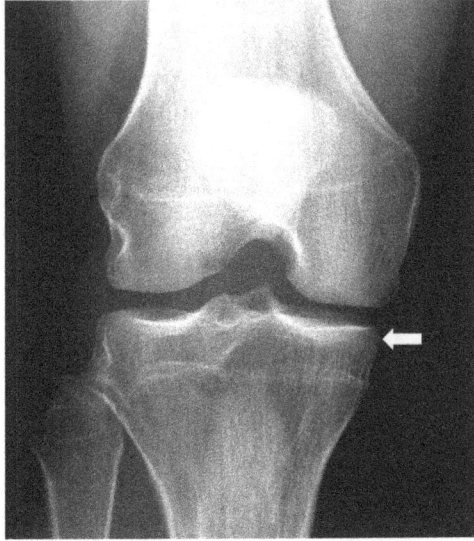

Fig. 7. AP radiograph of knee with KL score of 1. Note minimal osteophyte (arrow).

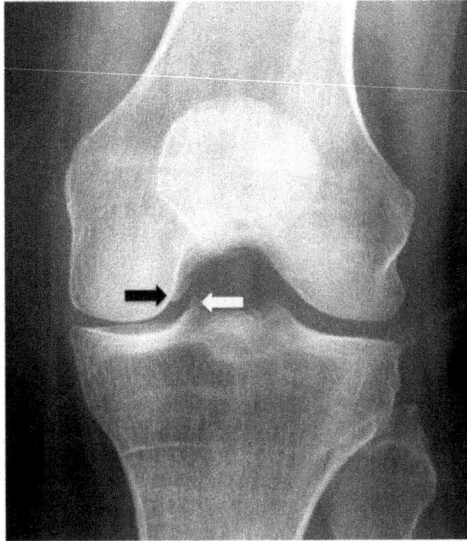

Fig. 8. AP radiograph of knee with KL score of 2. Note small osteophytes (arrows) but no joint space narrowing.

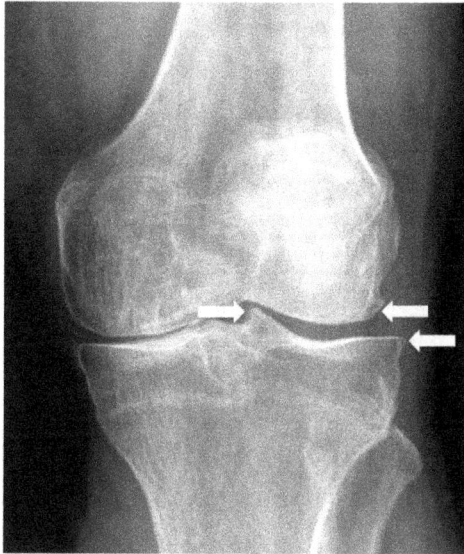

Fig. 9. AP radiograph of knee with KL score of 3. Note presence of medial joint space narrowing and osteophytes (arrows).

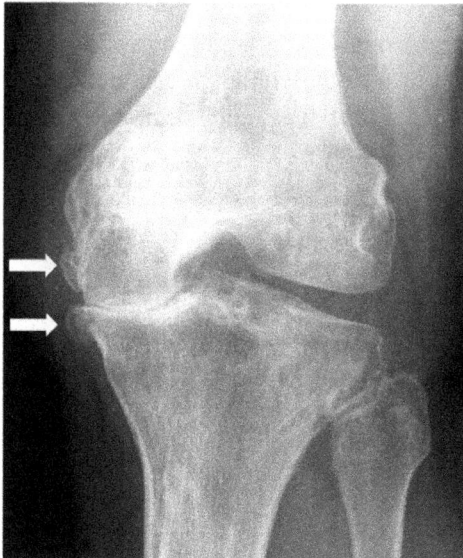

Fig. 10. AP radiograph of knee with KL score of 4. Note presence of severe medial joint space narrowing and multiple prominent osteophytes (arrows).

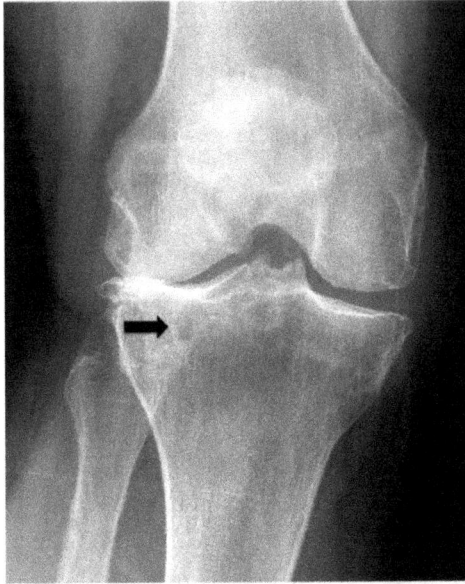

Fig. 11. AP radiograph of knee with KL score of 4. Note presence of severe lateral joint space narrowing and subchondral cyst (arrow).

in the joint by X-ray are late manifestations of the disease, leaving little room to intervene for the clinician. Magnetic Resonance Imaging, discussed in later chapters, offers a much desirable alternative for imaging of osteoarthritis.

References

1. Ahlback S. Osteoarthrosis of the knee. A radiographic investigation. *Acta Radiol Diagn (Stockh)* 1968;Suppl 277:277–272.
2. Thomas RH, Resnick D, Alazraki NP, Daniel D, Greenfield R. Compartmental evaluation of osteoarthritis of the knee. A comparative study of available diagnostic modalities. *Radiology* 1975;116(3):585–594.
3. Resnick D, Vint V. The "Tunnel" view in assessment of cartilage loss in osteoarthritis of the knee. *Radiology* 1980;137(2):547–548.
4. Brandt KD, Fife RS, Braunstein EM, Katz B. Radiographic grading of the severity of knee osteoarthritis: relation of the Kellgren and Lawrence grade to a grade based on joint space narrowing, and correlation with arthroscopic evidence of articular cartilage degeneration. *Arthritis Rheum* 1991;34(11):1381–1386.
5. Egund N, Frost S, Brismar J, Gustafson T. Radiography and scintigraphy in the assessment of early gonarthrosis. *Acta Radiol* 1988;29(4):451–455.

6. Fife RS, Brandt KD, Braunstein EM, Katz BP, Shelbourne KD, Kalasinski LA, Ryan S. Relationship between arthroscopic evidence of cartilage damage and radiographic evidence of joint space narrowing in early osteoarthritis of the knee. *Arthritis Rheum* 1991;34(4):377–382.

7. Bauer GC, Insall J, Koshino T. Tibial osteotomy in gonarthrosis (osteo-arthritis of the knee). *J Bone Joint Surg Am* 1969;51(8):1545–1563.

8. Harris WR, Kostuik JP. High tibial osteotomy for osteo-arthritis of the knee. *J Bone Joint Surg Am* 1970;52(2):330–336.

9. Leonard LM. The importance of weight-bearing x-rays in knee problems. *J Maine Med Assoc* 1971;62(5):101–106.

10. Marklund T, Myrnerts R. Radiographic determination of cartilage height in the knee joint. *Acta Orthop Scand* 1974;45(5):752–755.

11. Johnson F, Leitl S, Waugh W. The distribution of load across the knee. A comparison of static and dynamic measurements. *J Bone Joint Surg Br* 1980;62(3):346–349.

12. Leach RE, Gregg T, Siber FJ. Weight-bearing radiography in osteoarthritis of the knee. *Radiology* 1970;97(2):265–268.

13. Messieh SS, Fowler PJ, Munro T. Anteroposterior radiographs of the osteoarthritic knee. *J Bone Joint Surg Br* 1990;72(4):639–640.

14. Rosenberg TD, Paulos LE, Parker RD, Coward DB, Scott SM. The forty-five-degree posteroanterior flexion weight-bearing radiograph of the knee. *J Bone Joint Surg Am* 1988;70(10):1479–1483.

15. Boegard T, Jonsson K. Radiography in osteoarthritis of the knee. *Skeletal Radiol* 1999;28(11):605–615.

16. Buckland-Wright JC, Wolfe F, Ward RJ, Flowers N, Hayne C. Substantial superiority of semiflexed (MTP) views in knee osteoarthritis: a comparative radiographic study, without fluoroscopy, of standing extended, semiflexed (MTP), and Schuss views. *J Rheumatol* 1999;26(12):2664–2674.

17. Davies AP, Calder DA, Marshall T, Glasgow MM. Plain radiography in the degenerate knee. A case for change. *J Bone Joint Surg Br* 1999;81(4):632–635.

18. Merchant AC, Mercer RL, Jacobsen RH, Cool CR. Roentgenographic analysis of patellofemoral congruence. *J Bone Joint Surg Am* 1974;56(7):1391–1396.

19. Laurin CA, Dussault R, Levesque HP. The tangential x-ray investigation of the patellofemoral joint: x-ray technique, diagnostic criteria and their interpretation. *Clin Orthop Relat Res* 1979(144):16–26.

20. Ficat P, Hungerford DS. *Disorders of the Patello-Femoral Joint*. Baltimore: Williams & Wilkins, 1977.

21. Bradley WG, Ominsky SH. Mountain view of the patella. *AJR Am J Roentgenol* 1981;136(1):53–58.

22. Hughston JC. Subluxation of the patella. *J Bone Joint Surg Am* 1968;50(5): 1003–1026.

23. Jacobsen K, Bertheussen K, Gjerloff CC. Characteristics of the line of Blumensaat. An experimental analysis. *Acta Orthop Scand* 1974;45(5):764–771.

24. Jacobsen K. Landmarks of the knee joint of the lateral radiograph during rotation. *Rofo* 1976;125(5):399–404.

25. Butt WP, Lederman H, Chuang S. Radiology of the suprapatellar region. *Clin Radiol* 1983;34(5):511–522.

26. Engelstad BL, Friedman EM, Murphy WA. Diagnosis of joint effusion on lateral and axial projections of the knee. *Invest Radiol* 1981;16(3):188–192.

27. Hall FM. Radiographic diagnosis and accuracy in knee joint effusions. *Radiology* 1975;115(1):49–54.

28. Friedman AC, Naidich TP. The fabella sign: fabella displacement in synovial effusion and popliteal fossa masses. Normal and abnormal fabello-femoral and fabello-tibial distances. *Radiology* 1978;127(1):113–121.

29. Resnick D. Internal derangements of joints. In: Resnick D, editor. *Diagnosis of Bone and Joint Disorders*, Vol. 4. Philadelphia: W. B. Saunders Company, 2002, p. 3171.

30. Christensen P, Kjaer J, Melsen F, Nielsen HE, Sneppen O, Vang PS. The subchondral bone of the proximal tibial epiphysis in osteoarthritis of the knee. *Acta Orthop Scand* 1982;53(6):889–895.

31. Resnick D. Degenerative disease of extraspinal locations. In: Resnick D, editor. *Diagnosis of Bone and Joint Disorders*, 4th edn., Vol. 2. Philadelphia: W. B. Saunders Company, 2002. p. 1287.

32. Havdrup T, Hulth A, Telhag H. The subchondral bone in osteoarthritis and rheumatoid arthritis of the knee. A histological and microradiographical study. *Acta Orthop Scand* 1976;47(3):345–350.

33. Landells JW. The bone cysts of osteoarthritis. *J Bone Joint Surg Br* 1953;35-B(4):643–649.

34. Ondrouch AS. Cyst formation in osteoarthritis. *J Bone Joint Surg Br* 1963;45:755–760.

35. Jaffe HL. *Metabolic, Degenerative and Inflammatory Diseases of Bones and Joints*. Philadelphia: Lea & Febiger, 1972.

36. Trueta J. *Studies of the Development and Decay of the Human Frame*. Philadelphia: WB Saunders and Co, 1968.

37. Milgram JW. Morphologic alterations of the subchondral bone in advanced degenerative arthritis. *Clin Orthop Relat Res* 1983(173):293–312.

38. Crawford R, Sabokbar A, Wulke A, Murray DW, Athanasou NA. Expansion of an osteoarthritic cyst associated with wear debris: a case report. *J Bone Joint Surg Br* 1998;80(6):990–993.

39. Schmalzried TP, Akizuki KH, Fedenko AN, Mirra J. The role of access of joint fluid to bone in periarticular osteolysis. A report of four cases. *J Bone Joint Surg Am* 1997;79(3):447–452.

40. Ferguson AB Jr. The pathological changes in degenerative arthritis of the hip and treatment by rotational osteotomy. *J Bone Joint Surg Am* 1964;46:1337–1352.

41. Rhaney K, Lamb DW. The cysts of osteoarthritis of the hip; a radiological and pathological study. *J Bone Joint Surg Br* 1955;37-B(4):663–675.

42. Dieppe P, Kirwan J. The localization of osteoarthritis. *Br J Rheumatol* 1994;33(3):201–203.

43. Resnick D. *Diagnosis of Bone and Joint Disorders*, 4th edn. Philadelphia: WB Saunders, 2002, p. 26.

44. Resnick D. *Diagnosis of Bone and Joint Disorders*, 4th edn. Philadelphia: WB Saunders, 2002, p. 29.

45. Resnick D. *Diagnosis of Bone and Joint Disorders*, 4th edn. Philadelphia: WB Saunders, 2002, p. 28.

4

Introduction to Magnetic Resonance Imaging

by Roland Krug, Tobias D. Henning, Reinhard Meier
and Brian Hargreaves

Introduction

In 1946, Felix Bloch and Edward Purcell independently described the observation and theory underlying nuclear magnetic resonance (NMR) in a solid. This was the fundamental discovery that made MRI possible. As a result, in 1952, they were both awarded the Nobel Prize in Physics.

Bloch continued to extensively study NMR, establishing the framework for later developments that optimized the imaging technique. In essence, he described nuclear magnetism, the generation of a magnetic moment through the atomic nucleus' spin on an imaginary axis, which, is now known as the "Bloch equations." In the late 1960s, Raymond Damadian found an abnormal MR spectrum in malignant tissue. Finally, in the early 1970s, Damadian and Paul Lauterbur independently published the first MR images. Richard Ernst introduced the techniques of phase encoding and the Fourier transformation in 1975. Peter Mansfield developed the echo-planar imaging (EPI) technique. However, MR imaging did not gain clinical importance until the 1980s when improved hardware was available.

In contrast to X-ray imaging, which is based on the absorption of ionizing, electromagnetic radiation of high energy (20–150 keV), MRI uses the stimulation and subsequent emission of non-ionizing electromagnetic radiation of low energy (10^{-8}–10^{-6} eV) by biological tissue.

This chapter will provide the reader with a basic overview of the physical principles of MR imaging. Further, important problems will be covered more extensively and explained from a mathematical standpoint in order to provide a deeper understanding of the MR imaging technique. Furthermore, a "how to" section was added at the end of the chapter as a quick reference.

Overview

The principles of MRI are based on the fact that spinning charged nuclei behave like small magnetic dipoles when they are exposed to a magnetic field. A magnetic dipole can be viewed as a pair of magnetic charges with opposite signs but equal magnitude generating a magnetic moment analogous to a simple bar magnet (Fig. 1). In the presence of an external magnetic field, the magnetic dipoles align with the applied field, in a similar manner to small bar magnets. However, an additional factor is that they spin or precess about the field just like a gyroscope precesses around the earth's gravitational axis. The frequency of precession, known as the "Larmor frequency" ω_L, depends linearly upon the force of the magnetic field B_0 and a proportionality constant γ, called the gyromagnetic ratio, which is

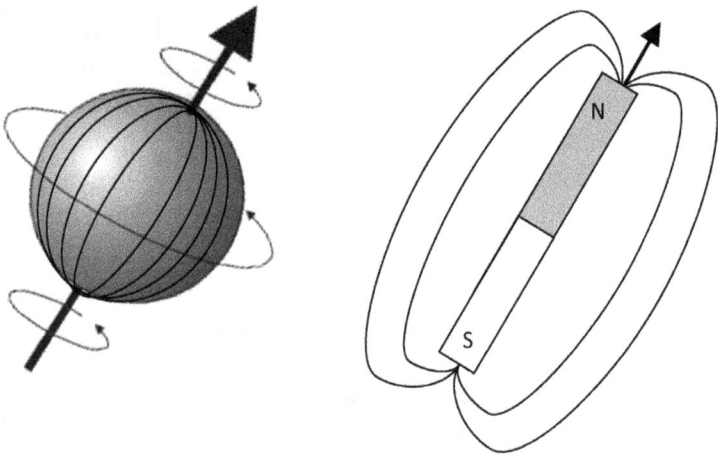

Fig. 1. Analogy between the magnetic fields resulting from a spinning nucleus and a bar magnet.

dependent upon the specific nucleus used for imaging:

$$\omega_L = \gamma \cdot B_z \tag{1}$$

where ω_L, Larmor frequency; γ, gyromagnetic ratio; B_z, magnetic field.

It should be noted that only charged nuclei, with an odd sum of nucleons (protons and neutrons) possess a nonzero intrinsic angular momentum or spin, which can be used for magnetic resonance imaging. The positively charged hydrogen nuclei represent approximately 80% of the atoms in the human body and hence are the main focus in MRI.

The orientation of each dipole causes a magnetic moment, $\vec{\mu}$, and can be described by a vector. The sum of all vectors yields the so-called net magnetization, $\vec{M}$. The individual nuclei spins precess with random phases around the applied magnetic field, commonly defined as the z-axis. The net transversal magnetization is therefore cancelled out and $\vec{M}$ in the xy-plane is zero. However, there is a nonzero net magnetization along the z-axis (Fig. 2).

It should be noted that spins in different longitudinal orientations, relative to the main magnetic field, have different energy levels. However, there are only two energy levels for the individual protons to assume: parallel (energetically favorable) and non-parallel (requires more energy) to the z-axis, the so-called Zeeman splitting. The state of the thermal equilibrium is dependent upon the temperature, T, the magnetic field strength, B_0, and the number of nuclear spins per unit volume. At a lower T and at a higher B_0 field, fewer spins reach the upper energy level. Under these conditions, the spin excess in the lower more favorable energy state increases and this leads to a higher MR signal.

Unfortunately, this explanation is not entirely comprehensive using the analogy of the gyroscope in classical physics. A more rigorous and accurate approach to the principles underlying the behavior of the individual spin requires the consideration of quantum mechanics. However, most MR effects can be described using classical physics because of the large amount of protons in consideration: a volume element (voxel) of 1 mm^3 of water contains more than 1.5×10^{19} protons. We will, therefore, refrain from a quantum mechanical description in this chapter because in practice we always deal with a bulk of spins per image voxel.

In order to acquire an MR signal, the randomly precessing spins at equilibrium have to be excited and this can be achieved by applying a

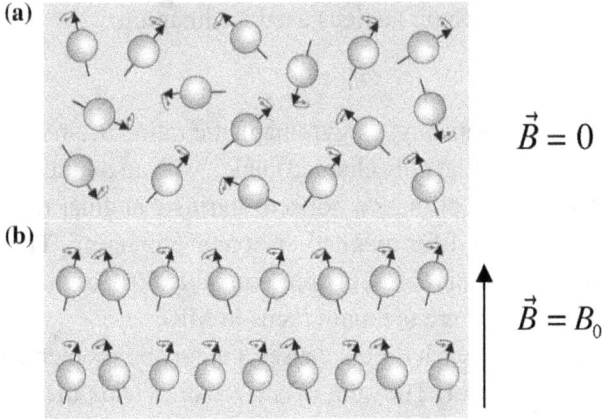

Fig. 2. Effect of an external magnetic field on spins. Without an external magnetic field spins do not have a preferential direction **(a)**. In an external magnetic field (B_0) spins align and precess around the axis of that field **(b)**. Depicted are only the excess protons with a spin parallel to the main magnetic field direction.

radiofrequency (rf) pulse. If the rf pulse is in resonance with the frequency of the precessing spins, energy can be transferred. This pulse synchronizes the phases of all spins to match that of the applied rf and a new transversal magnetization is created. This electromagnetic field, represented by the vector $\vec{M}$, can be collected or "received" by the same coil that was used to apply the rf pulse. This rf signal is called the free induction decay. When applying a longer rf pulse, an increasing number of protons will reach the non-parallel state while they continue to precess. The more protons at this higher energy level, the more "saturated" is the energetic state of the spin ensemble and the larger is the angle relative to the main magnetic field. This is called the *flip angle* (Fig. 3). To get a 90° transversal magnetization, the two energy states of the spin system have to be equally occupied. To invert the magnetization vector by a 180°-pulse, the higher energy state of the spin system has to be predominant.

Protons that spin at the same frequency are referred to as isochromats. Usually, multiple isochromats are present due to magnetic field inhomogeneities and applied magnetic gradients. By applying *selective* rf pulses, resonance frequencies in a narrower frequency bandwidth (e.g. 100 Hz) can be targeted. Thus only one group of isochromats would be in-resonance

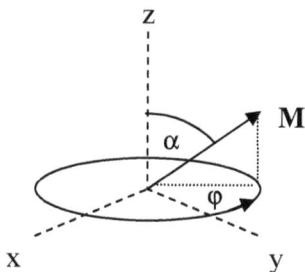

Fig. 3. Basic parameters of the spin. This figure depicts the bulk magnetization M, the flip angle α and the phase φ in a Cartesian coordinate system.

and emit the MR signal. For instance, this technique is used to suppress fat signals by only exciting water protons.

Eventually, the excited protons at the higher energy level (anti-parallel to the z-axis) flip back to their state of thermal equilibrium. The absorbed energy is thus released to the surroundings and this takes place along an exponential growth-course. The time point when exactly 63% of the maximum signal is reached is called the spin-lattice relaxation time or the $T1$ relaxation time. The $T1$ relaxation depends on the size of the molecules and their surroundings. The relatively small water-molecule has little possibility to release energy in the relaxed atom-fence of the liquid; the result is a long $T1$. Larger molecules will hand over their energy more quickly; the result is a short $T1$.

Concurrently, an additional process takes place in the transversal plane and thus overlaps the $T1$ effect. After the emission of an rf pulse, the originally synchronized spins gradually lose their phase coherence, resulting in attenuation and finally cancellation of the MR signal in the transversal plane (Fig. 4). This loss of the phase coherence is called the spin-spin relaxation or the $T2$ relaxation time, which denotes the point when only 37% of the maximal transversal magnetization is left. $T2$ is tissue-specific in a similar manner to $T1$. In the relatively dense atomic structure of a solid, the spins are continually exposed to locally fluctuating magnetic fields. Therefore, $T2$ is very short. In the less packed molecular structure of liquids, $T2$ is relatively long.

These two processes, alongside proton density, render it possible to distinguish between different tissue types and are thus the basic parameters

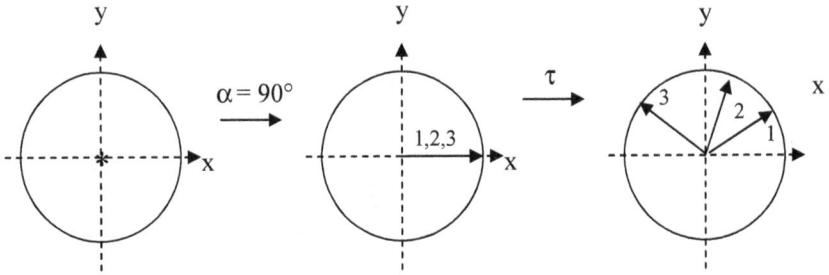

Fig. 4. $T2$-Dephasing. After having employed an rf pulse α, the originally synchronized isochromats (1,2,3) gradually lose their phase coherence, resulting in attenuation and finally cancellation of the MR signal in the transversal plane.

for image contrast. In addition, MRI can distinguish a broader range of tissue properties such as motion (diffusion and perfusion), elasticity, susceptibility and many more.

MR spatial resolution is achieved by superimposing gradient fields along all three planes of the main magnetic field. By applying these field gradients, the spins become spatially encoded through their different precession frequencies as defined by the Larmor equation. Further, at each acquisition time-point, all spins within the imaging region generate a certain phase pattern, i.e. spins related to different voxels of the image differ in their relative phases. These patterns are acquired using a coil detector and are consecutively digitally sampled. Since these patterns represent the essence of the Fourier transform, the original image can thus be obtained by applying the inverse Fourier transform. Of note, in contrast to other medical imaging modalities, resolution in MRI does not depend upon the transmitted wavelength (which is in meters). It is rather limited by the signal intensity, which is gained from the imaged voxel and the abilitiy to distinguish voxels which is limited by the strength of the magnetic field gradients.

Generally two units, Gauss [G] and Tesla [T], are used to describe magnetic field strength. Smaller field strengths like the field of rf pulses and magnetic gradients are commonly indicated in Gauss whereas the main magnetic field is often described in Tesla. This is partly historically motivated but also originates from the simple fact that Gauss is a much smaller unit (1 T equals 10^4 G) and thus more appropriate in order to quantify small field strengths.

MR Hardware

For MR imaging, three magnetic fields are required. The first is a large main magnet, which provides a strong (ideally) constant static magnetic field (B_0) that can be up to several thousand times stronger than the earth's magnetic field. The B_0 field is always operating due to the fact that it is usually generated by a superconducting magnet and thus does not require any power once turned on. However, superconducting magnets require liquid helium or liquid nitrogen in order to remain cool enough to maintain the superconducting state.

The gradient coils generate a second magnetic field used to spatially encode the object that is being imaged by modifying the main magnetic field strength at different locations. Their magnitude is generally in the order of a few Gauss per cm. Finally, the weakest magnetic field is the rf field, also called the B_1 field, and is created by rf coils. Magnetic resonance imaging and spectroscopy are both based on the use of rf pulses to manipulate magnetization. For example, $B_1 = 1/4$ G (Gauss) is typically applied to the head and often even less to the body. This is equivalent to half the field strength of the earth's magnetic field ($1/2$ Gauss). The B_1 field requires an average of approximately 2 kW (kilo Watt) of power at $B_0 = 1.5$ T (20 kW peak power). The majority of this power is dissipated within the subject and can raise the body temperature up to $3°$C, for any 1 g of tissue. Thus only about 1% of this energy has a direct impact on the spins. The rf power deposition is usually quantified as the specific absorption rate (SAR). The SAR is proportional to B_1 and to B_0 and must always be considered for any field strength higher than 1.5 T. It has to be maintained under the 3.2 W/kg US Food and Drug Administration (FDA) limit to ensure patient comfort and prevent scan interruptions. If electrons were used for imaging, an rf frequency in the range of microwaves would be necessary and, as a result, the energy deposition within the body would then be intolerably high.

Magnetic Resonance Condition

Living tissue consists of approximately 60% to 80% water. Thus, although other nuclei such as ^{23}Na and ^{31}P can also be used for MR imaging, the dominant nucleus used in MRI is the hydrogen nucleus (proton), as all other nuclei exist *in vivo* at much lower concentrations. As previously mentioned, nuclei with an even mass number (protons and neutrons) and even charge number have zero spin and cannot be used for magnetic resonance imaging. Transitions between energy states are associated with either the emission or absorption of photons. Their frequency corresponds to the difference in energy states and can be explained by the previously introduced Larmor equation [Equation (1)]. It has some advantages to introduce gamma-bar: $\bar{\gamma} = \gamma/2\pi$, with gamma and gamma-bar values both being nucleus specific. For example $\bar{\gamma} = 42.6$ MHz/Tesla for the hydrogen nucleus and $\bar{\gamma} = 10.71$ Hz/Tesla for the ^{13}C. In the classical description of the spin system as defined earlier, this frequency resembles the precession frequency in an external magnetic field. According to the above equation, a proton precesses with a frequency of approximately 64 MHz at 1.5 Tesla and the corresponding wavelength of the rf pulse is more than 4.5 m. For higher magnetic fields above 7.0 Tesla, the wavelength falls below 1 m signifying a higher energy state.

As explained earlier, in order to set the magnetization vector into precession, it must be tipped away from the external field direction. This is accomplished by applying an rf magnetic field for a short time perpendicular to the static field, a so-called "rf pulse," which is produced by a "transmit" coil. Classically, the magnetization vector is rotated away from its alignment along the longitudinal direction of B_0. But again, it is important that the rf pulse fulfils the mentioned resonance condition, i.e. it must be tuned to the Larmor frequency. Only then does the precessing spin (in the classic description of the system) gain the desired, continuously synchronized push in the transverse direction.

The Bloch Equation

The Bloch equation is a fundamental principle of MRI as it describes the time-dependent behavior of the bulk magnetization $\vec{M}$ within an external magnetic field. It is used to macroscopically describe the influence of a pulse sequence on a spin ensemble while taking into consideration the tissue specific and pulse sequence dependent parameters (e.g. relaxation times, flip angle, bandwidth, etc.). The following paragraph introduces the Bloch equation and its solution in a simplified manner. A more mathematical and rigorous derivation can be found in numerous MRI textbooks.

Having previously introduced the magnetic moment $\vec{\mu}$, the main magnetic field $\vec{B}$ and the constant γ, the basic Bloch equation can be written as:

$$\frac{d\vec{\mu}}{dt} = \gamma \cdot \vec{\mu} \times \vec{B} \tag{2}$$

where $\vec{\mu}$, magnetic moment; γ, constant; $\vec{B}$, magnetic field.

This describes the precession of the spins in an external magnetic field but neglects the interaction of protons with their environment. A summation of the magnetic moments of protons $\vec{\mu}$ per unit volume yields the bulk magnetization $\vec{M}$, which is written as:

$$\frac{d\vec{M}}{dt} = \gamma \cdot \vec{M} \times \vec{B} \tag{3}$$

where $\vec{M}$, bulk magnetization; γ, constant; $\vec{B}$, magnetic field.

This equation represents the precession of the bulk magnetization around a constant magnetic field B_0 with the Larmor frequency. On resonance, the rf pulse frequency is equal to the Larmor frequency. However, in order to simplify the mathematical concepts, a different reference system rotating with the Larmor frequency around the z-axis is commonly assumed (Fig. 5). Further, the precession due to the main magnetic field is not included in this coordinate system. Only the precession of the bulk magnetization M about the rotating x'-axis stemming from the rf pulse is depicted.

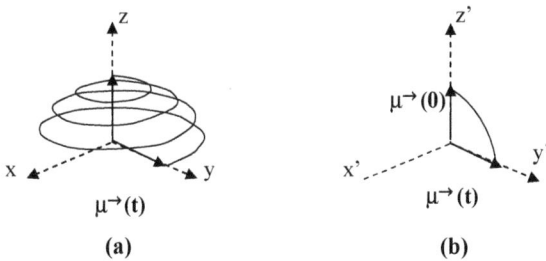

Fig. 5. On-resonance spin flip. The effect of an rf pulse on the bulk magnetization vector μ is depicted in the rotating frame. **(a)** Rotation about the x' axis) compared to the laboratory frame and **(b)** spiral.

The basic Bloch equation has to be further extended in order to describe the spin-lattice ($T1$) and spin-spin ($T2$) interactions of the protons with their surrounding atoms. Firstly, after tipping the magnetization vector $\vec{M}$ with an rf pulse to a certain flip-angle, the longitudinal magnetization returns to its equilibrium value M_0 due to spin-lattice interactions. As described by Curie's law, this equilibrium depends upon the absolute temperature T and the external field B_0, where C depends on the spin density ρ:

$$M_0 = C \cdot \frac{B_0}{T} \qquad (4)$$

where M_0, equilibrium of longitudinal magnetization; B_0, external magnetic field; T, absolute temperature.

Secondly, the transverse decay of $\vec{M}$ due to spin-spin interactions must also be considered. In essence, the spins lose their phase coherence due to field fluctuations stemming from surrounding spins and other field inhomogeneities and subsequently dephase. The relaxation times, $T1$ and $T2$, are tissue specific (see Table 1) and adding both relaxation phenomena, the Bloch equation yields:

$$\frac{d\vec{M}}{dt} = \gamma \cdot (\vec{M} \times \vec{B}) - \frac{\vec{M}_\perp}{T2} - \frac{\vec{M}_0 - \vec{M}_z}{T1} \qquad (5)$$

where $\vec{M}$, bulk magnetization; γ, constant; $\vec{B}$, magnetic field; $\vec{M}_\perp$, transversal magnetization vector; $\vec{M}_z$, momentary part of $\vec{M}_0$; $\vec{M}_0$, longitudinal magnetization vector.

The solutions of this differential equation are the following fundamental equations describing the change of the magnetization vectors M_z and $M_\perp$ over time t:

$$M_z(t) = M_z(0) \cdot e^{-t/T1} + M_0(1 - e^{-t/T1}) \qquad (6)$$

$$M_\perp(t) = M_\perp(0) \cdot e^{-t/T2} \qquad (7)$$

where $\vec{M}_z$, momentary part of $\vec{M}_0$; $\vec{M}_0$, longitudinal magnetization vector; $\vec{M}_\perp$, transversal magnetization vector.

As illustrated in Figure 6, the regrowth of longitudinal magnetization to its equilibrium M_0, as well as the decay of the transverse component occur according to exponential functions.

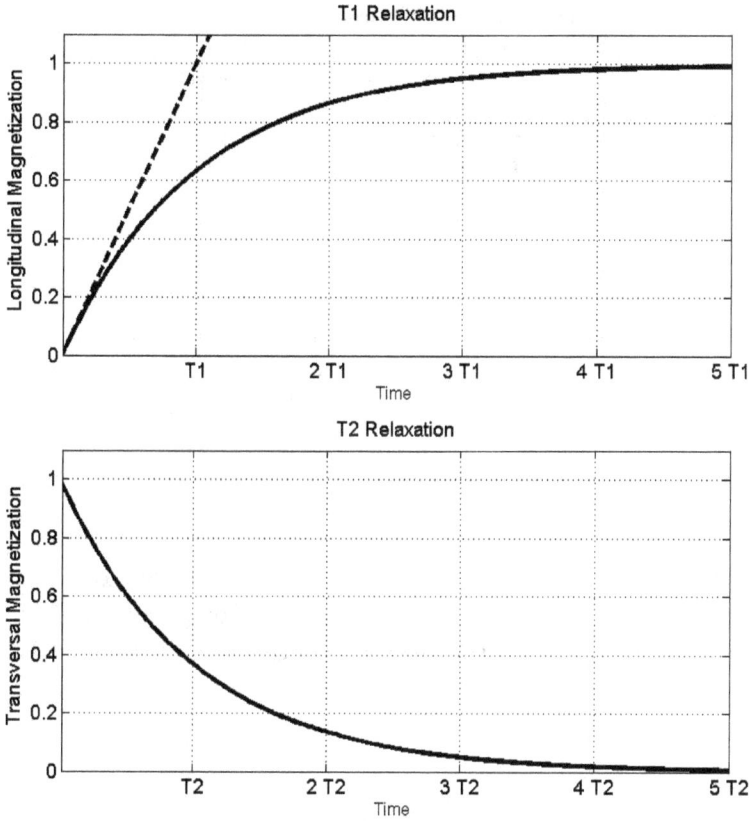

Fig. 6. Spin relaxation processes. The first figure demonstrates the exponential increase of the longitudinal magnetization to its initial equilibrium value. After the time $T1$, 63% of the maximum longitudinal magnetization is recovered. The slope (dashed) indicates the slope of the regrowth process depending on the remaining longitudinal magnetization from previous excitations. The figure below shows the decrease of transversal magnetization due to spin-spin interactions. After the time $T2$, 37% of the original transversal magnetization has decayed.

In the presence of B_0 field inhomogeneities, a much more rapid decay of the signal is observed and $T2$ has to be replaced by a smaller relaxation time represented as $T2^*$:

$$\frac{1}{T2^*} = \frac{1}{T2} + \frac{1}{T2'}. \tag{8}$$

Table 1. Relaxation parameters. Approximate relaxation parameters $T1$ and $T2$ in milliseconds for different human tissues at a static magnetic field of $B_0 = 1.5\,\text{T}$ and a temperature of $37°\text{C}$.

Tissue	$T1$ (ms)	$T2$ (ms)
Fat	250	60
Bone marrow	288	165
White brain matter	600	80
Grey brain matter	950	100
Cartilage	1060	42
Muscle	1130	35
Blood (venous)	1200	200
Synonvial fluid	2850	1210
Cerebrospinal fluid (CSF)	4500	2200

The additional dephasing characterized by $T2'$ is due to field inhomogeneities assuming exponential signal decay. However, by applying an additional rf pulse, this dephasing effect can be reversed by rephasing the spins using spin-echo type pulse sequences as we will discuss later in this chapter.

Spatial Encoding and Image Reconstruction

In order to fully understand how an image is created in MRI, a basic understanding of the Fourier transformation (FT) is necessary. Important image parameters like readout bandwidth or image distortions (e.g. wrapping artefacts) can only be fully appreciated within the Fourier or k-space domain of an image. We will develop, in this paragraph, the conceptual basics leading to a better understanding of the FT.

Every digital image can be thought of as a spatial distribution of grey values within a plane. In modern MR scanners, the dynamic range contains a maximum of 32 bit grey values. The number of pixels typically varies between 192 and 512 and more recently 1024 by 1024 pixels are more and more common. Radiologists normally use these grey value images for diagnosis, using only the magnitude of the complex pixel value (complex number z). The phase of each individual pixel is generally disregarded and only used for specific applications like the quantification of flow velocity where, for instance, the speed of blood can be encoded in the phase of the pixels. Thus, an MR image actually consists of two images, one representing the magnitude of the vector pixel and one representing its phase. In the following section we will further develop the important concept of how pixel values are represented by complex numbers.

Complex Numbers

Generally, a complex number z is written as:

$$z = a + ib \quad \text{where } i = \sqrt{-1} \tag{9}$$

where z, complex number; a, real part; b, imaginary part.

Alternatively, and more useful in MRI, z can be expressed as:

$$z = A \exp(-i\phi) = A(\cos \Phi + i \sin \Phi) \tag{10}$$

where z, complex number; A, amplitude; Φ, phase of the pixel vector.

Understanding can be enhanced by picturing a complex number as a pointer (vector), with a certain length (amplitude) and a certain phase (defined angle) as depicted in Fig. 7. The phase is typically but not

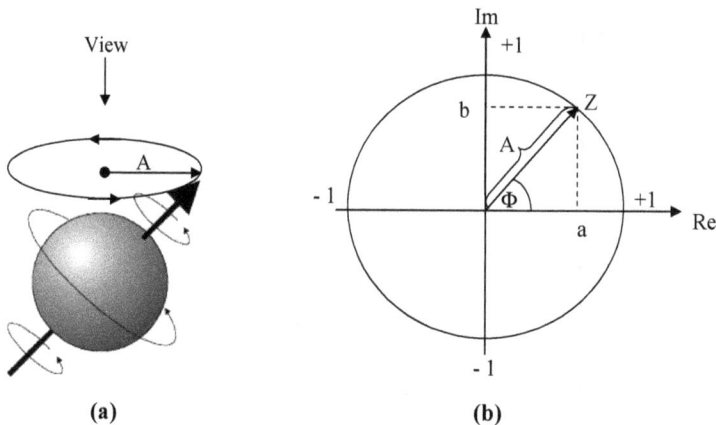

Fig. 7. Representations of complex numbers. Adopting an axial view **(b)**, the rotation of a spin **(a)** or a spin ensemble can be described by means of a complex number. A complex number Z can be represented by Cartesian coordinates a and b where a is usually called the real part and b the imaginary part of Z. Very often complex numbers are also represented in polar coordinates A and Φ where A is denoted the amplitude and Φ the phase of Z.

absolutely referenced with respect to the x-axis, where Φ is zero. The phase of an image vector plays a very important role in MRI as we will see further below.

From Fig. 7, it is clear that a rotating spin can be fully described by a complex number given its amplitude and its phase relative to the detecting coil. As already mentioned, in MRI we only consider the net (bulk) magnetization $\vec{M}$ of all spins in a voxel precessing with equal frequency (isochromats).

Discrete Sampling

While the spins precess, they constantly change their relative phase. Therefore, they will undergo different "phase combinations" during a single acquisition time. Although the precession of these isochromats is continuous, the final image will be discrete because of the discrete nature of computers. The process of sampling the received signal at discrete points is called digitization and is depicted in Fig. 8. At first glance, digitization may appear to represent an enormous loss of information. However, there are defined criteria regarding the sampling rate of the signal, which have to be met in order to preserve important structures and the integrity of an image.

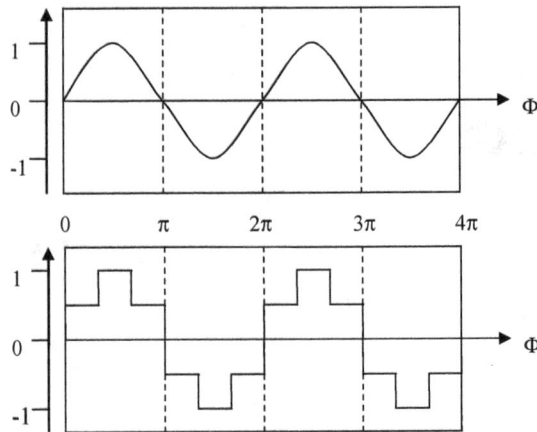

Fig. 8. Digitization of the received continuous signal. The received analogous signal from the receiver coil has to be sampled at discrete points in time. This process is called digitization or sampling. Certain criteria have to be fulfilled in order to not lose important information. Of note: Only the real part of the signal is depicted.

We will discuss this in more detail below as it is of paramount importance to understand the principles of image generation in MRI. All parameters used by an operator to enhance image quality (e.g. bandwidth, partial Fourier acquisition and no phase wrap) can only be fully comprehended once a basic understanding of spatial image encoding has been established.

Initially, the signal received by the coil consists of multiple superimposed signals from all isochromats, which by definition have equal phases at all times. By superimposing a so-called "linear magnetic field gradient" G on the static field B_0, we create different field strengths B at different spatial locations x according to:

$$B_x = G_x \cdot x \qquad (11)$$

where B_x, magnetic field in x direction; G_x, field gradient in x direction; x, different spatial locations.

Since the Larmor frequency of the spins depends linearly on the magnitude of the applied magnetic field, it is possible to locate the spins in a spatially varying field as a result of their different precession frequency. Now, the Larmor frequency of the spin depends linearly on its position.

As the precession frequency ω is directly proportional to B, different isochromats are created. The number of isochromats translates to an equal number of pixels. Immediately after employing a 90° rf pulse all spins are precessing in-phase in the transversal plane. At time $t = 0$ after the field gradient was turned on, all isochromats are still precessing in phase. If we look at the image again at the time Δt, the isochromats further away from the gradient center acquired a larger phase than the spins in the center of the applied magnetic gradient due to a higher B field. Spins towards the negative gradient acquired the same amount of phase but in the opposite direction. Spins in the center of the gradient field do not acquire any phase since they experience a B field of zero magnitude. If we go on in time, different phase patterns are projected on the image. The smallest structure which can be projected on an image with four isochromats is shown at time point $\Delta t = 4$. It is clear from Fig. 8, that this structure corresponds to a cosine sampled twice (two pixels) per repetition period 2π. A more detailed structure cannot be represented by an image using four pixels without distortions. This sample theorem is also known as the Nyquist theorem. It is important to notice that all structures at all eight different time points repeat themselves in the manner that $t = 4$ would correspond exactly to the formation of $t = 0$ and so on.

Fourier Transformation (FT)

The induction of different spin patterns by field gradients described above is nothing else than an inherent FT. As explained earlier, spins have to be encoded in order to yield different specific patterns on the image and thereby spatial information of the investigated object can be obtained. These patterns are the so-called basic functions of the FT. We will now translate this more phenomenological approach into a mathematical description.

The images used for diagnosis by radiologists are presented in the described spatial system using grey values. Although this is the most illustrative depiction regarding the perception of the human eye, the information inherent in an image can be depicted in different ways. One alternative image representation is the wave number or Fourier representation. Spatial and Fourier representation can be converted into each other without loss of information. They are both totally equivalent descriptions of a digital image and are transformed via the FT. In MRI the FT plays an important role in image reconstruction.

In essence, the FT is a complex multiplication of each pixel value with the FT kernel. The FT kernel is a complex number with the magnitude $A = 1$, which is only characterized by its phase (Fig. 7). In MRI, this multiplication is performed by applying a magnetic field gradient over the image and thus changing the precession frequency ω at each spatial position x. Merging Equations (1) and (11) we get:

$$\omega_L = \gamma G x \tag{12}$$

where ω_L, Larmor frequency; γ, gamma-bar; G, field gradient; x, different spatial locations.

The multiplication of ω_L with the time point t yields the exact phase of the precessing spins at this time point t. As mentioned above, a coordinate system that rotates with $f = \gamma B_0$ is commonly assumed in MRI (Fig. 5). Since all spins originally precess with this frequency there is no relative phase change due to B_0. Because of this, the incoming signal is always demodulated and the rotation stemming from B_0 is usually neglected (low pass filtered). Subsequently, the following equation gives us the phase of each isochromat depending on its location x:

$$\Phi = \gamma\, Gt = kx \tag{13}$$

where Φ, phase of the pixel vector; G, field gradient; x, different spatial locations; t, time; k, wave vector.

And thus $k = \gamma\, Gt$ for the wave vector yielding the following expression for the FT kernel:

$$W_x^t = \exp(i\phi) = \exp(-i\gamma\, Gxt) \tag{14}$$

where W_x^t, FT kernel; Φ, phase of the pixel vector; γ, constant; G, field gradient; x, different spatial locations; t, time.

W_x^t is a complex number (pointer) with variable phase Φ but constant amplitude $A = 1$ representing the FT kernel. Each isochromat can be represented by W_x^t at a specific time t and location x. Thus, by applying a certain gradient G over a certain time t, all basic functions needed for the FT can be generated. *Sampling time and magnetic field gradient are the two free fundamental variables the MR scanner adapts in order to yield a certain pixel size, FOV and image matrix.* The acquisition time is directly related to the readout bandwidth BW [Hz] chosen. Bandwidth is defined as the difference in frequency between neighboring isochromats. The gradient is then automatically adjusted to yield the desired imaging parameters.

Signal Equation

The signal response of all magnetic dipoles (spins) is detected by a receiver coil. Commonly, to generate the rotating B_1 field the same coil is being used as to acquire this signal. The precessing magnetization causes a change in flux in the coil inducing the free induction decay (FID), which is then recorded. At one recording point in time, the received signal $s(t)$ is a sum of all precessing transverse spin magnetization M_x in the volume of interest (voxel). This can be expressed by a summation over the total volume (for simplification purpose, we remain in one dimension):

$$S_t = c \cdot \sum_{x=0}^{N-1} M_x \cdot W_x^t, \quad 0 \le x \le N \tag{15}$$

where s_t, received signal; M_x, transverse spin magnetization; W_x^t, FT kernel; N, number of pixels.

Assuming an ideal case without field distortion and no field gradient applied ($t = 0$), all spins would be in-phase ($\Phi = 0$) and the real part of all voxels represented by W_x would be equal to one. In this case we would just sum up the magnitudes of the magnetization vector over the entire volume, which corresponds to the mean value of the image.

The above equation is equal to the discrete FT in one-dimension. All signals s_t correspond to the Fourier coefficients, which are the pixel values of the image in the Fourier space (or k-space). After having acquired all N Fourier coefficients, we have gained an equal representation of the original image, the so-called Fourier or k-space image. This is the image (signal) acquired by the coil and is usually "back Fourier transformed" (reconstructed) by an additional computer in order to gain the spatial image we are used to see on the screen. The image in Fourier space looks very different from the real image usually used for diagnosis and the k-values represent different spatial frequencies (wave number per meter) at each k-space point.

Two- and Three-Dimensional Encoding

Readout Direction

According to the signal equation above, the signal is detected (sampled) at different time points while the so-called "readout" gradient is applied during the time t. During the total readout time, the spins continue precessing with different Larmor frequencies and thus accumulating different phases ϕ at different time points.

Phase-Encoding Direction

In order to encode two-dimensional images, a second gradient is applied perpendicular to the readout gradient. This process is called phase-encoding and differs insofar as the second gradient is not employed during signal acquisition but before in order to prepare the phases of the spin in this direction (usually denoted as y-direction). The accumulation of phase depends again on the strength of the gradient and the duration time of the gradient similar to the readout process:

$$\Delta\phi_{(\gamma)} = \gamma \cdot \Delta G_y \cdot t_y \cdot \gamma = \Delta k_y \cdot \gamma \tag{16}$$

where Φ, phase of the pixel vector; γ, constant; G, field gradient; k, wave vector.

After switching off the so-called phase encoding gradient, all spins continue precessing with the initial Larmor frequencies but different phases in y-direction. These values are again related to the basic functions of the discrete FT described above.

Slice Selection

If the rf pulse is employed with only B_0 present, all spins in the volume are excited according to the sensitivity of the transmitting coil. In order to define more precisely the excited slice volume (slice selection), a spatially constant gradient is applied in the z-direction. Thus, corresponding to their resonance condition, the rf pulse only excites the spins within the same frequency spectrum around $\bar{\omega}_L$. Spins outside the defined frequency bandwidth are not interacting with the rf pulse.

Field of View and Aliasing (Phase Wrap)

As pointed out before, the smallest structure which can be depicted by a digital image must be sampled by at least two pixels in order to be represented without distortions (Nyquist theorem). Resulting from the signal sampling in time with appropriate time steps Δt, we get the field of view (FOV) of the image via:

$$\text{FOV} = \frac{2\pi}{\Delta k} = \frac{2\pi}{\gamma \cdot G_x \cdot \Delta t} \tag{17}$$

where k, wave vector; γ, constant; G, field gradient; t, time.

The so-calculated FOV is commonly depicted as a box on the user interface of the scanner. To avoid image distortion (aliasing or wrapping), the object has to fit the FOV. If there are overlaps, it means that the rf coil picked up signal from a region larger than the FOV. At these edges of the FOV the precession frequency of the spins is highest due to the high magnetic field of the employed gradients. Those overlapping parts of the object cannot be accurately sampled with the corresponding Δt and are mapped back into the FOV, because they have the same phase as the isochromats on the other side of the FOV. The resulting image is "aliased" which means that the one edge maps into the opposite side of the FOV. To increase the FOV, Δt has to be decreased resulting in a larger FOV according to the equation above. To avoid aliasing, the signal is commonly sampled in much shorter time intervals Δt. This process is called oversampling and is always performed in readout direction. The shortest possible sample times accomplished by modern scanners are in the order of a few microseconds. This technique does not require additional scan time, since only more data points are acquired during equal readout time. In contrast, to avoid aliasing in phase-encoding direction more sampling steps have to be added, increasing the total scan time. On the scanner, this approach is usually referred to as "no phase wrap."

Pulse Sequences

MRI is the medical image modality delivering the best soft tissue contrast. Since the main MRI parameters — $T1$, $T2$ and proton density — differ strongly between tissues, a wide variety of contrast can be acquired. In order to weight images according to these tissue properties, MRI parameters can be adjusted.

Echoes

In MRI an echo signal is commonly referred to as the maximal transversal signal resulting from a total phase coherence of precessing spins (e.g. at $t = 0$ directly after the excitation). The echo time TE is an important image parameter to change the contrast in an image. At TE, all spins are in phase. Immediately after excitation, the spins begin to dephase due to magnet field inhomogeneities as described in Fig. 9. However, the phase coherence can be re-established by applying a refocusing rf pulses at any time. This is mostly — but not necessarily — achieved by 180° pulses. Such generated echoes are called *spin echoes*. Using this method, any phase incoherence whether originating from field inhomogeneity or chemical shift etc. can be reversed. After having employed the rf pulse, the spins accrue the same

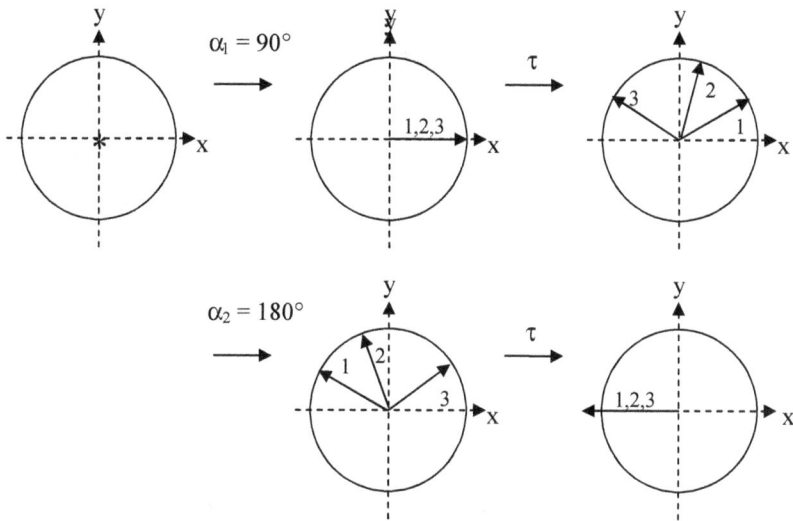

Fig. 9. Spin echo. A spin echo is generated by rephasing the asynchronized isochromats (1,2,3) by employing an rf pulse α_2. This is commonly but not necessarily done using a 180° rf pulse. Spins which experience higher local magnetic fields precess faster (3). After the inversion pulse α_2, these spins would regain the original phase and thus would synchronize with the slower spins that gained less phase in the same time τ.

amount of phase, only in the negative direction. Therefore, after the same time interval the spins all end up synchronized resulting in a so-called spin-echo.

In contrast to the spin-echo, the gradient-echo refers to a phase coherence due to the applied field gradients. After having superimposed a gradient field over the main magnetic field in order to encode the isochromats (Fig. 10), the original phase coherence can be established by just negating the applied gradient. However, field inhomogeneities can only be synchronized by applying a reversal rf pulse. Thus magnetic field gradients can only be used to rewind phases accumulated by previously applied magnetic field gradients. The so-established gradient echo usually refers to the center point in Fourier space, which represents the mean intensity value of the image. Therefore, spin-echo and gradient-echo should ideally coincide to yield maximum signal-to-noise ratio (SNR). This is the case using spin-echo sequences. MRI sequences of the gradient-echo type have usually their spin-echo immediately after the rf pulse and before

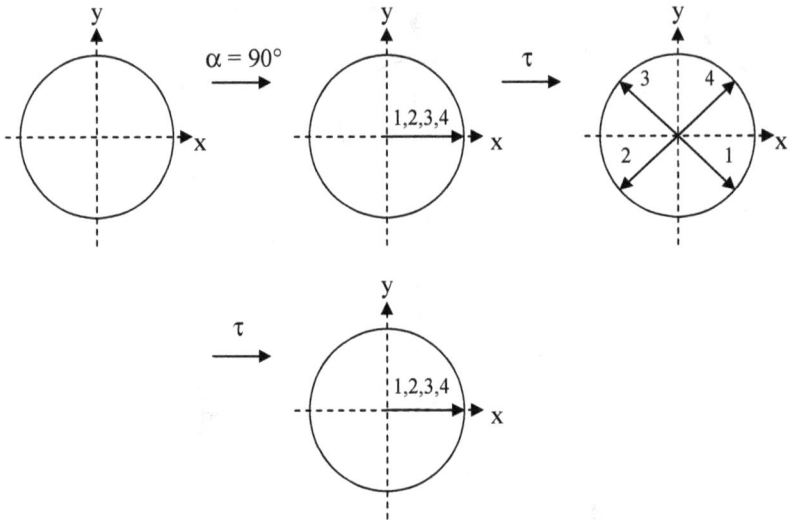

Fig. 10. Gradient echo. Since a gradient echo is generated by magnetic field gradients, the isochromats (1,2,3,4) are lineally distributed over all phases. These phase shifts can be easily reversed by employing the same gradient but inversely. However magnetic field inhomogeneities cannot be reversed by this method.

the gradient-echo occurs and thus show some signal loss due to field homogeneity-induced dephasing.

Spin- Versus Gradient-Echo Based Sequences

The imaging sequence is a protocol that describes the entire set of events generated by the MR system. All combined rf pulses and gradient waveforms are defined in such sequences. Basically, there are two types of sequences: The spin-echo sequence (Fig. 11) and the gradient-echo sequence. The main difference is the additional use of a refocusing pulse for the spin-echo type sequence. For a spin-echo sequence, this is managed by means of a rephasing rf pulse.

The gradient-echo sequence does not apply this pulse, but reverses the readout gradient polarity as described above. But while the gradient-echo refocuses the phase due to the application of the gradient, it does not refocus the dephasing induced to static-field inhomogeneities as the spin-echo does. Hence, problems caused by dephasing can occur more often. Note that a

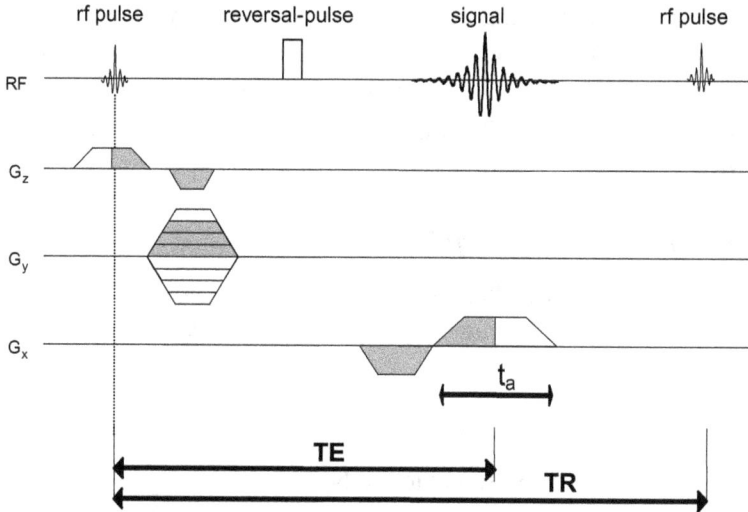

Fig. 11. Spin echo sequence. The first rf pulse generates the transverse magnetization. In order to specify an imaging slice, an encoding gradient is employed in the slice direction (commonly noted as the z-direction). After further preparation and y-encoding, a reversal pulse is applied in order to rephase all spins. Since this pulse is not used for gradient echo sequences, imaging time can be reduced. The signal is acquired during t_a when the readout gradient is turned on. The sequence recurs after each rf pulse, and a different value of the phase encode is played.

gradient-echo always has to occur in order to record the first basis function of the FT at $\Delta t = 0$. Additionally, using a spin echo (SE) sequence, both gradient-echo and spin-echo coincide yielding maximum signal at the echo time. Note, that a gradient-echo is always generated by these sequences in order to readout the k-space centre. Spin-echo based sequences generate an additional spin-echo where reversible magnetic field inhomogeneities are reversed. This behaviour generates a $T2$ contrast which is the most important contrast for clinical diagnosis.

How to Increase SNR

Field Strength

The primary noise source in MRI is of thermal origin. For instance, the Brownian motion or random movement of electrons within a conductor generates random electrical fluctuations. The subject in the scanner also generates similar fluctuating fields that are perceived by the receiver coil. From Equation (3), it is apparent that the SNR is directly proportional to the main magnetic field B_0 and inversely proportional to the temperature T. Accordingly, increasing the B_0 or decreasing the T will increase the SNR.

Number of Excitations/Acquisitions

When increasing the number of excitations (NEX) to two or more, the scanner automatically averages the signal amplitudes of two or more measurements:

$$\text{SNR} \propto \sqrt{\text{NEX}}.$$

The SNR is directly proportional to the NEX.

Readout Bandwidth

The readout time is defined as the time during which the signal is acquired. Increasing the readout time increases the SNR. Assuming that the readout time is inversely proportional to the readout bandwidth BW (which is true in most cases) the following relationship is true:

$$\text{SNR} \propto \frac{1}{\sqrt{\text{BW}}}.$$

Spatial Resolution

For a fixed readout time, the SNR in a voxel is proportional to its size $\Delta x \cdot \Delta y \cdot \Delta z$:

$$\text{SNR} \propto \Delta x \cdot \Delta y \cdot \Delta z.$$

Hence, decreasing the slice thickness by half requires a fourfold increase in NEX or readout time to maintain the same SNR.

Pulse Sequence and Tissue Properties

As previously discussed, the SNR depends on the specific MRI pulse sequence and sampling techniques used as well as the tissue parameters (e.g. proton density, $T1$ and $T2$ times).

How to Avoid Aliasing

According to the Nyquist sampling theorem, every signal has to be sampled twice per wavelength for exact reconstruction. In MRI, an object's signal outside the FOV is mapped incorrectly to a location inside the FOV but on the opposite side. This is called aliasing or phase wrap. Therefore, oversampling the signal usually avoids these aliasing artefacts. It is automatically performed in the readout direction. Oversampling in the phase encoding direction to avoid phase wrap results in longer scan times. Usually, when enabling this option, the scan time is kept constant but NEX and thus SNR is reduced. An alternative would be to increase the FOV or decrease the residual signal outside the FOV by using surface coils or saturation bands. Finally, sometimes readout and phase encoding directions can be changed to avoid infolding from one side.

How to Avoid Gibbs Ringing and Truncation Artefacts

This artefact appears as a series of lines in the MR image parallel to sharp changes in intensity. Undersampling of small structures in an image and thus truncation of the frequency domain results in Gibbs ringing. Fewer data points are sampled in the phase encoding direction and thus the effects are more pronounced in this direction. Since Gibbs ringing is primarily related to pixel size, smaller pixels would diminish the artefact, as would more samples.

How to Avoid Flow Artefacts

The MR signal is very sensitive to flow and motion. Flow and motion artefacts are similar in that spins change their location during spatial encoding leading to different phase accumulation. This results in signal loss due to dephasing, blur and displacement. Conversely, an increased signal can occur from previously unexcited blood flowing into the region of interest. The easiest way to compensate for phase-shifts is to weaken the signal of the flowing medium by placing saturation bands before the FOV. Also a "preparatory lobe" can be added to the readout gradient to compensate for velocity effects.

How to Avoid Motion Artefacts

Motion is the most prevalent source of MRI artefact. However, the motion that occurs is typically much slower than the rapid sampling process during readout time. For this reason, motion artefacts are usually more pronounced in the phase encoding direction thus resulting in blurring. To compensate for patient immobilization, navigator echoes can be employed to track motion during the scan and adjust for it.

How to Avoid Chemical Shift Artefacts

The protons in water perceive a different magnetic field from those in lipid due to small field variations at the molecular level. The difference in resonance frequency is 142 Hz/T between fat and water protons. The shift theorem of the FT states that a shift in frequency of the basic functions in the frequency domain results in a corresponding spatial shift. Thus the signal acquired from the fat protons is shifted relative to the water protons, i.e. the spins in the same voxel are encoded as being located in different voxels. The fat misregistration occurs along the readout direction and depends upon the readout bandwidth per pixel and the frequency difference between water and fat. For example, a readout BW of 250 Hz/pixel at 3 T field strength ($\Delta f = 426$ Hz/pixel) would result in a spatial shift of 1.7 voxel. Thus, in order to reduce chemical shift artefacts, the readout bandwidth has to be increased. It is important to note that missregistration only occurs in readout direction. In contrast to the readout gradient, which is applied during the readout time, the phase encoding gradient is only turned on for a brief moment to change phases and then switched off again. During the phase encoding time, there is a chemical shift between fat and water and a phase difference develops. However, since a new excitation is applied as we vary the strength of the gradient, the phase difference does not accumulate. The amount of chemical shift between fat and water does not change from one signal to the next. Thus the shift theorem does not apply and in the phase encoding direction, no chemical shift artefact is observed.

Abbreviations

BW	Bandwidth
FID	Free Induction Decay

FOV	Field of View
FT	Fourier Transformation
G	Gauss
Hz	Hertz
kW	kilo Watt
MHz	Megahertz
MR	Magnetic Resonance
MRI	Magnetic Resonance Imaging
NEX	Number of Excitations
NMR	Nuclear Magnetic Resonance
rf	Radiofrequency
SAR	Specific Absorption Rate
SE	Spin Echo
SNR	Signal-to-Noise Ratio
TE	Echo Time
T	Tesla

5

Current Magnetic Resonance Imaging Techniques for Clinical Diagnosis and Staging of Knee Osteoarthritis

by Ehsan Saadat, Thomas M. Link
and C. Benjamin Ma

Introduction

Although plain radiography of the knee is currently the most commonly used technique for radiographic diagnosis of knee osteoarthritis (OA), this technique has several limitations. Early and focal changes in the cartilage and other articular tissues are not directly visible using radiographs. Cartilage loss can only be indirectly inferred in X-rays by the development of joint-space narrowing. Because of the focal nature of the disease process, prominent findings are often readily apparent in one or two compartments of the joint and absent or mild in other compartments, despite pathologic abnormalities in those compartments. Although the most accurate appraisal of the compartmental distribution of the disease can be attained by direct visual inspection only (such as by arthroscopy), other non-invasive methods are also required. Magnetic Resonance Imaging (MRI) of the knee is currently the most promising technique. MRI offers superior soft tissue contrast, is capable of non-invasive evaluation of cartilage morphology as well as function, and does not cause ionizing radiation.

Articular cartilage is a complex anatomic structure with a biochemical make-up that directly dictates the fundamental characteristics of the tissue.

These include the presence of large amounts of proteoglycans, negatively-charged molecules attached to a complex, multi-layered collagen structure, which hold water in the tissue and impart to it the characteristic "reversible deformation" of articular cartilage. The water content of the tissue depends on a balance between the swelling pressure of the aggregated proteoglycans and the counter resistance of the fibrous collagen matrix. The MRI signal behavior of cartilage reflects its complex biochemistry and histology. Water constitutes 70% of the wet weight of normal articular cartilage, and therefore, water sensitive sequences such as $T2$-weighted are well suited to visualize cartilage.

This chapter introduces the two most commonly used MRI sequences for imaging of cartilage in the clinical setting and discusses the ability of each to evaluate findings in knee osteoarthritis. In addition, three MRI-based cartilage scoring systems commonly used in clinical research will be presented. This chapter will conclude with a discussion of MR imaging of articular cartilage repair. The technical details of the sequences discussed, their optimization, and other research-based MR imaging techniques for evaluation of articular cartilage morphology and function will be discussed elsewhere in the book.

Current MR Techniques for Imaging of Knee Osteoarthritis

A number of different clinically available pulse sequences can be used in MRI of cartilage, with each technique taking advantage of differing contrast characteristics of cartilage and adjacent soft tissue structure. Two pulse sequences are currently the mainstays of knee imaging: $T1$-weighted Spoiled Gradient Echo (SPGR) and $T2$-weighted Fast Spin-Echo (FSE).[1]

$T1$-weighted imaging provides visible distinction between cartilage and subchondral bone, though contrast between cartilage and synovial fluid is poor. Three-dimensional $T1$-weighted SPGR acquisitions provide high-resolution contiguous thin-slice images with reasonable scan times. Fat-suppressed SPGR images show good contrast between bright cartilage and the relatively dark bone, muscle and synovial fluid.[2] The adjunct use of fat suppression with SPGR and other clinical imaging sequences (such as FSE) increases the dynamic range of signal intensity throughout the image, and allows for better detection of signal intensity alterations.[3,4] In 3D SPGR imaging, cartilage abnormalities are seen as morphologic abnormalities of cartilage contour.

For cartilage, fat-suppressed $T2$-weighted and intermediate-weighted imaging is particularly valuable and routinely acquired as it yields good contrast with the synovial fluid at the cartilage surface, permitting identification of cartilage surface lesions. FSE imaging of cartilage also benefits from inherent magnetization transfer effects within normal cartilage, which may increase the conspicuity of cartilage abnormalities.[5,6] Both intermediate- and $T2$-weighted FSE imaging have been advocated in the clinical assessment of articular cartilage.[7–12] Importantly, FSE imaging sequences are also valuable for examination of other intra-articular structures, such as ligaments, menisci and subchondral bone. FSE acquisitions primarily produce two-dimensional data sets, with relatively coarse resolution in the slice direction, limiting the possibilities for multiplanar reformatting of the curved surfaces.

Three-dimensional imaging with gradient echo acquisitions, particularly with fat suppression via water-selective excitation, can generate isotropic image volumes with high cartilage signal intensity relative to surrounding tissues. The thinner slices and reformatting capabilities result in high sensitivity and specificity for identification of cartilage defects and the potential for accurate quantitative volume measurements.[13] The cost is a relatively long scan time and the possibility of motion artifacts during that time.

Numerous variations of these imaging techniques exist, with imaging parameters and acquisitions varying between centers depending on user preferences and the available hardware platforms. In general, for evaluation of hyaline articular cartilage, a typical MR protocol will include proton density, $T1$, $T2$ and fat-suppressed images with fast spin-echo-based techniques such as Fast Spin-Echo (FSE), which give a comprehensive picture of the morphologic changes associated with injury and subsequent degenerative processes.[14] Images are commonly acquired in all three planes. Supplemental acquisitions, or reformatting of high-resolution 3D data may further optimize the evaluation of patellar cartilage and central weight-bearing aspects of femoral condyles and tibial plateau.

MRI Findings in Cartilage Lesions of Knee Osteoarthritis

Early degenerative disease may be seen on MRI as early alterations in cartilage contour morphology (fibrillation, surface irregularity); changes in cartilage thickness; or signal intensity changes of the cartilage which may reflect pre-morphologic cartilage damage manifesting as collagen degradation and increased water content of cartilage. Advanced lesions typically represent as multiple areas of cartilage thinning or varying depth and size, usually seen on opposing articulating surfaces. These may be associated with increased signal intensity on $T2$-weighted images in the subchondral bone, representing subchondral edema or cyst formation. Advanced cartilage lesions may also be associated with decreased signal intensity in the subchondral bone, representing fibrosis or trabecular sclerosis. Central and marginal osteophytes, joint effusion and synovitis are other joint abnormalities present in advanced osteoarthritis and detectable using MRI.[2] The findings above stand in contrast to traumatic cartilage lesions, which manifest as solitary focal lesions with acutely angled margins. Linear cartilage clefts or fissures of varying depth may also be seen.

A careful evaluation of a knee MRI for osteoarthritis should include the examination of the articular cartilage, menisci, ligaments, subchondral bone and the synovium. Each will be discussed in detail below.

Articular Cartilage

Because of its excellent contrast resolution, high spatial resolution, and the multiplanar capabilities, MR imaging is an excellent method for assessment of articular cartilage. In practice, however, the usefulness of this technique in providing clinically important information regarding the integrity of the articular cartilage is uncertain. Several chondral lesions, such as full-thickness defects and denudation of the articular surface are delineated with MRI.

MRI — Normal articular cartilage

Layers or laminae of varying signal intensity are the characteristic feature of MR images of normal articular cartilage (Figs. 1 to 7). Recht and

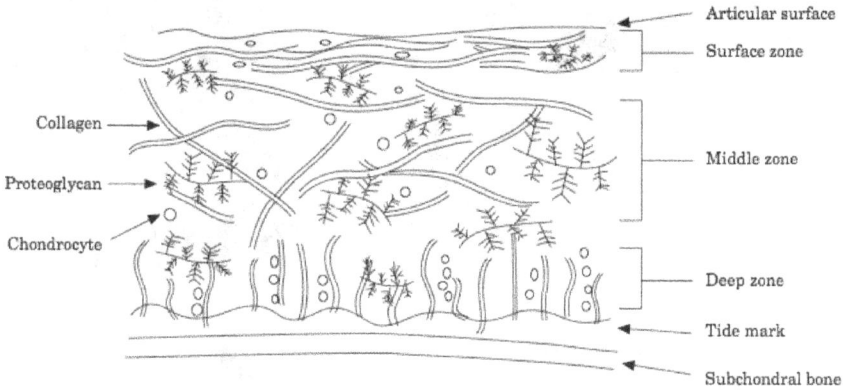

Fig. 1. Schematic diagram demonstrating the three-layer organization of collagen fibrils in articular cartilage.[88]

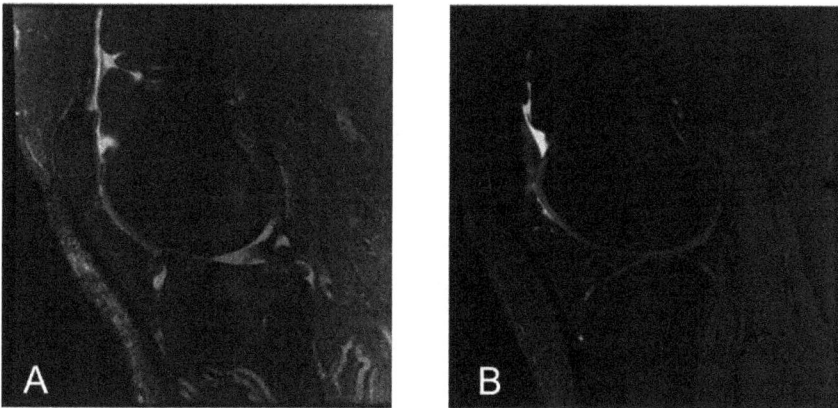

Fig. 2. **(A)** Sagittal fat-saturated FSE image of severely degenerative knee OA, with full thickness cartilage loss at femur and tibia and maceration of the posterior horn of lateral meniscus. **(B)** Corresponding sagittal image of a healthy knee for comparison.

collaborators[15] in a study of cadaveric knees, found that when images are acquired with the articular surface perpendicular to the main magnetic field, a higher-signal-intensity mid zone separates the lower-signal-intensity superficial and deep zones. This trilaminar appearance was later confirmed by Rubenstein and collaborators[16] using spin-echo MR imaging sequences in the analysis of bovine articular cartilage. These layers reflect the continuous variation of $T2$ times across the thickness of the tissue. Results

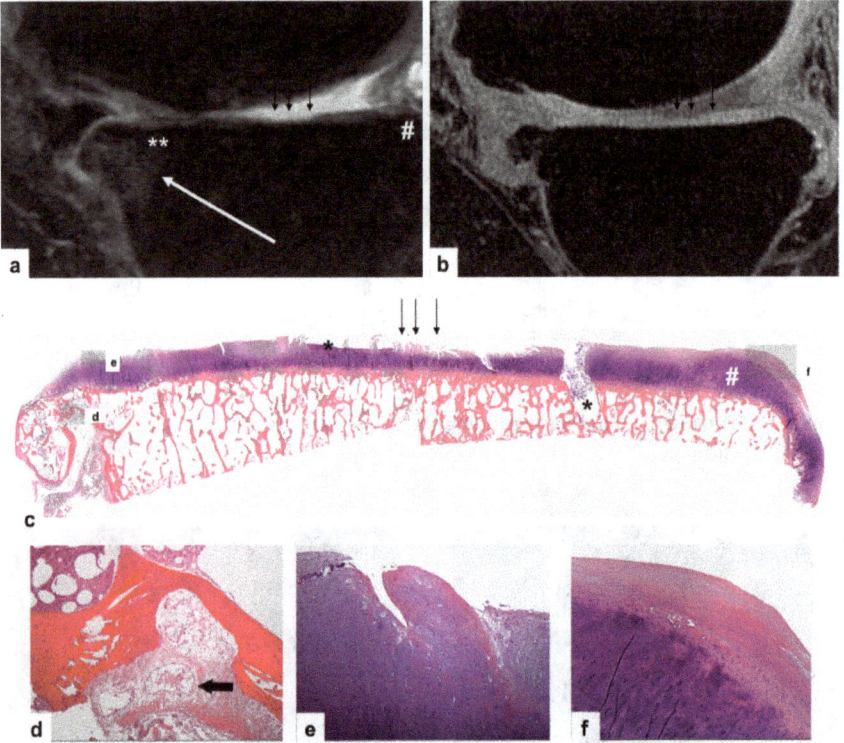

Fig. 3. Sagittal fat-saturated FSE **(a)** and SPGR **(b)** images of the medial joint compartment and corresponding tibial histological section (H&E) **(c)** in a 54-year-old female patient. ∗ in (c) indicates sectioning and folding artifacts. Magnified histological areas demonstrate osteophyte **(d)**, fibrocartilage overlying the osteophyte **(e)** and synovial (pannus) tissue overlying normal cartilage **(f)**. An area of bone marrow edema pattern is identified at the anterior part of the tibia (large arrow) in the region of the osteophyte (a), which corresponds to an area of fibrovascular tissue in the histological section (c, d). Increased fibrovascular tissue ingrowth (arrow in d) within the bone marrow of the osteophyte leads to increased osteoclast resorption. Fibrocartilage overlying the osteophyte (e) corresponds to an area of increased signal in (∗∗ in a). Black arrows in (a, b, c) indicate less than 50% thinning and surface fraying of the cartilage in the central tibia. Synovial (pannus) tissue in (c, e) corresponds to an area of bright signal in the FSE image (# in a and c).[89]

of polarized light microscopy of histologic specimens confirmed the three zones and transmission electron microscopy showed different collagen arrangement in the zones. Collagen fibrils are oriented in parallel arrays perpendicular to the subchondral bone in the deep zone of cartilage, and horizontal to the surface in the superficial zone. The mid zone of cartilage

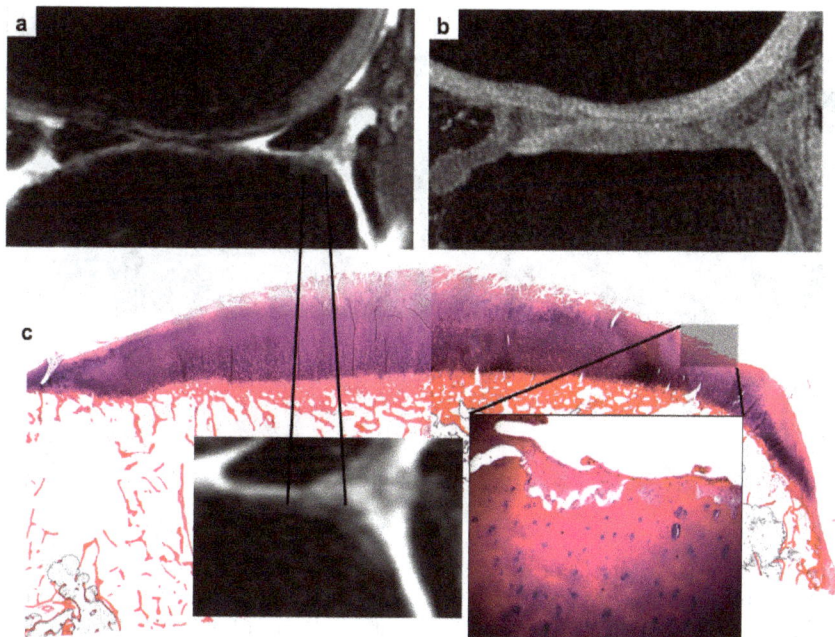

Fig. 4. Sagittal fat-saturated FSE **(a)** and SPGR **(b)** images of the lateral joint compartment and corresponding tibial histological section (H&E) **(c)** in a 51-year-old male patient. On the histological image (c) fraying with fibrillation involving less than 50% of the cartilage surface is shown centrally and posteriorly at the tibia. Magnification shows minor synovial tissue ingrowth in the posterior part, degrading the superficial cartilage layer. Corresponding findings on the FSE MR image (a), however, are relatively subtle. The superficial cartilage surface irregularity at the posterior tibial cartilage (highlighted and magnified region) and less well pronounced centrally are demonstrated. Surface irregularities are not appreciated in the SPGR images (b).[89]

consists of randomly oriented fibrils and separates the superficial and deep zones (Fig. 1).

The fibrillar collagen immobilizes the protons belonging to water molecules in the tissue and promotes dipole-dipole interactions among them, increasing $T2$ relaxation time and therefore signal decay. Articular cartilage $T2$ varies from the superficial to mid and deep zones of cartilage, and this variation can be explained by the heterogeneous distribution of collagen in the tissue as well as the orientation of collagen fibrils relative to the static magnetic field $(B0)$.[16−18] The "magic angle" phenomenon accounts for $T2$ anisotropy in cartilage, with decreased signal decay in

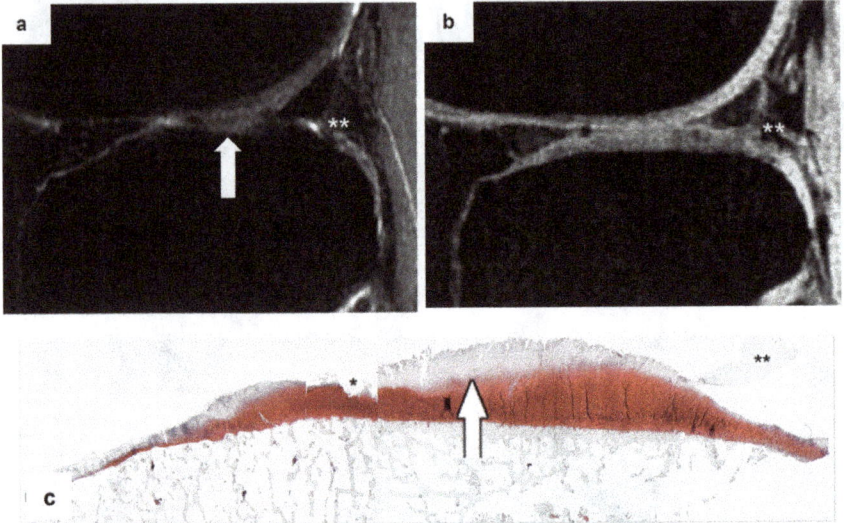

Fig. 5. Sagittal fat-saturated FSE **(a)** and SPGR **(b)** images of the lateral joint compartment and corresponding tibial histological section (Saf-O) **(c)** in a 74-year-old x patient. Cutting artifacts (∗) are demonstrated in the anterior part of the tibia (c). The FSE image (a) shows a $T2$ signal increase (arrow) and height reduction in the central region of the tibial cartilage which relates to cartilage thinning, fibrillation and proteoglycan loss by a 50% reduction in red-staining in the Saf-O staining (c, arrow). SPGR image does not clearly demonstrate these findings, yet shows some signal inhomogeneity. Signal inhomogeneity at the surface of the posterior tibia indicates pannus tissue floating on the cartilage surface (∗∗ in a, b, c).[89]

regions where the collagen fibrils are oriented at 55° to $B0$. Therefore, the mid zone of cartilage will have a mildly elevated signal intensity.

MRI — Abnormal articular cartilage

With MR imaging, two fundamental findings of abnormal articular cartilage include altered thickness and modified signal intensity. Cartilage thinning is the pathologic *sine qua non* of osteoarthritis. However, it must be noted that thickening, not thinning, of articular cartilage may occur after injury, a finding repeatedly documented in animal models in which the knee has been rendered unstable with surgical techniques.[19,20] Cartilage, like other connective tissues, swells when injured; however, the cause of post-traumatic cartilage thickening is not well-established; an increase in proteoglycan content, water, or both, may be important in the pathogenesis

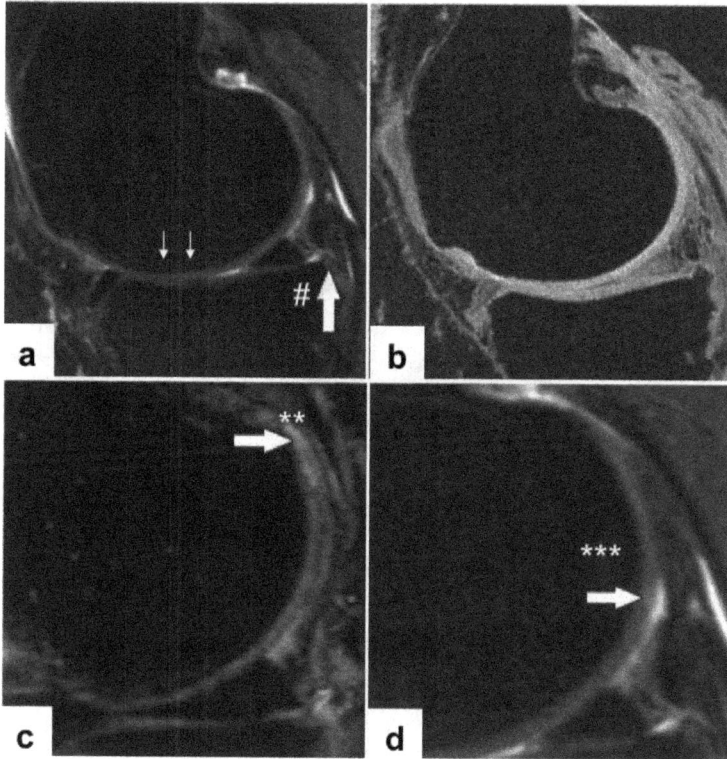

Fig. 6. Sagittal fat-saturated FSE **(a, c, d)** and SPGR **(b)** MR images of a 68-year-old female patient and complete histological reconstruction of the corresponding sagittal knee section (**e, f, i** = H&E staining; **g, h** = Safranin-O staining) at the medial joint compartment (*sectioning and folding artifacts). Cartilage thickness and surface appear generally well maintained in MR and histological images, yet a number of pathologies are depicted in the histological section that are only partially visualized in the MR images: (I) Deep (>50%) fissures/clefts in the cartilage (two small black arrows) in (e) are not visualized in corresponding FSE (a) and SPGR (b) images (two small arrows). (II) Osteophyte (arrow, # in a and e, f) with increased bone marrow signal/bone marrow edema pattern in (a) and fibrovascular tissue with multiple large vascular sinuses within the marrow indicating increased vascular flow (e, f). (III) In (** in e, g) a small area of thick fibro-cartilage, with reduced Safranin-O red staining indicating reduced proteoglycan content and increased matrix water content is shown. This is not visualized in the corresponding MR images (a, b), but in a neighboring section an area of increased cartilage signal intensity was demonstrated (arrow and ** in c). (IV) In (i) necrotic chondrocytes with myxoid degeneration of the surrounding matrix (Weichselbaum's lacunae) are demonstrated in the vicinity of a cartilage lesion (h), however, there is no corresponding pathology identified on the MR images. (V) In (h) horizontal cartilage delamination with reduced PG (Saf-O) content in the separated cartilage layer is shown (*** in e). The corresponding finding in the MR image (d) is a subtle line of increased signal intensity (***) at the posterior femoral condyle.[89]

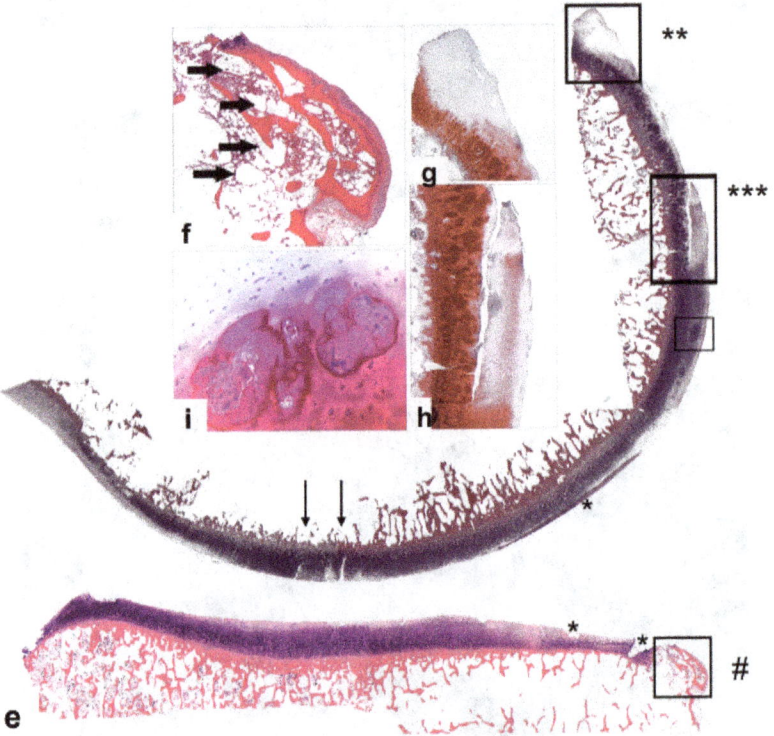

Fig. 6. (*Continued*)

of cartilage thickening.[19,21] Long-term studies in such knees have indicated that cartilage breakdown and loss may follow the stage of cartilage thickening.[22] Similarly, thickening of articular cartilage may represent an early manifestation of osteoarthritis in humans, and progressive loss of articular cartilage may indicate more advanced disease.

The second fundamental finding of cartilage abnormality is intracartilaginous signal intensity alterations. The clinical significance of this finding, however, in the absence of alterations in cartilage thickness or surface irregularities is unclear. In a recent study[11] cartilage signal pattern (signal homogeneity versus inhomogeneity, independent of cartilage thickness and surface abnormalities) in intermediate-weighted FSE images was not adequately suited to characterize articular cartilage degeneration as validated by histology. Other studies[15,23] have used signal hypo- or

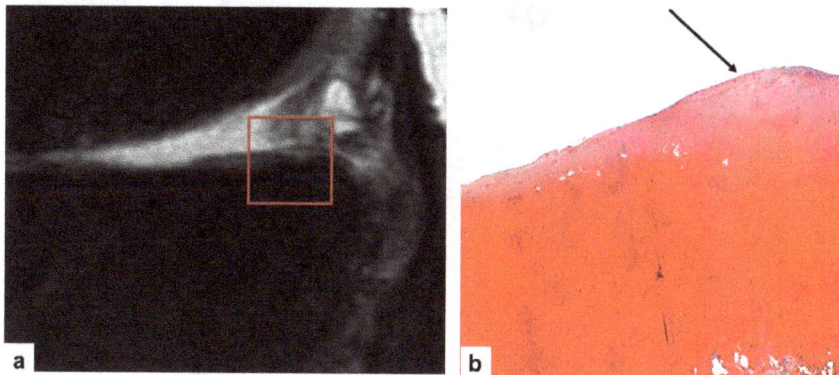

Fig. 7. Sagittal fat-saturated FSE **(a)** of the medial joint compartment and corresponding tibial histological section (Saf-O) **(b)** in a 54-year-old female patient. Cartilage tickening/swelling at the posterior aspect of the tibia with high signal intensity region (highlighted area in a). The corresponding Saf-O staining (b) shows an area of cartilage thickening due to synovial overgrowth (pannus tissue) with proteoglycan loss.[89]

hyper-intensity to characterize the intracartilaginous signal pattern, but these did not allow assessment of the clinical significance of this grade of abnormality in the absence of cartilage surface or thickness abnormalities.

Subchondral Bone Marrow

Subchondral bone abnormalities are often present as occult injuries in MR images of osteoarthritic knees. Changes are appreciated in the distal portion of the femur and the proximal portion of the tibia, are often a result of forces that lead to impaction of one articular surface against another, and are frequently accompanied by insults to menisci and ligamentous structures of the knee. Concurrent with the changes in articular cartilage, there is rebuttressing and sclerosis of the underlying cancellous bone. MR imaging documents alterations in signal intensity within the subchondral marrow, which is referred to as "bone bruise" or "bone marrow edema."[2,24] The precise histologic correlates of a "bone bruise" are not definitively established, though subchondral ingrowth of fibrovascular tissue and increased bone remodeling were observed in histologic sections correlated to *in-vivo* MRI's of patients with OA of the knee prior to total knee replacement surgery in a recent study.[11]

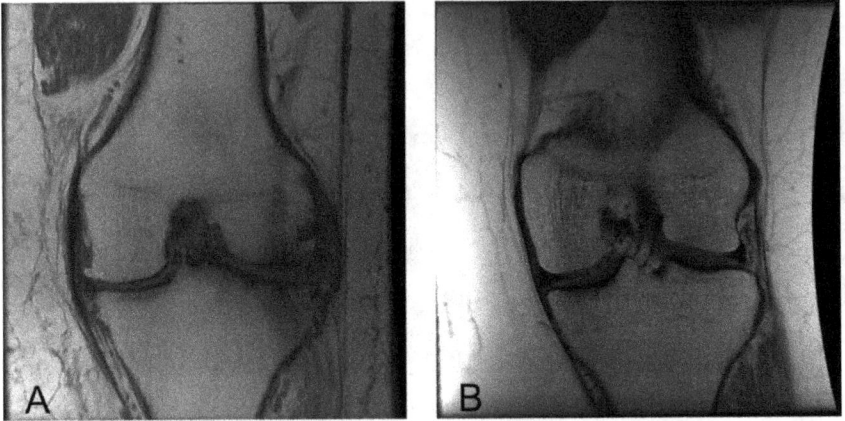

Fig. 8. **(A)** Coronal MRI section of a severely degenerated knee with OA. There is evidence of medial meniscal extrusion and lateral meniscal maceration with multiple osteophytes and medial joint space narrowing. **(B)** Corresponding coronal section of a healthy knee for comparison.

Menisci

The association of meniscal abnormalities and degenerative disease is complex (Fig. 8). The occurrence of degenerative alterations in the menisci and osteoarthritis of the knee is well recognized. The prominent role played by the menisci in maintaining joint stabilization by promoting joint congruence, stress reduction and shock absorption suggest that damage to these structures may result in detrimental changes to the surrounding articular cartilage.[25-27] Underscoring the value of maintaining as much meniscal function as possible is the recent trend in arthroscopic surgery of the knee to remove as little meniscus as possible or possibly repair the meniscus, thereby avoiding the subsequent deterioration of the hyaline articular cartilage and osteoarthritis.

MRI — Normal menisci

The normal morphology of a meniscus is characterized by a triangular appearance and a sharp central tip.[28,29] This appearance is apparent in both the coronal and sagittal sections. Typically, a normal meniscus is characterized by low signal intensity, though regions of intermediate signal intensity are often encountered in asymptomatic individuals. Stoller and colleagues provided the first full description of inhomogeneous signal intensities that may be observed in normal menisci.[30] In the sagittal plane, in peripheral sections, the anterior and posterior horns of the menisci combine and form a structure that is shaped like a bow tie.[31] In central sections, menisci normally have a rhomboid shape. In the coronal plane, very posterior sections show the menisci as broad and elongated structures extending far into the central portion of the joint. The medial collateral ligament is seen adjacent to the mid portion of the medial meniscus, with an interface apparent between it and the outer portion of the meniscus. On both sagittal and coronal images, the course of the popliteus tendon and its sheath, and their intimacy with the posterior horn of the lateral meniscus are appreciated.

MRI — Torn menisci

Most reports have indicated an 85% to 90% sensitivity, specificity and accuracy of MR imaging in detection of meniscal tears.[32–36] The two MR imaging criteria for diagnosis of a meniscal tear are intramensical signal intensity that extends to a meniscal surface and abnormal meniscal morphology. The sagittal plane and $T1$- and intermediate-weighted spin-echo sequences are more valuable in this diagnosis than are coronal and axial planes and $T2$-weighted spin-echo sequences. Although some meniscal tears will fill with fluid and appear as regions of very high signal intensity on intermediate-weighted FSE sequences, most do not. When fluid is observed within a meniscal tear and leads to high signal intensity on such images, a unstable meniscal tear is often present.[37]

Alterations in the morphology of torn menisci take several forms. The inner portion of the meniscus may appear blunted in coronal or sagittal MR images. The meniscus may have a normal triangular shape but appear too small. Diagnosis of tears of the free edge of the meniscus often requires careful analysis of both sagittal and coronal MR images so that subtle blunting or poor definition of the involved portion of the meniscus is recognized.[38]

The notch sign[39] is an abrupt change in contour or a focal deformity of the meniscus, and is an important indicator of a meniscal tear. The notch sign is a definitive indicator of meniscal tear when it is accompanied by abnormalities in intrameniscal signal intensity.

Radial tears of the menisci may be difficult to recognize.[40,41] Such tears are oriented perpendicular to the long circumferential axis of the meniscus, may be of full or partial thickess, and may be straight or obliquely oriented.[41]

Displacement of normal or torn menisci is recognizable using MRI and is of three classic types: bucket-handle tears[42] (displaced longitudinal tears), parrot-beak tears (displaced radial or oblique tears), and flap tears[43] (displaced horizontal tears). Several situations can cause displacement of the meniscus without a tear.[44,45] Posterior displacement of the posterior horn of the lateral meniscus related to anterior translation of the tibia is a sign of anterior cruciate ligament tear. Peripheral displacement of the medial meniscus is associated with joint effusions, osteophytes and osteoarthritis.

Ligaments

The primary role of the ligaments about and within the knee is to provide stability in more than one degree of freedom, as well as to restrain the motion of the knee in response to an externally-applied force. Injury to ligaments of the knee, among other things, result in the application of abnormal forces to the knee that result in varus or valgus angulation, internal or external rotation, hyperflexion or hyperextension, anterior or posterior dislocation, axial loading or a combination of these forces. Injury to any one of the supporting structures changes the knee kinematics. Complete disruption of one or more ligaments leads to knee instability. MR imaging can be successfully applied to determine the extent of soft-tissue abnormalities, including injuries to the ligaments of the knee. Damage to the Anterior Cruciate Ligament (ACL) and the Medial and Lateral Collateral Ligaments (MCL and LCL, respectively) have been associated with the development of osteoarthritis of the knee and are commonly seen in this condition.

Anterior cruciate ligament

As with menisci of the knee, spin-echo or fast spin-echo MR imaging is the most popular method to assess the ACL (Fig. 9). The best plane for analysis of ACL is the sagittal plane, but coronal and axial planes can supply additional data valuable in diagnosis and increase sensitivity and specificity.[46]

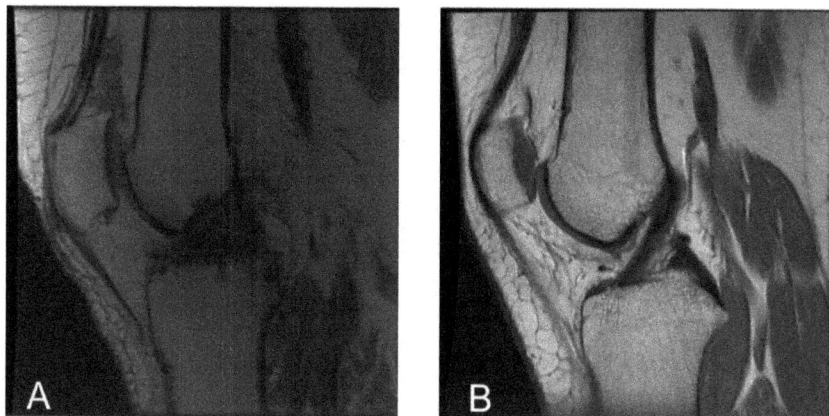

Fig. 9. (**A**) Sagittal MRI section of severe knee OA, demonstrating degeneration of ACL in severe OA with tear of ACL, diffuse cartilage loss at patella, and osteophytes. (**B**) Corresponding sagittal section of a healthy knee for comparison.

MRI — Normal ACL: In evaluating the ACL on sagittal MR images, it is useful to start with the section that displays the intercondylar roof of the femur as a straight line of low signal intensity. In this section, the anterior cruciate ligament appears as a straight band of low signal intensity whose course parallels or is steeper than that of the intercondylar line. The dominant pattern of signal intensity in a normal ACL is low, and increases somewhat in elderly persons for unclear reasons.[47]

MRI — Torn ACL: MR imaging is a sensitive (90 to 98%), specific (90 to 100%) and accurate (90 to 98%) method for identifying tears of the ACL.[46,48−51] The MR imaging diagnosis of injuries to the anterior cruciate ligament relates to the documentation of 1) abnormalities in the ACL itself; 2) alterations in the appearance of other structures related to the abnormal alignment of the tibia and femur that results from an ACL tear; 3) abnormalities that result from bone impaction and other forces that occur in the course of injury itself or are caused by an ACL tear; and 4) miscellaneous abnormalities.[52−56] In patients with knee pain and a known chronic tear of the ACL, MR imaging may be indicated to determine the cause of the pain. In such patients, meniscal tears are common and have a predilection for the medial meniscus.[57] Abnormalities of the articular cartilage, which are most frequent in the medial femorotibial and patellofemoral compartments, can also be identified with MR imaging of such knees. Only MRI abnormalities of the ACL itself will be discussed here.

The two major alterations occurring within the ligament itself are 1) changes in its morphology or course and 2) changes in its signal intensity.[46,49–51,58] A complete tear of the ACL is accompanied by disruption of all the fibers and an irregular contour. These findings are more apparent on sagittal sections. On sagittal sections, the course of a completely torn ACL may appear depressed, with a decrease slope of residual fibers extending almost parallel to the tibial surface rather than at an angle to this surface and parallel to the intercondylar roof. With acute or chronic tears of some but not all the fibers of the ACL, the ligament may appear attenuated or small, and its course may not be altered.

The presence of increased signal intensity within the ACL on intermediate- or $T2$-weighted FSE images usually indicates an acute or subacute injury resulting in complete or partial disruption of the ligament. This pattern of increased signal intensity reflects edematous soft tissue, not joint fluid.[59]

Medial collateral ligament (MCL)

Tears of the MCL may be classified as acute, subacute or chronic, or classified according to severity, from a ligament sprain (grade I) to partial (grade II) or complete (grade III) rupture. A knee with grade I sprain is clinically stable, though microscopic tearing of ligaments have occurred. A knee with grade II sprain is unstable yet has a firm end point on stress testing and a grade III sprain is unstable with a soft endpoint on stress testing and has suffered a full thickness rupture of the MCL.[60]

MRI — Normal MCL: The coronal plane is the best imaging plane for viewing and evaluation of the MCL. In the coronal plane, the superficial longitudinal fibers of the MCL appear as a smooth structure of low signal intensity that extends from the medial epicondyle of the femur superiorly to the proximal metaphysis of the tibia inferiorly. At the level of the joint line, the medial collateral ligament is separated from the periphery of the medial meniscus by a bursa and surrounding fat.[61]

MRI — Abnormal MCL: The MR imaging characteristics of injured MCL depend on the severity of injury and its acuity[62] (also see above discussion).

With acute injuries, subcutaneous edema or hemorrhage, and possibly joint effusions, are present. With chronic injuries, edema and hemorrhage are not present. Sprains of the MCL may lead to slight contour irregularity or thickening of the ligament, but no discontinuity of its fibers. In acute sprains, subcutaneous edema is present but signal intensity of the MCL itself is normal. Partial tears are associated with increased signal intensity of the ligament itself and complete tears are associated with frank discontinuity of all MCL fibers.[63]

Lateral collateral ligament complex (LCL)

MR imaging is an effective technique for assessment of the LCL.[64–66]

MRI — Normal LCL: On posterior MR images in the coronal plane, a normal biceps femoris muscle is seen in the lateral aspect of the leg, above the knee. On coronal images just anterior to those that show the biceps femoris muscle and tendon, the LCL is seen arising from the fibula and extending superiorly and anteriorly to attach to the epicondyle in the distal potion of the femur, and has low signal intensity.

MRI — Abnormal LCL: Disruption of the LCL is appreciated on MR images as interruption or waviness of the tendon or regions of high signal intensity on T2-weighted spin-echo MR images within or adjacent to the ligament.[62]

Synovium

In normal joints, small amounts of fluid is present to coat the numerous folds of synovial membrane and to lubricate the articular surfaces, as well as to provide nutrients to the resident chondrocytes via diffusion from the synovium through the avascular articular cartilage. In the normal state, the volume of fluid is never sufficient to distend the joint or to separate the redundant surfaces of the synovium.[67] MR imaging is extremely sensitive to the presence of intra-articular fluid, which appears with low signal intensity on T1-weighted spin-echo sequences and with high intensity on T2-weighted spin-echo MR images. Detection of a knee effusion with MR imaging is aided by differences in the signal intensity of fluid and that of the adjacent soft-tissue structures. In particular, in the region of the suprapatellar recess, the synovial membrane is intimate with three fat bodies: the anterior and posterior suprapatellar fat bodies and the infrapatellar fat body. These fat bodies are intracapsular but extrasynovial. The presence of a bland knee effusion (one resulting from trauma or internal derangement) typically does not lead to a distortion of the interface between these fat bodies and the adjacent fluid.[68] The presence of a proliferative effusion (one associated with synovial proliferation) may lead to scalloping, truncation or displacement of these fat bodies and obstruction of the interface between them and the adjacent fluid.[69]

MRI-Based Cartilage Scoring Systems

Recht Scoring System

Among the earliest systems to quantify cartilage changes in osteoarthritis was a system developed by Recht *et al.*, which utilized the Noyes classification[70] modified to MR imaging.[71] In this system, five grades (0–4) are assigned to the cartilage depending on the thickness of cartilage defects: grade 0 is the absence of cartilage lesion; grade I lesions are defined as areas with signal inhomogeneity on high-resolution SPGR sequences; grade II lesions are cartilage defects involving less than half of the articular cartilage thickness; grade III lesions are cartilage defects involving more than half of the cartilage, but less than full thickness; and lesions of grade IV expose the bone.

Whole Organ Magnetic Resonance Imaging Score (WORMS) of the Knee in OA

As discussed in Chapter 2, the precise structural determinants of pain and mechanical dysfunction in OA, though not well understood, are believed to involve multiple interactive pathways.[72–74] OA can appropriately be modeled as a disease of organ failure, where injury to one compartment facilitates the failure of other compartments. As such, development and utilization of a broader panel of imaging markers for degenerative joint disease may improve the assessment of disease and disease-modifying therapies and also illuminate new potential areas for improvement in therapy. One such system, the Whole Organ Magnetic Resonance Imaging Score (WORMS) of the knee in OA was proposed recently by Peterfy *et al.*[75] This semi-quantitative system offers an initial instrument for performing multi-feature assessment of the knee using conventional MRI, taking into account multiple features believed to be relevant to pathophysiology of OA. These include cartilage signal and morphology, subarticular bone marrow abnormality, subarticular cysts, subarticular bone attrition and marginal osteophytes. Each articular region of the knee joint is divided into subdivisions and each of the five variables are assessed in each subdivision of the joint. The ligaments of the knee, as well as the menisci are also assessed individually: the ACL, PCL, MCL and LCL are independently scored as intact or torn; and the anterior horn, body segment and posterior horn of the medial and lateral menisci are also graded separately using sagittal and coronal sections. Additionally, this scoring system accounts for synovial thickening and joint effusion, loose bodies in synovial cavity as well as synovial cysts or bursal collections.

Arthroscopic Evaluation of Articular Cartilage

Knee arthroscopy is a minimally-invasive surgical procedure performed under anesthesia in which small arthroscopes are inserted into the knee joint in order to directly visualize the articular surfaces on a computer screen. Arthroscopy is able to provide a direct, magnified view of all six articular surfaces of the knee. Direct visualization through an arthroscope is more sensitive and specific than plain radiography or MRI in detecting cartilage lesions.[76] Indeed, arthroscopy is so sensitive and specific in the evaluation of hyaline articular cartilage that it has been called the gold standard of reference for assessment of articular cartilage, whereby other methods will be judged.[77] However, it must be noted that while arthroscopy is able to visualize surface lesions well (since the technique is only capable of visualizing surfaces if subchondral bone is exposed), it is inherently inaccurate in estimating cartilage thickness and the depth of lesions.

Several researchers have used arthroscopy to quantify the severity of chondropathy in studies to follow cartilage lesions over time; to assess the effectiveness of surgical techniques in correcting abnormalities; or to assess the diagnostic performance of cartilage imaging techniques. Articular cartilage lesions can be defined by three baseline parameters: depth, size and location. The most widely-used scoring systems include the "Outerbridge" system and the "Noyes" classification. These two will be presented below.

Outerbridge Scoring System

The Outerbridge scoring system[78] (Table 1) subdivides cartilage lesions into four grades: grade I — softening and swelling of cartilage without fissuring (true chondromalacia); grade II — fragmentation and fissuring with a diameter of half an inch or less; grade III — fragmentation and fissuring with a diameter of greater than half an inch; and grade IV — erosion of cartilage with exposure of subchondral bone (Fig. 10). This

Table 1. The Outerbridge scoring system.

Surface description of articular cartilage	Diameter
I — softening and swelling	I — none
II — fragmentation and fissuring	II — <1/2 inch
III — fragmentation and fissuring	III — >1/2 inch
IV — erosion of cartilage down to bone	IV — none

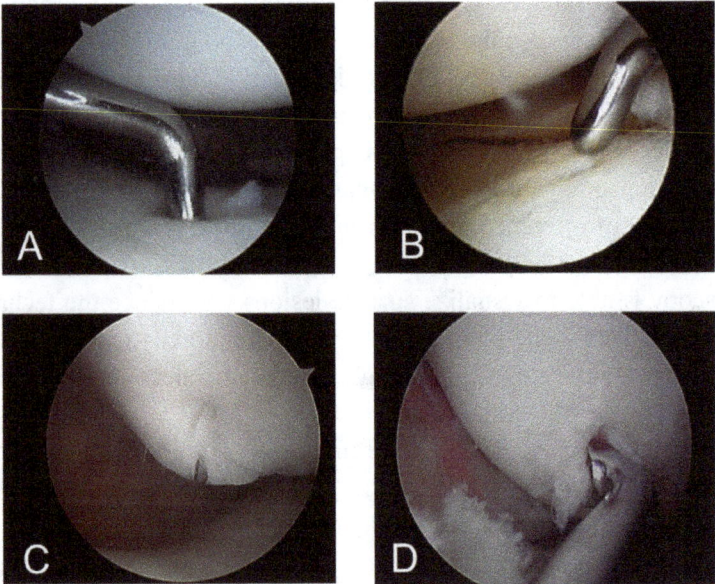

Fig. 10. Arthroscopic images demonstrating articular cartilage lesions of varying degrees of severity as classified by the Outerbridge scoring system. (A) grade 1, (B) grade 2, (C) grade 3, and (D) grade 4.

system has been used for classifying patients in cross-sectional studies[77] but appears inadequate for accurate outcome measurement of chondropathy since the size of lesions in grades I and IV is not evaluated, and the size of lesions in grades II and III is not a continuous variable.

Noyes Scoring System

In 1989, Noyes and Stabler proposed a system for grading articular cartilage lesions at arthroscopy which separates the description of the surface appearance, depth of involvement, and the diameter and location of the lesions[70] (Table 2). This scoring system distinguishes three surface grades: grade 1 — articular cartilage intact; grade 2 — open lesion at cartilage surface; and grade 3 — bone exposed. Each grade is then divided into subtypes A or B based on the depth of involvement. The lesions are reported on a knee diagram, and the diameter of each lesion is estimated by the examiner in millimeters using a graduated probing hook. Depending on the diameter and the depth of the lesions, a point scaling system is used to calculate the score of chondropathy for each compartment, and finally, an overall joint score is calculated.

In the Noyes system, a lesion less than 10 mm in diameter is not considered clinically significant and no points are subtracted. This may reduce the sensitivity of the system, since in monitoring the effect of drug or surgical interventions on articular cartilage, even the smallest lesions must be carefully evaluated.

MR Imaging of Cartilage Repair

Corrective surgical procedures for cartilage, such as autologous osteochondral transplantation (AOT) and autologous chondrocyte implantation (ACI) are being conducted more widely and post-operative imaging of cartilage to monitor the success of such procedures is of increasing importance. Due to its ability to visualize all tissues in a diarthroidal joint, MRI is a promising tool for post-operative evaluation and monitoring of cartilage repair.

Autologous Osteochondral Transplantation

Autologous osteochondral transplantation involves the use of cylindrical osteochondral plugs of various sizes acquired from minimally

Table 2. The Noyes classification of articular cartilage lesions.

Surface description	Extent of involvement	Diameter	Location	Degree of knee flexion

Cartilage surface intact	A. Definite softening with some resilience remaining
	B. Extensive softening with loss of resilience (deformation)
		<10
		≤20
		≤25
		>25
			Patella
			A. Proximal 1/3
			  Middle 1/3
			  Distal 1/3
			B. Odd facet
			  Middle facet
			  Distal facet
			Trochlea
			  Medial femoral condyle
			  a. anterior 1/3
			  b. middle 1/3
			  c. posterior 1/3
			Lateral femoral condyle
			  a. anterior 1/3
			  b. middle 1/3
			  c. posterior 1/3
			Medial tibial condyle
			  a. anterior 1/3
			  b. middle 1/3
			  c. posterior 1/3
			Lateral tibial condyle
			  a. anterior 1/3
			  b. middle 1/3
			  c. posterior 1/3
				Degree of knee flexion where the lesion is in weight-bearing contact (e.g., 20–45 degrees)

Cartilage surface damaged: cracks, fissures, fibrillations or fragmentation	A. <1/2 thickness B. ≥1/2 thickness			
Bone exposed	A. Bone surface intact B. Bone surface cavitation			

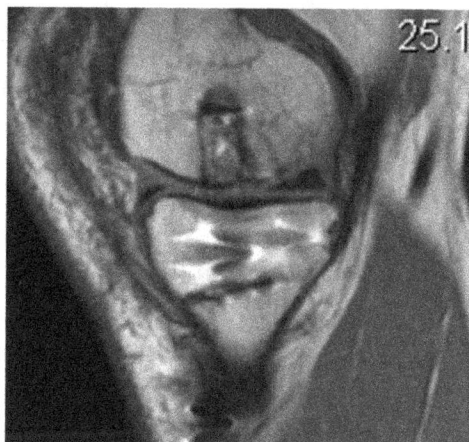

Fig. 11. Sagittal MRI section of knee after mosaicplasty of medial femoral condyle, demonstrating osteotomy of proximal tibia, bone core and overlying cartilage with good result and satisfactory cartilage coverage.

weight-bearing areas of the joint to fill chondral defects in weight-bearing areas (Fig. 11).[79,80] The chondral defect being repaired is debrided down to the subchondral bone and the osteochondral plugs are transplanted into the defect site perpendicular to the bone surface, with the goal of producing a congruent cartilage surface. If one edge of the plug is raised or recessed relative to the surrounding native cartilage, abnormal mechanical forces created in the area will cause worse outcomes.[81] Spaces between the plugs will typically fill with a fibrocartilaginous grout stimulated by abrasion or sharp curretage of the base of the defect. The goal of MR imaging after autologous osteochondral transplantation is to evaluate graft incorporation and defect filling, morphology and signal characteristics. Initial studies show that MRI can identify the transplanted plugs and repair tissue, and evaluate the spatial positioning of the plug (bone-bone and cartilage-cartilage interfaces) with regards to the surrounding tissues.[82] When surface irregularity or incongruity is present, MRI can demonstrate reasons for such problems, such as improper graft positioning, subsidence, or graft displacement or rotation.

Animal studies of AOT have shown that graft revascularization begins as early as six to 14 weeks[83,84] and the signal intensity changes seen on MRI appear to parallel this process. The grafts show a normal, fat-like marrow signal at two weeks and an edema-like signal change is seen within the marrow of the graft and surrounding bone by four to six weeks,[85] believed to be due to fibrovascular reactive and inflammatory agents. The signal returns to normal in six to nine months, believed to indicate graft incorporation. A large, persistent, peri-graft edema-like signal or formation of cyst-like regions are worrisome signs of poor graft incorporation.

Autologous Chondrocyte Implantation

ACI is a cell-based two-stage surgical treatment for deep articular cartilage defects.[86] Briefly, the first stage of treatment is arthroscopic assessment of cartilage defect and harvestation of a small amount of cartilage from a non-weight-bearing region of the joint. The cells from this biopsy tissue are then removed from the extracellular matrix by enzymatic digestion and grown in culture until appropriate numbers of cells are generated.[87] In the second stage, an open arthrotomy is performed during which the defect is debrided with avoidance of the subchondral bone, covered with periosteal tissue taken from the tibia or femur, and sealed with fibrin glue. The harvested and cultured cells are subsequently injected in the covered defect to grow. The repair tissue should restore the contour of the cartilage surface and fill the cartilage defect to the same level as that of the adjacent articular cartilage, regardless of the depth of the defect.

In the post-operative evaluation of autologous chondrocyte implantation, MRI is a reliable tool for detecting and often characterizing graft hypertrophy. MRI can also identify partial and complete graft delamination.[82] Areas of high signal intensity in the bone marrow of patients following autologous chondrocyte implantation are often observed on $T2$ images. Advanced cartilage imaging techniques that depict biochemical composition of cartilage (such as $T_{1\rho}$ mapping, discussed in a later chapter) may allow for evaluation of the maturation of the osteochondral autograft and to monitor whether new hyaline cartilage has formed following autologous chondrocyte implantation procedures.

Conclusions

MRI is a tool of unprecedented capabilities for evaluation of joint diseases. It offers superior soft tissue contrast, lacks ionizing radiation, and can offer high spatial resolution. These characteristics allow it to evaluate a joint as a whole organ and OA as a disorder of organ failure, rather than just of articular cartilage. Especially exciting are new advances in MR imaging that allow identification of compositional changes in soft tissues in addition to simple morphology, a topic that will be discussed in detail in later chapters of this book. MRI has the potential to provide very sensitive and specific markers for disease progression, to monitor treatment and help in the development of new strategies for controlling the progression of osteoarthritis.

References

1. Link TM, Stahl R, Woertler K. Cartilage imaging: motivation, techniques, current and future significance. *Eur Radiol* 2007;17(5):1135–1146.
2. Recht MP, Goodwin DW, Winalski CS, White LM. MRI of articular cartilage: revisiting current status and future directions. *AJR Am J Roentgenol* 2005;185(4):899–914.
3. Chandnani VP, Ho C, Chu P, Trudell D, Resnick D. Knee hyaline cartilage evaluated with MR imaging: a cadaveric study involving multiple imaging sequences and intraarticular injection of gadolinium and saline solution. *Radiology* 1991;178(2):557–561.
4. Totterman S, Weiss SL, Szumowski J, Katzberg RW, Hornak JP, Proskin HM, Eisen J. MR fat suppression technique in the evaluation of normal structures of the knee. *J Comput Assist Tomogr* 1989;13(3):473–479.
5. Gray ML, Burstein D, Lesperance LM, Gehrke L. Magnetization transfer in cartilage and its constituent macromolecules. *Magn Reson Med* 1995;34(3):319–325.
6. Wolff SD, Chesnick S, Frank JA, Lim KO, Balaban RS. Magnetization transfer contrast: MR imaging of the knee. *Radiology* 1991;179(3):623–628.
7. Bredella MA, Tirman PF, Peterfy CG, Zarlingo M, Feller JF, Bost FW, Belzer JP, Wischer TK, Genant HK. Accuracy of T2-weighted fast spin-echo MR imaging with fat saturation in detecting cartilage defects in the knee: comparison with arthroscopy in 130 patients. *AJR Am J Roentgenol* 1999;172(4):1073–1080.
8. Broderick LS, Turner DA, Renfrew DL, Schnitzer TJ, Huff JP, Harris C. Severity of articular cartilage abnormality in patients with osteoarthritis: evaluation with fast spin-echo MR vs. arthroscopy. *AJR Am J Roentgenol* 1994;162(1):99–103.
9. Mohr A. The value of water-excitation 3D FLASH and fat-saturated PDw TSE MR imaging for detecting and grading articular cartilage lesions of the knee. *Skeletal Radiol* 2003;32(7):396–402.
10. Potter HG, Linklater JM, Allen AA, Hannafin JA, Haas SB. Magnetic resonance imaging of articular cartilage in the knee. An evaluation with use of fast-spin-echo imaging. *J Bone Joint Surg Am* 1998;80(9):1276–1284.
11. Saadat E, Jobke B, Chu B, Lu Y, Cheng J, Li X, Ries MD, Majumdar S, Link TM. Diagnostic performance of *in vivo* 3-T MRI for articular cartilage abnormalities in human osteoarthritic knees using histology as standard of reference. *Eur Radiol* 2008;18(10):2292–2302.

12. Sonin AH, Pensy RA, Mulligan ME, Hatem S. Grading articular cartilage of the knee using fast spin-echo proton density-weighted MR imaging without fat suppression. *AJR Am J Roentgenol* 2002;179(5):1159–1166.

13. Disler DG, McCauley TR, Wirth CR, Fuchs MD. Detection of knee hyaline cartilage defects using fat-suppressed three-dimensional spoiled gradient-echo MR imaging: comparison with standard MR imaging and correlation with arthroscopy. *AJR Am J Roentgenol* 1995;165(2):377–382.

14. Gold GE, Hargreaves BA, Beaulieu CF. Protocols in sports magnetic resonance imaging. *Top Magn Reson Imaging* 2003;14(1):3–23.

15. Recht MP, Kramer J, Marcelis S, Pathria MN, Trudell D, Haghighi P, Sartoris DJ, Resnick D. Abnormalities of articular cartilage in the knee: analysis of available MR techniques. *Radiology* 1993;187(2):473–478.

16. Rubenstein JD, Kim JK, Morova-Protzner I, Stanchev PL, Henkelman RM. Effects of collagen orientation on MR imaging characteristics of bovine articular cartilage. *Radiology* 1993;188(1):219–226.

17. McCauley TR, Disler DG. MR imaging of articular cartilage. *Radiology* 1998;209(3):629–640.

18. Dardzinski BJ, Mosher TJ, Li S, Van Slyke MA, Smith MB. Spatial variation of T2 in human articular cartilage. *Radiology* 1997;205(2):546–550.

19. Braunstein EM, Brandt KD, Albrecht M. MRI demonstration of hypertrophic articular cartilage repair in osteoarthritis. *Skeletal Radiol* 1990;19(5):335–339.

20. Vignon E, Arlot M, Hartmann D, Moyen B, Ville G. Hypertrophic repair of articular cartilage in experimental osteoarthrosis. *Ann Rheum Dis* 1983;42(1):82–88.

21. Adams ME, Brandt KD. Hypertrophic repair of canine articular cartilage in osteoarthritis after anterior cruciate ligament transection. *J Rheumatol* 1991;18(3):428–435.

22. Brandt KD, Braunstein EM, Visco DM, O'Connor B, Heck D, Albrecht M. Anterior (cranial) cruciate ligament transection in the dog: a bona fide model of osteoarthritis, not merely of cartilage injury and repair. *J Rheumatol* 1991;18(3):436–446.

23. Conway WF, Hayes CW, Loughran T, Totty WG, Griffeth LK, el-Khoury GY, Shellock FG. Cross-sectional imaging of the patellofemoral joint and surrounding structures. *Radiographics* 1991;11(2):195–217.

24. Mink JH, Deutsch AL. Occult cartilage and bone injuries of the knee: detection, classification, and assessment with MR imaging. *Radiology* 1989;170(3 Pt 1):823–829.

25. Dandy DJ, Jackson RW. Meniscectomy and chondromalacia of the femoral condyle. *J Bone Joint Surg Am* 1975;57(8):1116–1119.

26. Fukubayashi T, Kurosawa H. The contact area and pressure distribution pattern of the knee. A study of normal and osteoarthrotic knee joints. *Acta Orthop Scand* 1980;51(6):871–879.

27. Walker PS, Erkman MJ. The role of the menisci in force transmission across the knee. *Clin Orthop Relat Res* 1975;(109):184–192.

28. Kaplan PA, Dussault RG. Magnetic resonance imaging of the knee: menisci, ligaments, tendons. *Top Magn Reson Imaging* 1993;5(4):228–248.

29. Kursunoglu-Brahme S, Resnick D. Magnetic resonance imaging of the knee. *Orthop Clin North Am* 1990;21(3):561–572.

30. Stoller DW, Martin C, Crues JV 3rd, Kaplan L, Mink JH. Meniscal tears: pathologic correlation with MR imaging. *Radiology* 1987;163(3):731–735.
31. Beltran J, Noto AM, Mosure JC, Weiss KL, Zuelzer W, Christoforidis AJ. The knee: surface-coil MR imaging at 1.5 T1. *Radiology* 1986;159(3):747–751.
32. Boeree NR, Watkinson AF, Ackroyd CE, Johnson C. Magnetic resonance imaging of meniscal and cruciate injuries of the knee. *J Bone Joint Surg Br* 1991;73(3):452–457.
33. Crues JV 3rd, Mink J, Levy TL, Lotysch M, Stoller DW. Meniscal tears of the knee: accuracy of MR imaging. *Radiology* 1987;164(2):445–448.
34. Glashow JL, Katz R, Schneider M, Scott WN. Double-blind assessment of the value of magnetic resonance imaging in the diagnosis of anterior cruciate and meniscal lesions. *J Bone Joint Surg Am* 1989;71(1):113–119.
35. Reicher MA, Hartzman S, Duckwiler GR, Bassett LW, Anderson LJ, Gold RH. Meniscal injuries: detection using MR imaging. *Radiology* 1986;159(3):753–757.
36. van Heuzen EP, Golding RP, van Zanten TE, Patka P. Magnetic resonance imaging of meniscal lesions of the knee. *Clin Radiol* 1988;39(6):658–660.
37. van de Berg BC, Poilvache P, Duchateau F, Lecouvet FE, Dubuc JE, Maldague B, Malghem J. Lesions of the menisci of the knee: value of MR imaging criteria for recognition of unstable lesions. *AJR Am J Roentgenol* 2001;176(3):771–776.
38. Resnick D. Internal derangement of joints. In: Resnick D, editor. *Diagnosis of Bone and Joint Disorders.* 4th edn., Vol. 4. Philadelphia: W. B. Saunders Company, 2002, p. 3206.
39. Davis SJ, Teresi LM, Bradley WG, Burke JW. The "notch" sign: meniscal contour deformities as indicators of tear in MR imaging of the knee. *J Comput Assist Tomogr* 1990;14(6):975–980.
40. Firooznia H, Golimbu C, Rafii M. MR imaging of the menisci. Fundamentals of anatomy and pathology. *Magn Reson Imaging Clin N Am* 1994;2(3):325–347.
41. Tuckman GA, Miller WJ, Remo JW, Fritts HM, Rozansky MI. Radial tears of the menisci: MR findings. *AJR Am J Roentgenol* 1994;163(2):395–400.
42. Singson RD, Feldman F, Staron R, Kiernan H. MR imaging of displaced bucket-handle tear of the medial meniscus. *AJR Am J Roentgenol* 1991;156(1):121–124.
43. Ruff C, Weingardt JP, Russ PD, Kilcoyne RF. MR imaging patterns of displaced meniscus injuries of the knee. *AJR Am J Roentgenol* 1998;170(1):63–67.
44. Breitenseher MJ, Trattnig S, Dobrocky I, Kukla C, Nehrer S, Steiner E, Imhof H. MR imaging of meniscal subluxation in the knee. *Acta Radiol* 1997;38(5):876–879.
45. Miller TT, Staron RB, Feldman F, Cepel E. Meniscal position on routine MR imaging of the knee. *Skeletal Radiol* 1997;26(7):424–427.
46. Fitzgerald SW, Remer EM, Friedman H, Rogers LF, Hendrix RW, Schafer MF. MR evaluation of the anterior cruciate ligament: value of supplementing sagittal images with coronal and axial images. *AJR Am J Roentgenol* 1993;160(6):1233–1237.
47. Hodler J, Haghighi P, Trudell D, Resnick D. The cruciate ligaments of the knee: correlation between MR appearance and gross and histologic findings in cadaveric specimens. *AJR Am J Roentgenol* 1992;159(2):357–360.
48. Ha TP, Li KC, Beaulieu CF, Bergman G, Ch'en IY, Eller DJ, Cheung LP, Herfkens RJ. Anterior cruciate ligament injury: fast spin-echo MR imaging with arthroscopic correlation in 217 examinations. *AJR Am J Roentgenol* 1998;170(5): 1215–1219.

49. Lee JK, Yao L, Phelps CT, Wirth CR, Czajka J, Lozman J. Anterior cruciate ligament tears: MR imaging compared with arthroscopy and clinical tests. *Radiology* 1988;166(3):861–864.

50. Mink JH, Levy T, Crues JV 3rd. Tears of the anterior cruciate ligament and menisci of the knee: MR imaging evaluation. *Radiology* 1988;167(3):769–774.

51. Remer EM, Fitzgerald SW, Friedman H, Rogers LF, Hendrix RW, Schafer MF. Anterior cruciate ligament injury: MR imaging diagnosis and patterns of injury. *Radiographics* 1992;12(5):901–915.

52. Brandser EA, Riley MA, Berbaum KS, el-Khoury GY, Bennett DL. MR imaging of anterior cruciate ligament injury: independent value of primary and secondary signs. *AJR Am J Roentgenol* 1996;167(1):121–126.

53. Gentili A, Seeger LL, Yao L, Do HM. Anterior cruciate ligament tear: indirect signs at MR imaging. *Radiology* 1994;193(3):835–840.

54. Kaye JJ. Ligament and tendon tears: secondary signs. *Radiology* 1993;188(3):616–617.

55. Liu SH, Osti L, Dorey F, Yao L. Anterior cruciate ligament tear. A new diagnostic index on magnetic resonance imaging. *Clin Orthop Relat Res* 1994(302): 147–150.

56. Robertson PL, Schweitzer ME, Bartolozzi AR, Ugoni A. Anterior cruciate ligament tears: evaluation of multiple signs with MR imaging. *Radiology* 1994;193(3):829–834.

57. Allen CR, Wong EK, Livesay GA, Sakane M, Fu FH, Woo SL. Importance of the medial meniscus in the anterior cruciate ligament-deficient knee. *J Orthop Res* 2000;18(1):109–115.

58. Tung GA, Davis LM, Wiggins ME, Fadale PD. Tears of the anterior cruciate ligament: primary and secondary signs at MR imaging. *Radiology* 1993;188(3):661–667.

59. Vahey TN, Broome DR, Kayes KJ, Shelbourne KD. Acute and chronic tears of the anterior cruciate ligament: differential features at MR imaging. *Radiology* 1991;181(1):251–253.

60. Resnick D. Internal derangement of joints. In: Resnick D, editor. *Diagnosis of Bone and Joint Disorders*. 4th edn., Vol. 4. Philadelphia: W. B. Saunders Company, 2002, p. 3223.

61. De Maeseneer M, Lenchik L, Starok M, Pedowitz R, Trudell D, Resnick D. Normal and abnormal medial meniscocapsular structures: MR imaging and sonography in cadavers. *AJR Am J Roentgenol* 1998;171(4):969–976.

62. Garvin GJ, Munk PL, Vellet AD. Tears of the medial collateral ligament: magnetic resonance imaging findings and associated injuries. *Can Assoc Radiol J* 1993;44(3):199–204.

63. Resnick D. Internal derangement of joints. In: Resnick D, editor. *Diagnosis of Bone and Joint Disorders*. 4th edn., Vol. 4. Philadelphia: W. B. Saunders Company, 2002, p. 3225.

64. LaPrade RF, Gilbert TJ, Bollom TS, Wentorf F, Chaljub G. The magnetic resonance imaging appearance of individual structures of the posterolateral knee. A prospective study of normal knees and knees with surgically verified grade III injuries. *Am J Sports Med* 2000;28(2):191–199.

65. Miller TT, Gladden P, Staron RB, Henry JH, Feldman F. Posterolateral stabilizers of the knee: anatomy and injuries assessed with MR imaging. *AJR Am J Roentgenol* 1997;169(6):1641–1647.

66. Recondo JA, Salvador E, Villanua JA, Barrera MC, Gervas C, Alustiza JM. Lateral stabilizing structures of the knee: functional anatomy and injuries assessed with MR imaging. *Radiographics* 2000;20 Spec No:S91–S102.

67. Harris EDJ. Biology of the joint. In: Kelley WN, Harris ED Jr, Ruddy S, Sledge CB, editors. *Textbook of Rheumatology*, 2nd edn. Philadelphia: W. B. Saunders Company, 1985, p. 254.

68. Resnick D. Internal derangement of joints. In: Resnick D, editor. *Diagnosis of Bone and Joint Disorders*, 4th edn., Vol. 4. Philadelphia: W. B. Saunders Company, 2002, p. 3172.

69. Schweitzer ME, Falk A, Pathria M, Brahme S, Hodler J, Resnick D. MR imaging of the knee: can changes in the intracapsular fat pads be used as a sign of synovial proliferation in the presence of an effusion? *AJR Am J Roentgenol* 1993;160(4):823–826.

70. Noyes FR, Stabler CL. A system for grading articular cartilage lesions at arthroscopy. *Am J Sports Med* 1989;17(4):505–513.

71. Recht MP, Piraino DW, Paletta GA, Schils JP, Belhobek GH. Accuracy of fat-suppressed three-dimensional spoiled gradient-echo FLASH MR imaging in the detection of patellofemoral articular cartilage abnormalities. *Radiology* 1996;198(1):209–212.

72. Felson DT, Chaisson CE, Hill CL, Totterman SM, Gale ME, Skinner KM, Kazis L, Gale DR. The association of bone marrow lesions with pain in knee osteoarthritis. *Ann Intern Med* 2001;134(7):541–549.

73. Hirasawa Y, Okajima S, Ohta M, Tokioka T. Nerve distribution to the human knee joint: anatomical and immunohistochemical study. *Int Orthop* 2000;24(1):1–4.

74. Summers MN, Haley WE, Reveille JD, Alarcon GS. Radiographic assessment and psychologic variables as predictors of pain and functional impairment in osteoarthritis of the knee or hip. *Arthritis Rheum* 1988;31(2):204–209.

75. Peterfy CG, Guermazi A, Zaim S, Tirman PF, Miaux Y, White D, Kothari M, Lu Y, Fye K, Zhao S, Genant HK. Whole-Organ Magnetic Resonance Imaging Score (WORMS) of the knee in osteoarthritis. *Osteoarthr Cartil* 2004;12(3):177–190.

76. Blackburn WD Jr, Bernreuter WK, Rominger M, Loose LL. Arthroscopic evaluation of knee articular cartilage: a comparison with plain radiographs and magnetic resonance imaging. *J Rheumatol* 1994;21(4):675–679.

77. Fife RS, Brandt KD, Braunstein EM, Katz BP, Shelbourne KD, Kalasinski LA, Ryan S. Relationship between arthroscopic evidence of cartilage damage and radiographic evidence of joint space narrowing in early osteoarthritis of the knee. *Arthritis Rheum* 1991;34(4):377–382.

78. Outerbridge RE. The etiology of chondromalacia patellae. *J Bone Joint Surg Br* 1961;43-B:752–757.

79. Hangody L, Fules P. Autologous osteochondral mosaicplasty for the treatment of full-thickness defects of weight-bearing joints: ten years of experimental and clinical experience. *J Bone Joint Surg Am* 2003;85-A(Suppl 2):25–32.

80. Recht M, White LM, Winalski CS, Miniaci A, Minas T, Parker RD. MR imaging of cartilage repair procedures. *Skeletal Radiol* 2003;32(4):185–200.

81. Duchow J, Hess T, Kohn D. Primary stability of press-fit-implanted osteochondral grafts. Influence of graft size, repeated insertion, and harvesting technique. *Am J Sports Med* 2000;28(1):24–27.

82. Trattnig S, Millington SA, Szomolanyi P, Marlovits S. MR imaging of osteochondral grafts and autologous chondrocyte implantation. *Eur Rad* 2007;17:103–118.

83. Dew TL, Martin RA. Functional, radiographic, and histologic assessment of healing of autogenous osteochondral grafts and full-thickness cartilage defects in the talus of dogs. *Am J Vet Res* 1992;53(11):2141–2152.

84. Lane JM, Brighton CT, Ottens HR, Lipton M. Joint resurfacing in the rabbit using an autologous osteochondral graft. *J Bone Joint Surg Am* 1977;59(2):218–222.

85. Sanders TG, Mentzer KD, Miller MD, Morrison WB, Campbell SE, Penrod BJ. Autogenous osteochondral "plug" transfer for the treatment of focal chondral defects: postoperative MR appearance with clinical correlation. *Skeletal Radiol* 2001;30(10):570–578.

86. Brittberg M, Lindahl A, Nilsson A, Ohlsson C, Isaksson O, Peterson L. Treatment of deep cartilage defects in the knee with autologous chondrocyte transplantation. *N Engl J Med* 1994;331(14):889–895.

87. Minas T, Peterson L. Advanced techniques in autologous chondrocyte transplantation. *Clin Sports Med* 1999;18(1):13–44, v-vi.

88. Setton LA, Elliott DM, Mow VC. Altered mechanics of cartilage with osteoarthritis: human osteoarthritis and an experimental model of joint degeneration. *Osteoarthr Cartil* 1999;7(1):2–14.

89. Saadat E, Jobke B, Chu B, Lu Y, Cheng J, Li X, Ries MD, Majumdar S, Link TM. Diagnostic performance of *in vivo* 3-T MRI for articular cartilage abnormalities in human osteoarthritic knees using histology as standard of reference. *Eur Radiol* 2008;18(10):2292–2302.

6

Quantitative Morphological Imaging of the Knee Joint

by Julio Carballido-Gamio and Felix Eckstein

Preview

Hyaline cartilage, which lines the bearing surface of diarthrodial joints, displays unique morphological and biomechanical properties to meet complex mechanical demands without undergoing tear and wear.[1-3] Cartilage destruction and loss are, however, common pathophysiological elements of osteoarthritis (OA) of the knee.[4] Therefore there has been a great demand for quantitative parameters of cartilage macro-morphology and cartilage loss. Although joint space narrowing (JSN) on weight-bearing radiographs remains as the current surrogate marker for demonstrating structural changes by regulatory agencies,[5-8] radiography is a projectional technique, which collapses three-dimensional anatomy (3D) into 2D images. It has been reported that before the first radiographic abnormalities appear knee cartilage defects are frequently observed.[9] Also, a substantial portion of subjects with normal radiographs displayed advanced OA at arthroscopy, whereas femoro-tibial JSN was common in participants with normal cartilage status at arthroscopy.[10] Although JSN is often viewed as a surrogate of cartilage thinning, it is also strongly confounded by meniscal pathology, in particular extrusion or subluxation.[11-13] Magnetic resonance imaging (MRI), in contrast to radiography, is a 3D tomographic imaging technique capable of directly visualizing the articular cartilage and providing semi-quantitative and quantitative imaging endpoints.

In this chapter, we examine the main topics associated with quantitative morphological imaging of the knee joint with MRI. Image acquisition, quantitative imaging analysis techniques, accuracy and precision of morphological measures, as well as their clinical utility as demonstrated by cross-sectional and longitudinal OA studies are presented in that order. Although they can be presented in other ways, this approach simplifies their explanation and understanding since it follows the natural pathway of imaging-based cartilage analysis.

Magnetic resonance (MR) advantages as well as challenges for cartilage quantitative morphological imaging are discussed in conjunction with current and potential pulse sequences used for measures of cartilage morphology. Because specific structures (the cartilage) in distinct anatomic regions of interest need to be identified before morphological measures can be computed, a brief overview of the segmentation techniques used in this field is presented. Cartilage morphological measures are defined and explained in conjunction with image analysis techniques to compute them. More sophisticated approaches to compare corresponding regions of interest in longitudinal and cross-sectional studies are addressed, and the technical accuracy and precision of these measures, as well as their importance for designing and interpreting OA studies are presented for human studies. Beyond that, the clinical utility of cartilage morphology-based measures using MRI is reviewed with results from cross-sectional and longitudinal OA studies.

MR Pulse Sequences for Quantitative Analysis of Cartilage Morphology

MRI offers unique advantages in comparison to other imaging modalities for quantification of cartilage morphology. MRI is a non-ionizing imaging technique capable of non-invasively imaging knee articular cartilage *in vivo* and at different imaging planes. Because MRI is a 3D technique, consecutive slices are contiguous and spatially aligned so 3D parameters can be obtained that characterize cartilage appropriately.[14] These advantages together with the excellent soft tissue contrast provided by MRI make it an attractive and powerful technique for semi-quantitative or quantitative assessment of articular cartilage.[15] However, the imaging requirements imposed by the physical dimension, geometry, anatomic location, and biochemical composition of cartilage also become a challenge for MRI.

Pulse Sequence Requirements

A pulse sequence suitable for quantitative morphological imaging of cartilage should have high signal to noise ratio (SNR), high contrast to noise ratio (CNR), high-spatial resolution, should be fast, should minimize artifacts at the bone-cartilage interface, and must have short echo times (TE). These challenges are more evident when dealing with subjects with knee OA since there are signal changes, cartilage surface fibrillation, tissue thinning, appearance of repair tissue, osteophytes,[16] and motion artifacts due to pain, which make cartilage delineation even more difficult.

High SNR and CNR are needed to clearly distinguish articular cartilage from the background signal, and from surrounding structures such as bone, muscle and ligaments, respectively. Cartilage segmentation becomes an easier, less subjective process, and consequently more accurate, when the bone-cartilage interface and articular surface are clearly depicted. High-spatial resolution is required so that cartilage is represented by sufficient number of pixels throughout the joint surface including areas with thin cartilage coverage, thus enabling accurate and precise morphological delineation. Involuntary or not, motion of patients during image acquisition could result in substantial data contamination because of the particular size and geometry of knee cartilage, so short image acquisition and total scanning times should be considered when designing an OA protocol to maintain patient comfort in addition to containing costs. The differences in magnetic susceptibility of bone and cartilage, and the presence of fat in the bone marrow, makes the bone-cartilage interface prone to experience artifacts; for this reason pulse sequences that minimize image distortions at this anatomic location are required. Because cartilage has short transverse relaxation time (T_2), pulse sequences with short echo times are needed to acquire the signal soon after proton excitation.

Most of the scanning parameters controlling the factors mentioned above, however, are interdependent, meaning that optimizing one of them usually involves a loss in another. The first step to guarantee high SNR in quantitative morphological imaging of the joint is the usage of high field magnets (≥ 1.0 Tesla). Although high fields also accentuate possible image artifacts, the benefits (at least up to 3 Tesla) outweigh the disadvantages, because high fields also enable higher spatial resolutions, CNR, or shorter acquisition times. Improvement of CNR and minimization of artifacts at the bone-cartilage interface, as well as elimination of the chemical shift artifact is usually accomplished by avoiding signal from the bone marrow. This is achieved with frequency-selective spectral fat-suppression by a pre-pulse, or with frequency-selective water excitation techniques.[17–19] As a result of this process, the dynamic range between cartilage and surrounding voxel signal intensities is increased.

In a systematic study, where SNR and CNR were sacrificed at the expense of higher in-plane spatial resolution, Hardy *et al.*[20] reported significantly larger precision errors for femoral and tibial cartilage volume measurements derived from the lower-resolution images (0.55×0.55 mm) than for those from the higher-resolution (0.28×0.28 mm). In another study by Link *et al.*[21] where artificial lesions were created in rabbit joints, a similar finding was reported. Higher spatial resolution enabled detection of small lesions at the expense of lower SNR. Investigators have also studied the effects of out-plane spatial resolutions on cartilage volume with phantoms and human subjects, however results have not been as conclusive as for the in-plane spatial resolution. While some authors have reported negative effects when slice thickness is increased, others have not.[20,22–24] However, since mean thickness of cartilage layers in healthy human knees is in the range of 1.3 to 2.5 mm, and even thinner in knees with OA, in-plane spatial resolutions of ≤ 0.3 mm, and slice thickness of ≤ 1.5 mm is recommended to minimize partial volume effects. Slice thickness of 1.5 mm and 1.0 mm are common for 1.5 Tesla and 3.0 Tesla acquisitions, respectively.[25] Proper patient positioning and immobilization in the scanner help to reduce motion artifacts, however pulse sequences of < 15 minutes and total imaging sessions of < 75 minutes are strongly recommended. Shorter acquisition times for morphologic imaging also would allow for scans looking at cartilage physiology[26–28] and biochemistry.[29,30] Imaging techniques using water excitation to avoid signal from fat usually allow shorter TE than fat-suppression pulse sequences, since no pre-pulse is necessary.

Current and Prospective Pulse Sequences

T_1-weighted spoiled gradient echo sequences such as spoiled gradient recalled acquisition at steady state (SPGR), also known as fast low angle shot (FLASH), are sequences that fulfill most of the above-mentioned requirements. These types of sequences are therefore most commonly used in quantitative morphological imaging of the knee joint, and they have also shown to be accurate for detecting arthroscopically verified cartilage lesions.[31–33] In these sequences, cartilage shows bright signal, joint fluid low signal, and bone shows low (background like) signal, since signal from fat is eliminated with fat suppression or water excitation techniques. Another advantage of sequences like SPGR/FLASH is that they are widely available on virtually all clinical MRI systems with ≥1.0 Tesla.

Although the SPGR/FLASH sequences are most commonly used and have shown high accuracy and precision,[34–39] they have two main disadvantages: lack of reliable contrast (a) between cartilage and fluid that outlines surface defects, (b) between the cartilage and the synovium at the level of Hoffa's fat pad, and (c) between the cartilage of the posterior femoral condyle and the posterior capsule; also they required relatively long imaging acquisition times. Although the latter can be ameliorated with parallel imaging techniques (special pulse sequences that in combination with hardware properties and coil sensitivity information acquire images faster),[40,41] other pulse sequences are available for potential contrast improvement. Furthermore, since SPGR uses spoiling at the end of each repetition time (TR) to reduce artifacts and achieve near T_1-weighting, this reduces the signal efficiency compared with steady-state techniques.[15]

Driven equilibrium Fourier transform (DEFT) is another pulse sequence that has been proposed for cartilage imaging. DEFT provides a contrast dependent on the ratio of T_1 / T_2 of a given tissue. DEFT enhances the signal from synovial fluid rather than attenuating cartilage signal as in T_2-weighted sequences. DEFT provides greater cartilage to fluid contrast than SPGR at short TR.[42] However, quantitative cartilage analysis has not been performed to date using this sequence.

Balanced steady-state free precession (bSSFP) MRI is an SNR efficient method for obtaining 3D MR images. This method, also known as true fast imaging with steady precession (FISP), looks promising in the field. Variants of this technique such as fluctuating equilibrium magnetic resonance (FEMR) have also been tested. Although FEMR and other bSSFP-based techniques have a well-known disadvantage of being sensitive to off-resonance artifacts, modern shimming technology to improve field homogeneity makes this less of a problem. Iterative decomposition of water and fat with echo asymmetry and least squares estimation (IDEAL) in combination with bSSFP has shown, however, to be relatively insensitive to field variations.[15] The superior SNR, fast acquisition times, and contrast similar to DEFT make this combination a strong candidate for morphological imaging of knee cartilage, but again, no quantitative cartilage data has yet been presented.

MR images for morphological assessment of cartilage in the Osteoarthritis Initiative (OAI; http://www.oai.ucsf.edu), which is a multi-center, longitudinal, prospective observational study of knee OA, include sagittal double echo steady-state with water excitation[43,44] (DESS-WE) and coronal FLASH-WE. DESS images have been proposed to provide higher SNR efficiency (SNR per unit of time) than SPGR,[45,46] with contrast similar to that of DEFT where signal from fluid shows higher than that of cartilage, thus providing high fluid-to-cartilage contrast. A cross-calibration study showed consistent results between DESS-WE and FLASH,[46] similar test retest precision in an independent[46] and pair-wise reading[47,48] of repeat scans, and a similar sensitivity to change of DESS as FLASH,[48] albeit only in a very small pilot cohort. However, two recent studies from the OAI, one using sagittal DESS-WE,[49] and one using coronal FLASH-WE,[50] found very similar rates of change for both protocols.

There is no current consensus in terms of which image orientation is best for morphological imaging of cartilage, since no face-to-face studies of accuracy, precision or sensitivity have been performed. While sagittal images depict all cartilage plates of the knee, including the femoro-patellar and femoro-tibial compartments, coronal images optimally delineate the femoro-tibial joint, and axial images the patella with little partial volume effects. Figure 1 shows fat-suppressed sagittal and coronal examples of 3.0 Tesla SPGR acquisitions, while Fig. 2 shows representative sagittal DESS-WE and coronal FLASH-WE images of the OAI.

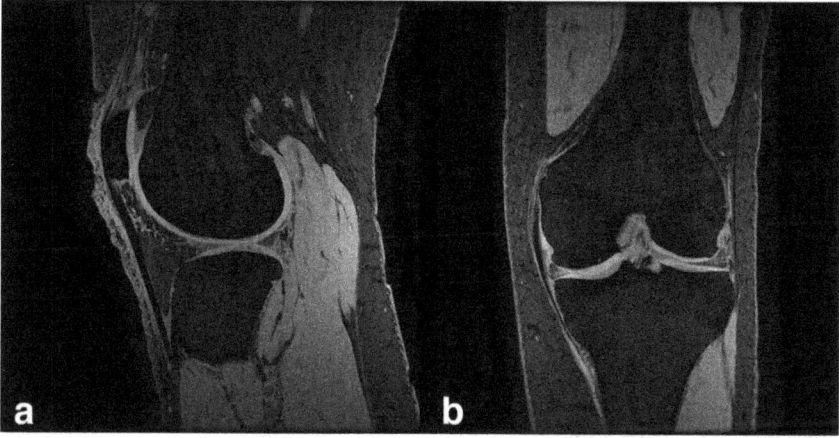

Fig. 1. Fat-suppressed SPGR images of the knee joint at 3.0 Tesla. **(a)** Sagittal orientation with in-plane spatial resolution of 0.312×0.312 mm and slice thickness of 1.00 mm. **(b)** Coronal orientation with in-plane spatial resolution of 0.312×0.312 mm and slice thickness of 1.50 mm.

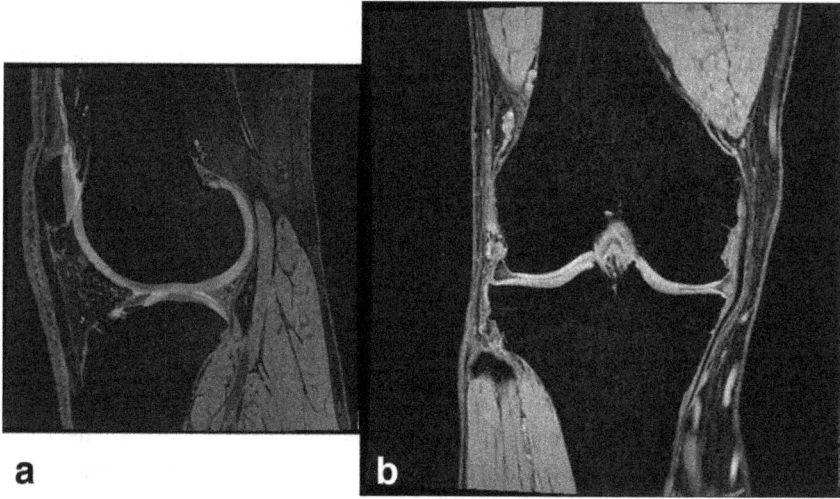

Fig. 2. MR images of the knee joint at 3.0 Tesla from the OAI. **(a)** Sagittal DESS-WE with in-plane spatial resolution of 0.365×0.456 mm and slice thickness of 0.7 mm. **(b)** Coronal FLASH-WE with in-plane spatial resolution of 0.312×0.312 mm and slice-thickness of 1.5 mm.

Quantitative Imaging-Based Measures of Cartilage Morphology

In contrast to categorical variables of semi-quantitative scoring systems of cartilage morphology (i.e. WORMS,[51] KOSS[52] or BLOKS[53]), quantitative imaging-based measures offer continuous variables that are easier to handle from the statistical point of view and that may be less subjective and more sensitive to change.[54] The nomenclature used in this section follows that proposed by a group of experts in the field.[55]

Parameters

Cartilage volume (VC; units of volume) and cartilage thickness (ThC; units of distance) are the most common imaging-based measures of cartilage morphology derived from MRI. Additional measures include cartilage surface area (AC; units of area), total subchondral bone (or bone interface) area (tAB; units of area), denuded subchondral bone area (dAB; units of area), and cartilaginous subchondral bone area (cAB; units of area), which are indicated on MR images in Fig. 3. Each of these parameters should be computed independently because it has been shown that ThC and AC are not strongly associated in healthy joints,[56,57] and that gender differences in AC are substantially larger than those of ThC,[58,59] a finding that is not possible to infer from measuring VC alone.[60] Furthermore, since VC scales with bone size,[61] VC may be reported additionally normalized by tAB yielding a composite metric (VCtAB; units of distance), which has shown to perform better than VC in differentiating subjects with and without OA.[62] It has also been suggested that ThC should be reported as either ThCtAB, which includes dAB (0 mm thickness), or as ThCcAB, which only includes regions with cartilage coverage (Fig. 3). Although ThCtAB and VCtAB represent different ways for measuring thickness, it is recommended that both variables be reported independently, because values may not be identical due to different computational approaches applied. Morphological measures of the knee joint are usually reported with mean, median, minimum, maximum, and standard deviation values.

Since VC can remain constant even if there are focal changes in ThC and dAB, researchers have also implemented techniques to quantify the depth,

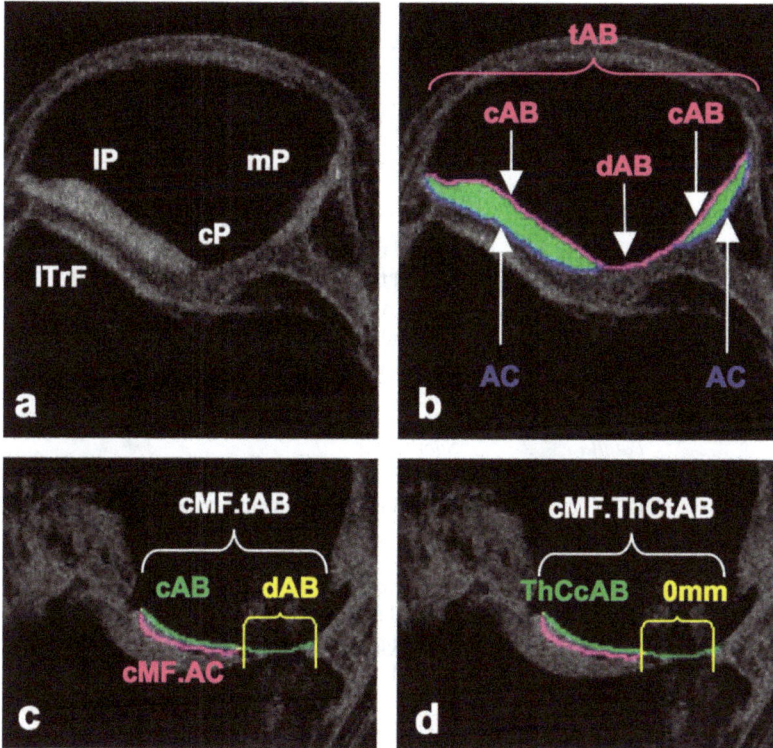

Fig. 3. (a) Anatomical labels of knee joint cartilage plates and (b) cartilage morphology labels for measurements of areas on axial images. This example displays an area of denuded cartilage in the center of the patella. (c) Cartilage morphology labels for measurements of areas and (d) for measurements of cartilage thickness in the medial femoral condyle. This example displays an area of denuded cartilage in the external aspect of the medial femoral condyle. Note that the peripheral osteophyte is not included in the measurement of tAB. When reporting values for cartilage thickness, it is important to differentiate whether or not the values include denuded areas (dAB) as areas of 0 mm cartilage thickness. The group recommends the use of ThCtAB for measurements including dAB (0 mm cartilage thickness) and ThCcAB for those only including cartilage. This figure and label have been reproduced with permission from Ref. 55. Copyright © 2006 OsteoArthritis Research Society International Published by Elsevier Ltd. Refer to Table 1 for additional details of anatomical nomenclature.

diameter, area, and volume of cartilage lesions from cartilage thickness maps.[63] The accuracy of these measurements was validated using a porcine experimental model as well as with arthroscopic evaluation of cartilage lesions,[64] and using experimental defects in human cartilage.[65] These

Table 1. Anatomical labels of the knee joint.

Label	Explanation
Knee	
K	Knee, total (P + MT + LT + F)
P	Patella
T	Tibia (MT + LT)
MT	Medial tibia
LT	Lateral tibia
F	Femur, total (TrF + MF + LF)
TrF	Femoral trochlea
MF	Medial femoral condyle
LF	Lateral femoral condyle
Patella	*Subregions*
lP	Lateral aspect of patella
mP	Medial aspect of patella
cP	Central aspect of patella
Trochlea	*Subregions*
cTrF	Central aspect of trochlea
mTrF	Medial aspect of trochlea
lTrF	Lateral aspect of trochlea
Femoral condyle	*Subregions*
cMF	Central medial femoral condyle
pMF	Posterior medial femoral condyle
cLF	Central lateral femoral condyle
pLF	Posterior lateral femoral condyle

Source: Adapted from Ref. 55.

metrics are consequently focal, opposite of those previously described, which are global.

When the articular cartilage surfaces are nonconforming, the phenomenon is called joint incongruity. Morphological imaging of the knee joint with MRI also enables its quantification.[29,66] This metric is particularly useful in surgery and computer modeling of joint biomechanics.[67,68]

Segmentation

In order to quantify the above-mentioned parameters, cartilage and/or other anatomic structures must be segmented. Although MR images show good cartilage contrast with respect to other tissues, its delineation is challenging even to the trained human eye, especially in knees with OA and at specific regions such as the patello-femoral and femoro-tibial articulations, and posterior part of the femoral condyles. This task is most of the times performed manually on a section-by-section basis, which makes it a time consuming process, generally requiring one to several hours per knee data set, by a trained reader. A sagittal scan of the knee joint with slice thickness of 0.7 mm, such as a DESS-WE of the OAI, involves approximately 120 slices from which femoral, tibial and patellar cartilage have to be carefully segmented. Currently, there is no fully automatic cartilage segmentation technique. For this reason, literature related to image analysis techniques that aim to minimize user interaction for cartilage segmentation while maintaining accuracy and precision, is vast. Since MR images of cartilage morphology yield in general good cartilage boundaries in most regions, most of the segmentation approaches rely on edge information, and most of them perform on a slice-by-slice basis propagating the segmentation of one slice as the initialization of a contiguous one. Stammberger and colleagues[69] implemented a quadratic B-spline with a scale-space approach and three energy terms to guide the segmentation. An internal energy term controlled the rigidity of the contour, an external energy term attracted the contour to the cartilage edges, and a coupling force enforced smooth changes from one slice to another. In another 2D approach, Lynch *et al.*[70] combined expert knowledge with cubic splines and image processing algorithms reporting better reproducibility and less user interaction than region growing techniques. There have been also 3D approaches such as those of Grau *et al.*[71] Pakin *et al.*[72] and Warfield and colleagues.[73] Grau *et al.*[71] extended the watershed technique to examining difference in class probability of neighboring pixels. Pakin *et al.*[72] used a region growing method with prior knowledge. Warfield and colleagues[73] developed an adaptive, template moderated, spatially varying statistical classification method, which consisted of an iterative technique between classification and template registration. The template was used to moderate the segmentation of the statistical classification. However, the manual editing required in the context of semi-automated cartilage segmentation some times is more cumbersome and time-consuming than segmentation approaches that are exclusively manual.

Quantitative Analysis

The easiest morphological measure to compute after segmentation is VC since it only involves a sum of the total number of voxels representing cartilage, followed by corresponding scaling according to the voxel dimensions. Voxels, however, are usually highly anisotropic with in-plane spatial resolutions three times higher or more than the slice thickness. A common approach to deal with this issue, particularly when extending analyses to surface areas and cartilage thickness, is the usage of interpolation techniques to obtain isotropic voxels.[74,75] Although interpolation is not equivalent to acquiring images with higher spatial resolutions, it smoothes jaggy boundaries and minimizes differences between measures obtained from different imaging planes: sagittal, coronal, and axial. Interpolation can be either based on gray-level values or based on shape. The disadvantage of using gray-level interpolation techniques is that it substantially increases the number of sections to be segmented in a knee data set. This is the main reason why shape-based interpolation is usually preferred. Figure 4a shows a 3D example of shape-interpolated knee cartilage plates, where commonly used compartments have been color-coded.

In terms of ThC, researchers have used different approaches and most of them have computed this metric in 3D. As with VC, shape-based interpolation has also been proposed as an intermediate step for ThC calculations.[74,76] The most common approach to compute cartilage thickness is based on 2D or 3D minimum Euclidean distances.[74,76,77] For

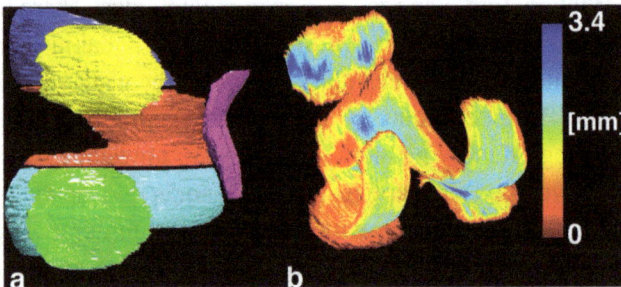

Fig. 4. (a) Bottom view of shape-interpolated knee cartilage compartments: blue = medial femoral compartment; red = trochlea; cyan = lateral femoral compartment; yellow = medial tibia; green = lateral tibia; and magenta = patella. (b) Knee cartilage color-coded thickness map calculated in 3D.

each point on the bone-cartilage interface or articular surface, the closest point on the opposite surface is computed. Another 3D approach consists on computing normal vectors on one surface (articular or bone-cartilage interface), and finding the intersection of the vectors on the opposite surface.[66,78] The average of the minimum distances or length of the vectors, respectively, is reported as the average cartilage thickness. Figure 4b shows a 3D knee articular cartilage thickness map, where thickness values have been color-coded. Surface area calculations are usually performed by representing the surface in question with triangles (a process called triangulation) followed by the sum of the individual triangle areas.[75]

Because global metrics are insensitive to small focal/regional changes that affect only small portions of the cartilage surface, it is common to report them by compartment. Femoral cartilage is commonly divided into three compartments: medial femoral condyle, lateral femoral condyle, and trochlea.[55] Tibial cartilage is reported as the lateral and medial tibia plateaus. The subdivision of patellar cartilage into smaller units is possible, but not common. Figures 3 and 5 and Table 1 indicate the suggested nomenclature for MRI-based measures of articular cartilage in OA by a group of experts.[55]

However, investigators have also developed techniques to monitor focal changes over time. Kshirsagar *et al.*[79] suggested that sub-volume analysis within the joint surface could reduce precision errors versus total VC, a finding that was confirmed by Koo and colleagues.[80] Techniques to perform this kind of comparisons are, however, more sophisticated. Since there is patient motion between scans, images at different time points need to be aligned, a process known as image registration.

To obtain an impression of the spatial distribution of change (between time points) across the entire cartilage surface, image registration is required. For this purpose some investigators have used the bone-cartilage interface[81–84] while others have used the total bone shape.[76,85] Once shapes have been aligned, matching of cartilage thickness patterns can be performed at a local level. Because there is an increasing interest in performing regional comparisons of cartilage properties at specific anatomic locations between different populations for a better understanding of OA, techniques have also been developed for this purpose.[76,86] For inter-subject comparisons, shapes have to be registered prior to any comparison,

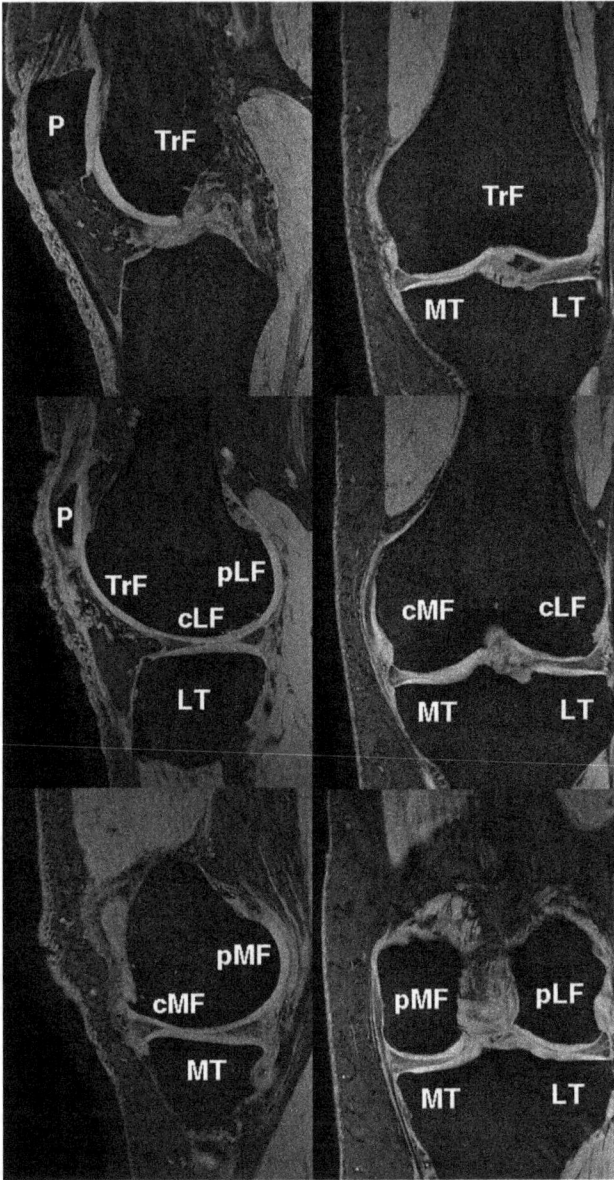

Fig. 5. Anatomical labels of knee joint cartilage plates. Sagittal images (left column), and coronal images (right column). Refer to Table 1 for the meaning of anatomical labels.

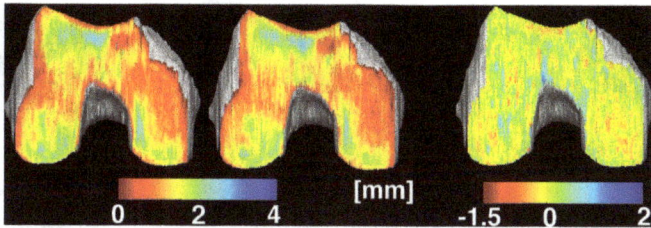

Fig. 6. Longitudinal point-to-point comparison of femoral knee cartilage thickness values: baseline thickness map (left), follow-up thickness map (center), follow-up minus baseline based on bone shape matching (right).

but in this case, scale factors as well as nonlinear differences between shapes have to be considered. The bone shape, and not only the interface, has recently been proposed for this type of matching.[76] Figure 6 shows an intra-subject longitudinal example of cartilage thickness matching using the technique described by Carballido-Gamio and colleagues, which can also be applied for inter-subject comparisons of cartilage properties.[76]

Other techniques to analyze cartilage on anatomically based sub-regions have also been developed that eliminate the need for spatial registration between data sets and can also be applied to cross-sectional studies.[77,80,84,87,88] Several longitudinal studies have recently reported the spatial pattern of cartilage loss within the femoro-tibial joint and have found that the rate of change in some sub-regions (i.e. central) exceeds that in other sub-regions.[84,89–91] Figure 7 shows two different approaches for regional comparison of cartilage thickness of different subjects.

Accuracy of Quantitative Measurements

Accuracy (validity) of morphological measures, not to be confused with the surrogate validity of the marker in predicting patient-relevant outcome, has been addressed by several investigators, specifically with SPGR/FLASH sequences. It is important to note that whenever a new segmentation/analysis technique is developed, validation against independent, established methods is recommended. Ideally, validation should be based not only on phantoms, but the actual biological structure of interest since some MRI artifacts occur only when the actual tissue is placed in the magnetic field.

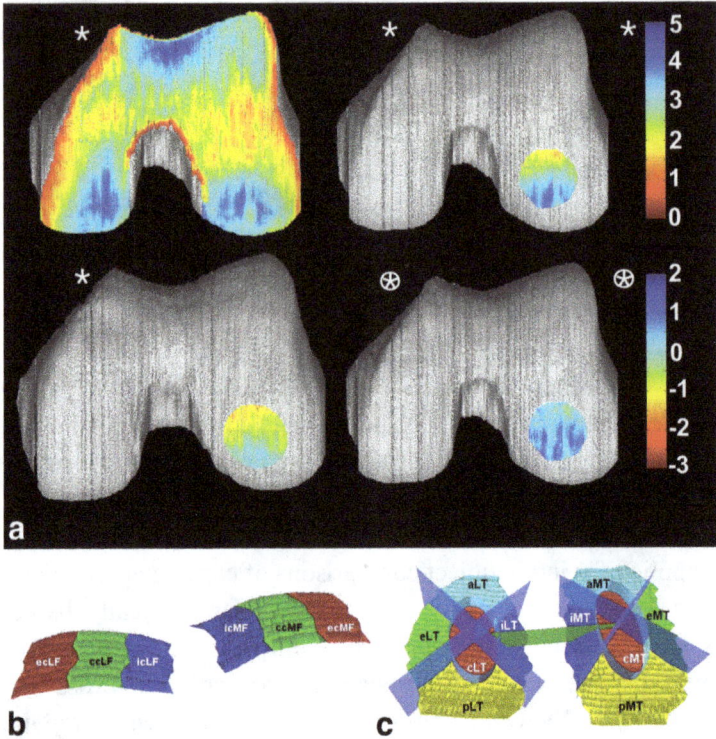

Fig. 7. Inter-subject sub-regional comparison of cartilage thickness values. **(a)** Inter-subject cartilage thickness comparison of a small region of interest. Top row: Source cartilage thickness map and its matched region. Bottom left: Target cartilage thickness region. Bottom right: Source minus target thickness region of interest. Color bars are in mm. This figure and label have been reproduced with permission from Ref. 76, copyright © 2007 Elsevier B.V. **(b)** Three-dimensional reconstruction of the femoral subchondral bone (lateral femur left, medial femur right; view from inferior). Sub-regions are color-coded. **(c)** Three-dimensional reconstruction of the tibial subchondral bone (lateral tibia left, medial tibia right; view from inferior). The figure also shows the surfaces used for the subdivision and indicates the line connecting the centers of gravity of both tibial plates by the green plane through the cartilage. Sub-regions are color-coded. Figures 7b and 7c, and their labels, have been reproduced with permission from Ref. 88 © 2008 IEEE.

Validation studies have been carried out in comparison with various established methods considered as gold standards. VC and ThC are perhaps the cartilage morphological metrics that have received more attention. Amputated joints, unselected cadaveric joints, and knee joints of patients undergoing total knee arthroplasty (TKA) present unique opportunities for validation of these parameters.[34,35,60,92] In these situations, MR images of the intact joint can be obtained, followed by cartilage removal and quantification with water displacement methods (by weight or volume),[34,38,39] anatomical sections obtained with high-precision band saws,[36,92–94] or stereophotogrammetry.[66] Comparisons to other imaging modalities techniques such as A-mode ultrasound and computed tomography (CT) arthrography have also been implemented.[37,95,96] Most of the validation studies in the scientific literature have yielded high agreement between the reference methods and MRI.[16]

Precision of Quantitative Measurements

If repeated measurements of a parameter that is assumed to remain constant are taken, there are differences due to random variations. This type of error is known as precision error. Morphological changes in knee cartilage due to OA are small and occur over long periods of time. In order to detect changes with these characteristics with statistical significance, highly reproducible techniques are required. It is important to note however, that precision errors in imaging-based morphological quantification of the knee depends on factors associated to both image acquisition and image analysis. As accuracy, precision plays a key role in OA trials since techniques that are highly reproducible translate in trials that required less number of subjects and consequently of less duration to detect possible drug effects on cartilage changes. This fact is of special importance from the ethical and economic point of view, because participants are exposed for shorter periods of time to an investigational drug, and delayed entry into the market is shortened.

When reporting technical reproducibility it is important to differentiate under which conditions the precision study was performed. There are four determinant factors to be considered: (1) Is the analysis performed on the same image set? (2) Is the analysis performed in the same session? (3) Is the same person doing all the analysis? (4) Were the images taken in the same scanner? It is important to note here that on the image analysis side, segmentation is a key component on morphological measures. So when the same image set is analyzed repeatedly in the same session, the error part corresponding to the image acquisition does not exist. This kind of studies measured what is called technical precision. When the same image set is analyzed repeatedly in different sessions, then a measured of the re-segmentation precision is obtained. Most of the reproducibility studies in the literature are of the inter-scan precision type, where measurement of at least two image sets that were acquired within the same imaging session but with subject repositioning between repeated acquisitions is performed. Precision errors of this category are expected to be larger since the orientation of image sections is different between sets. Long-term precision errors refer to the same conditions of short-term errors except for the fact that images were acquired during different imaging sessions. The overall precision refers to the combination of short- or long-term acquisitions with analysis being done in different sessions. Inter-observer and inter-scanner precision errors are those due to different observers doing the analysis, and image acquisitions done at different scanners, respectively. It is highly recommended to avoid inter-observer errors in any study by assigning only one reader for image analysis of pairs of baseline and follow-up acquisitions. It is also important to be aware of the fact that precision errors are likely to increase with subjects with OA when compared to studies involving only healthy subjects.

Reproducibility errors are usually reported as coefficients of variation (CV%) by dividing the standard deviation (SD) by the mean value of the measurements. However, one should be careful when reporting reproducibility studies involving multiple measurements for multiple individuals. Reporting the mean CV% or mean SD (which sometimes is also used to report reproducibility) underestimates the true precision error in the population. Instead, according to Glüer et al.,[97] one should report the squared root of the mean of the variances or the square root of the mean of the squared CV%, giving more weight to large precision errors. These values can also be reported as percentages.

The tomographic advantage of MRI yielding aligned consecutive slices is an important factor in precision error improvement when compared to other imaging modalities. Individual studies have been performed in terms of plane orientations yielding precision values between 1% and 5% for both VC and ThC measurements.[98] Although lower precision errors have been found for the femoro-tibial articulation using coronal images,[99] no direct comparisons with other imaging planes have been performed. MRI at 3T has been shown to display somewhat smaller precision errors than 1.5 T systems.[100,101]

Pulse sequences coming from different vendors such as FLASH and SPGR have yielded similar precision errors,[102] and a recent multi-center clinical trial of the precision of quantitative cartilage morphology using 3.0 Tesla MRI reported root mean square (RMS) CVs% for thickness and volume ranging from 2.1% to 2.9%, and 2.4% to 3.3%, respectively.[103]

Clinical Utility of Cartilage Morphology

In order to be considered of clinical utility, any imaging-based marker needs to lie on the disease pathway in question, and the technique for its quantification should be accurate and precise. Accuracy and precision of quantitative MRI (qMRI) cartilage morphology was covered in the previous section. In this section, we will start with a brief review of cross-sectional and longitudinal studies highlighting the potential of morphological cartilage measures as imaging-based biomarkers of OA. OA studies comparing qMRI of cartilage morphology with radiography, and studies of cartilage morphology and its relationship with clinical symptoms will also be discussed. The last sub-section will contain material related to risk factors of cartilage morphology change in OA.

MRI Cross-Sectional Studies

Hudelmaier and colleagues[104,105] studied cross-sectional data from elderly healthy subjects without history of knee joint symptoms, trauma, or surgery (50–78 years; 11 men, 12 women), relative to a cohort of young, healthy subjects who met the same criteria (20–30 years; 49 men, 46 women), to estimate cartilage thinning during normal aging. An estimated 0.3% to 0.5% reduction of cartilage thickness per annum for all knee compartments was reported, with women showing higher differences (between elderly and young) than men in the patella. No gender differences (of these differences) were found in other knee compartments. Beattie *et al.*,[106] in a study of 119 healthy individuals (female = 73, male = 47), assessed medial tibial cartilage morphology with a peripheral MRI at 1.0 Tesla. The authors reported lower baseline tibial cartilage volume (1.50 vs. 1.77 μl/mm^2) and thickness (1.45 vs. 1.71 mm) in females than in males, as also previously reported by other authors in all knee compartments,[58,59] even when adjusting for body height and weight.[59]

Jones *et al.*[107] suggested that MRI might be superior to radiography at detecting early knee OA based on a cross-sectional study involving 372 subjects, where grade 1 medial JSN was reported to be associated with reductions in MRI tibial and patellar cartilage volume (11%–13%), while grade 1 osteophytosis was associated with substantial increases in tibial surface area (10%–16%), but no change in cartilage volume. Differences in tibial bone area were not related to JSN, and differences in cartilage volume were not related to osteophytosis. These findings, however, were not entirely reproduced in a recent study.[108]

The advantage of normalizing the cartilage volume by the bone interface area was seen in studies of Burgkart *et al.*[62] and Hunter and colleagues.[109] The first study showed better discrimination between patients with an indication to correction osteotomy or TKA and normal healthy subjects; and the second one reported that this normalized measure yielded the best discrimination between patients with radiographic OA of the femoro-tibial joint and non-radiographic OA participants in the Framingham cohort. Also, normalizing cartilage volume to the bone interface area increased the correlation of cartilage morphometry with knee alignment in a cross-sectional study.[110] Burgkart *et al.*[62] were the first to apply T- and Z-scores for quantification of cartilage loss in OA as they are used in osteoporosis. A recent cross-sectional study of the minimum joint space width (JSW) and tibial cartilage morphology in knee of healthy individuals by Beattie and colleagues,[106] suggested that for radiographic measurements there may be no need to differentiate a T-score and a Z-score in OA diagnosis, because cartilage thickness and JSW may remain constant throughout life in the absence of OA.

In a recent study of the Framingham cohort, Reichenbach and colleagues[111] reported that median WORMS scores were higher in subjects with mild OA than in non-OA, but that regional cartilage volume (VC) and thickness (ThCtAB) were not different between mild OA versus non-OA. Hellio Le Graverand *et al.*[108] reported greater cartilage thickness in Kellgren-Lawrence grade[112] (KLG) 2 participants (osteophytes, no JSN) compared with healthy women, indicating that cartilage may undergo swelling or hypertrophy in early radiographic OA, as indicated by several animal models.[113–117] In a recent study, Andreisek and colleagues[118] evaluated cartilage thickness (ThC) and subchondral bone area (tAB) of the operated and contra-lateral non-operated (healthy) knees in patients with anterior cruciate ligament (ACL)-reconstruction seven years after surgery using a quantitative and regional cartilage MR imaging technique. The authors reported changes in tAB and femoral shape between the operated and contra-lateral operated knees, but no side-to-side differences in sub-regional ThC. Lateral femoral tAB was significantly lower (−9.2%), and medial tibial tAB was significantly larger (+2%) in the operated versus the non-operated knee; and significantly flattened and broader shapes of medial femoral condyles were found in operated knees.

MRI Longitudinal Studies

Longitudinal studies of knee cartilage have been performed on both, healthy subjects and patients with OA.

Healthy Subjects

Wluka *et al.*[119] reported a significant change in cartilage volume in healthy postmenopausal women without knee pain ($n = 57$) over a period of 2.5 years. Total tibial cartilage decreased 2.4% in average per year, between 1.5% and 3.2%. Similarly, Hanna *et al.*,[120] in a two-year follow-up study of a cohort of 28 healthy men, reported a mean reduction in tibial cartilage volume per year of 162 μl, equivalent to a 2.8% reduction in total tibial cartilage per year. In a recent multi-center study of Hellio Le Graverand and colleagues,[90] 145 women were recruited, from which 86 were non-obese and had no symptoms and no radiographic OA, and 55 were obese and had symptoms and radiographic OA based on KLG ($n = 27$ with KLG $= 2$; and $n = 28$ with KLG $= 3$). Coronal MRI at 3.0 Tesla was obtained at six months, one year, and two years; while Lyon schuss (LS) and fixed flexion (FF) radiographs were obtained at baseline, one year, and two years. MRI cartilage morphology was assessed as sub-regional femoro-tibial cartilage thickness, and the minimum JSW was measured in the medial femoro-tibial compartment of radiographs. The standardized response mean (SRM), which is the mean change divided by the standard deviation change, was used to evaluate longitudinal changes. The authors reported small cartilage thickness changes in controls, and observed that at six-month follow-up, the greatest reduction in cartilage thickness in the control group was in the central medial tibia and central sub-region of the central weight-bearing medial femur. Over one year, no relevant changes ($\leq 0.2\%$) were reported in ThCtAB in controls using qMRI or radiography. At two-year follow-up, authors reported that only small-annualized changes ($\leq 0.5\%$) in ThCtAB of the medial femoro-tibial compartment were found in healthy controls.

OA Subjects

Wluka *et al.*[121] examined a cohort of 123 subjects with OA over the course of two years, detecting a mean total tibial articular cartilage decreased of 5.3% per year. The authors reported that an increased baseline cartilage volume was the factor most strongly affected with increased cartilage loss, and suggested that cartilage loss may be more rapid early in the disease.

In a study on the association between sex, age and rate of change on knee cartilage volume in adults, Ding and colleagues[122] studied 325 (mean age 45 years, range 26–61 years) subjects (17% with radiographic OA) for approximately two years. The authors observed a knee cartilage volume decreased of 1.5% to 4.2% per year with women showing higher rates of change than males (medial tibia, lateral tibia, and patella). Age was significantly associated with annual change in knee cartilage volume (medial tibia, lateral tibia, and patella), with stronger associations in women. A recent study on a first release of the OAI progression subcohort, however, did not confirm an association of cartilage loss with sex or age.[50]

Hellio Le Graverand *et al.*,[90] in contrast to the study of Wluka *et al.*,[121] reported cartilage thickness changes over two years to be substantially faster in participants with KLG = 3 (osteophytes and joint space narrowing) than in those with KLG = 2 (osteophytes, but no joint space narrowing). Cicuttini and colleagues[123] analyzed a subcohort of 110 subjects from the study of Wluka *et al.*,[121] reporting an annual percentage loss of patellar cartilage of 4.5% with no association between change in patellar cartilage volume and change in either medial or lateral tibial cartilage volume. The authors observed higher rate of patellar cartilage loss in women (5.3%) than in men (3.5%), and higher loss in subjects with higher body mass index (BMI) and pain scores at baseline. Wang *et al.*,[124] in the same sample, reported that the medial and lateral tibia plateau areas increased over a two-year period 2.2% and 1.5% per year, respectively. This was confirmed not only in OA participants, but also in healthy participants over a three-month period using 3 Tesla MRI.[103] Wang *et al.*[124] also observed that the increases at the medial tibia were stronger in males, in subjects with high BMI, and in subjects with higher baseline grade of medial JSN. In another study, the ratio of the medial and lateral tibial plateau area was found to depend on knee alignment, and alignment was significantly associated with the rate of increase of the medial and lateral femoral subchondral bone areas.[125]

The variability of annual loss of cartilage volume reported in earlier studies was large with annual rates going from −0.3% to 7.4% in the medial tibia, showing the heterogeneity of knee OA progression.[16] Gandy and colleagues[126] even reported no loss of MRI cartilage volume over three years in patients with knee OA ($n = 11$). More recent studies have generally reported, on average, lower rates of change per annum[49,50,89–91] than earlier studies.

The OAI [http://www.oai.ucsf.edu], which involves longitudinal MR images of 4800 participants, promises further cartilage morphological investigation and better understanding of knee OA. Hunter *et al.*[49] reported initial results of changes in cartilage morphology in a sample of 160 subjects of the progression cohort of the OAI. Cartilage morphology was longitudinally studied (baseline and 12-month follow-up) using the sagittal DESS-WE sequence in terms of cartilage volume, normalized cartilage volume (VCtAB), and percent bone denuded area (dAB). Results were given in terms of absolute and percentage changes from baseline at one year, and using the SRM. Results indicated small-annualized rates of change with the central medial femur showing the greatest consistent change. Eckstein *et al.*[50] and Wirth *et al.*[89] reported similar rates of change and SRMs in the same cohort using the FLASH-WE sequence, although it was not always the same knee, but sometimes the contra-lateral side, that was studied.

Frobell *et al.*[127] investigated changes in the knee during the first year after acute rupture of the anterior cruciate ligament (ACL), and reported that an ACL reconstruction performed within a mean of six weeks from injury was associated with increased ThCcAB and VC in cMF and decreased AC in TrF, compared to knees treated without reconstruction. As suggested in the study of Hellio Le Graverand *et al.*,[108] this could be potentially a sign of cartilage swelling/hypertrophy in early OA.

Cartilage Morphology and Radiography

Magnetic resonance imaging, technologically speaking, is certainly a more sophisticated imaging technique than radiography; however, in terms of its sensitivity in morphological quantification of knee OA, its superiority has yet to be established. Gandy *et al.*,[126] studied 11 patients with well-established OA based on radiographic scores, and followed them over a period of three years. Results showed an average decrease in medial tibio-femoral JSW of -0.21 ± 0.37 mm, but no significant change of MRI cartilage volume in any compartment assessed at 1.0 Tesla.

Cicuttini and colleagues[128] studied 252 subjects and compared MRI tibial cartilage volume with radiographic assessment of the tibio-femoral joint. JSN of the medial and lateral femoro-tibial joints was inversely associated with the corresponding tibial cartilage volume. The inverse relationship was strengthened after adjusting for age, sex, BMI, and bone size. For every increase in JSN grade (0–3), medial and lateral tibial cartilage volume was reduced by 257 and 396 mm^3, respectively. This association was stronger than that between osteophytes and cartilage volume. In another study involving 28 subjects, the same group found moderate significant association of JSN with MRI tibial and femoral cartilage volume in the medial femoro-tibial compartment at baseline, but no significant correlation between JSN and longitudinal change of cartilage volume over two years.[129] With respect to the patello-femoral joint, the study of Cicuttini *et al.*[130] indicated better diagnostic performance with MRI-based measures than radiographic measures of cartilage morphology.

Raynauld *et al.*[131] found no significant correlation between cartilage volume loss and radiographic changes in 31 patients followed over two years at six-month intervals, but they reported significant cartilage loss at all follow-up points. While 27 of the 31 patients showed MRI medial cartilage loss over two years, 50% of the patients with JSW measurement at both baseline and year 2 showed a decrease in the minimum JSW. However, the mean JSW change among the 19 patients with primary medial disease and an osteophyte at baseline was -0.13 mm, indicating the importance of considering this subgroup when measuring medial progression by JSW. The authors suggested that MRI might be more sensitive to change than standardized radiography since loss of cartilage volume in the knee was detected as early as six months. In another study, Cicuttini *et al.*[129]

measured JSW in 28 subjects with knee OA using standing radiographs in full extension. MRI femoral, tibial, and combined femoral and tibial cartilage volumes were also computed. Follow-up radiographs and MR scans were done approximately two years after baseline. No correlation between longitudinal change of medial tibio-femoral cartilage volume and JSW was reported, despite a modest correlation between these measures at baseline.

Bruyere *et al.*,[132] in a one-year longitudinal study, investigated the relationship between X-ray and MRI findings in patients with knee OA ($n = 62$). MRI cartilage thickness and volume of the medial tibia, lateral tibia, and femur, were computed at baseline and one year. Lateral and medial femoro-tibial JSW were digitally assessed from fixed-flexion, postero-anterior radiographs. The authors reported moderate significant association between changes in JSW and changes in cartilage thickness or volume. One-year changes were as follows: medial femoro-tibial JSW 6.7%, medial cartilage volume 0.4%, and medial cartilage thickness 2.1%. Pelletier *et al.*[84] reported a strong correlation on a symptomatic knee OA cohort ($n = 107$) between the JSN and the loss of cartilage over the span of 24 months in the central area of the medial femoral condyle and, to a lesser extent, with the loss on the medial central tibial plateau. In a multi-center study involving seven clinical sites, Hellio Le Graverand and colleagues[90] had the objective of directly comparing MRI sub-regional cartilage thickness change at 3.0 Tesla with radiographic progression of JSN in OA and non-OA subjects. Results showed that both, MRI and LS radiography were able to detect significant changes in patients with KLG = 3, but not in KLG = 2. Although MRI showed greater sensitivity to change than FF radiography at one year and two years in patients with KLG = 3, this was not the case with respect to LS radiography.

Cartilage Morphology: Clinical Symptoms and Clinical Outcome

Studies investigating the association of clinical symptoms with cartilage morphology have yielded diverse results over time. In a cohort study, 110 subjects with OA were studied by Cicuttini *et al.*[123] over approximately two years to investigate patellar cartilage changes, showing that subjects with higher pain scores at baseline or higher BMI, showed higher cartilage loss than those with lower scores. Link and colleagues,[133] however, based on a cross-sectional study reported that in patients with OA only the degree of cartilage pathology seen in MR images was associated with clinical symptoms, while image features determined from MR images or conventional radiographs were not. The same year, in a different cross-sectional study by Hunter *et al.*,[134] a significant negative association of patellar cartilage volume with WOMAC score[135] was observed. The studied was performed in 133 postmenopausal women with a fat-saturated T_2-weighted sagittal gradient echo sequence. Raynauld and colleagues[131] supported those findings in a longitudinal study, reporting a faster progression for subjects with more pain at baseline, but no significant correlation between worsening of symptoms and cartilage volume change. In contrast, Wluka *et al.*[136] with 132 patients with symptomatic early knee OA reported no significant associations between symptoms at baseline and subsequent cartilage loss, but a weak association between tibial cartilage volume and symptoms given by WOMAC at baseline. One of the most recent studies investigating the association between longitudinal cartilage loss (increase in cartilage lesions) and change in symptoms (WOMAC) was performed by Phan *et al.*[137] indicating no association in a group of 40 subjects.

The assessment of cartilage volume or thickness loss appears to be a valid indicator of particular clinical outcomes such as the likelihood of progression to knee replacement surgery.[138] Cicuttini and colleagues followed 113 subjects for a period of four years. Individuals who were in the top tertile of rate of cartilage loss over two years, had a seven-fold increased risk of progressing to a TKA within four years, compared with those in the lower tertile.[139] For every 1% increase in the rate of tibial cartilage loss there was a 20% increased risk of undergoing TKA at four years. Radiographic scores of OA were no significant predictors of TKA. Similar to the previous study, Cicuttini *et al.*[129] reported a trend towards a significant association between change in medial tibio-femoral cartilage volume and TKA at four years (odds ratio (OR) $= 9.0$, $p = 0.07$), but not change in medial tibio-femoral JSW (OR $= 1.1$, $p = 0.92$). Together these findings indicate that the protection of articular cartilage morphological integrity and structure modification in knee OA could be valuable in the treatment of the disease because it may delay TKA.

Risk Factors of Cartilage Morphology Change (Progression) in OA

Different investigators[140–143] have studied the relationship between knee cartilage morphology and the menisci. Berthiaume *et al.*[140] in a 24-month follow-up study at six-month intervals, investigated the relation between meniscal structural damage and cartilage degeneration. Thirty-two patients were included in the study where highly significant difference in global cartilage volume loss was observed between severe medial meniscal tear and absence of tear. Similarly, a difference was found between the presence of a medial meniscal extrusion and loss of medial compartmental cartilage volume. Raynauld *et al.*[141] followed 107 patients over a period of two years, and reported that severe meniscal extrusion, severe medial tear, medial and/or lateral bone edema, high BMI, weight, and age, were predictors of fast progressors, which were defined as those with knee cartilage volume loss of −13.2%. Two hundred and ninety-four non-osteoarthritic subjects were followed on a two-year longitudinal study to investigate the associations between meniscal extrusion, knee structure, radiographic changes and risk factors for OA.[142] MRI cartilage morphology was studied in terms of tibio-femoral defect scores, tibio-femoral volume, and tibial plateau bone area. The authors reported that meniscal extrusion at baseline was associated with a greater rate of loss of medial tibio-femoral cartilage volume. Sharma and colleagues[143] studied the independent predictive capability of meniscal damage, meniscal extrusion, malalignment, and joint laxity on subsequent tibio-femoral cartilage loss of 251 knees of 153 subjects. Progression was defined as cartilage loss of more than twice the CV for each plate. Cartilage morphology in each plate was quantified based on cartilage volume, denuded bone area, and thickness. In the medial compartment, medial meniscal damage and varus malalignment predicted tibial cartilage volume loss; medial meniscal damage and varus malalignment predicted tibial and femoral denuded bone increase; and varus malalignment predicted tibial thickness loss. In the lateral compartment all outcomes were predicted by the meniscal damage. In contrast to the previous study, meniscal extrusion had inconsistent effects, similar to laxity. The qualitative approach, assessed as worsening of cartilage scores using a WORMS scoring system,[51] was less sensitive in identifying significant risk factors compared to the quantitative measures of cartilage morphology.

The relationship between knee trabecular bone and cartilage morphology was investigated by Lindsey *et al.*[144] and Blumenkrantz *et al.*,[145] who reported that cartilage loss on one side of the knee joint was related to trabecular bone loss on the opposite side of the knee joint. Lindsey *et al.*[144] studied 21 healthy volunteers and 53 patients with varying degrees of knee OA as given by KLG.[112] Authors also observed that patients with varus OA revealed correlations between medial tibia and medial femoral cartilage degeneration, and loss of bone structure in the lateral tibia and lateral condyle. In addition, significant correlations existed between the compartmental differences (lateral minus medial) of cartilage thickness and bone structure. The authors suggested that malalignment of the knee due to cartilage degeneration is associated with bone formation in the diseased condyle and bone resorption in the opposite compartment. The two-year longitudinal study of Blumenkrantz *et al.*[145] on 38 patients established a positive relationship between cartilage changes and localized bone changes closest to the joint line, and a negative relationship between cartilage changes and global bone changes farthest from the joint line.

Cicuttini and colleagues[146] performed the first study on knee alignment and progression. They studied the relationship between knee angle at baseline, and the rate of cartilage loss in knee-OA patients. For this purpose, 117 subjects with knee OA were studied based on standing radiographs and MRI at baseline and 1.9 year follow-up. Results indicated that for every one-degree increase in baseline varus angulation, there was an average annual loss of medial femoral cartilage of $17.7\,\mu$l. In the previously mentioned study of Sharma *et al.*,[143] varus malalignment was a predictor of medial tibial cartilage volume and thickness loss, as well as of femoral denuded bone increase. Eckstein *et al.*[91] studied the same cohort and confirmed a very strong effect of knee alignment on the ratio of medial versus lateral cartilage thickness loss, but did not detect differences in the sub-regional pattern of cartilage loss between varus and neutral knees, and valgus and neutral knees, respectively. In a more recent study of Teichtahl *et al.* and colleagues,[147] change in knee angle was also found to influence the rate of medial tibial cartilage volume loss. Their study consisted on 78 adults, followed over a period of 4.5 years, to determine whether a change in knee alignment between baseline and two years was associated with a change in knee cartilage volume in knee OA in the subsequent 2.5 years. The authors found that progressive change toward genu valgum reduced the annual rate of medial tibial cartilage volume loss in people with knee OA, and suggested that since their measures of change in alignment and cartilage volume were continuous, their results implied that there was an associated increase in the rate of annual medial tibial cartilage volume loss in progressive change toward genu varum. Change in knee angle did not significantly affect the rate of loss of the lateral tibial cartilage volume. The author concluded that their findings might suggest that the reduction of varus malalignment may delay the progression of medial tibio-femoral OA warranting further investigation. The relationship of varus and valgus alignment with the size of the subchondral bone areas has been addressed above.[125]

The relationship between bone marrow lesions (BMLs) and cartilage morphology has been studied by several authors.[148–150] Hunter *et al.*[148] performed a 30-month longitudinal study on 217 patients with primary knee OA observing that enlarging BMLs were strongly associated with more cartilage loss (modified WORMS score), and that any change in BML was mediated by limb alignment. Raynauld and colleagues,[149] using quantitative MRI, observed 107 patients with knee OA over a period of two years, and reported that size change of BMLs was strongly and independently associated with medial cartilage volume loss. In the study of Wluka *et al.*[150] 271 asymptomatic subjects having no history of knee injury, knee pain or clinical knee OA were recruited. MRI of the dominant knee at baseline and two years later was performed to assess the relationship between the presence of BMLs at baseline and change in tibio-femoral cartilage defects and tibial cartilage volume. With respect to cartilage volume, the authors reported that the presence of very large BMLs indicated a trend for increased annual tibial cartilage volume loss.

The presence of cartilage defects has been associated with cartilage volume loss[151,152] among asymptomatic individuals, a reason why it may represent early OA.[138,152,153] Cicuttini and colleagues,[151] prospectively, cross-sectionally, and longitudinally studied the association of cartilage defects with knee cartilage loss in healthy, middle-age adults. The population consisted of 86 subjects with mean age 53.8 years (± 8.8 years), for which MR images were taken at baseline and two-year follow-up. A reduction of 25%, 15%, and 19% in medial tibial cartilage volume, lateral tibial cartilage volume, and total femoral cartilage volume, respectively, was observed in subjects with cartilage defects relative to those with no cartilage defects. In fact, the authors suggested that in the absence of radiographic knee OA, the presence of asymptomatic, non-full thickness medial tibio-femoral cartilage defects might identify healthy individuals most likely to lose knee cartilage. Result of this study were supported by Ding *et al.*[154] on a cross-sectional study of 372 subjects, where cartilage defects were also associated with lower cartilage volume.

Summary

In this chapter, we have discussed what we consider a series of relevant topics with respect to MRI quantification of knee cartilage morphology. Key information can be summarized as follows: In terms of MR pulse sequences for quantitative analysis of cartilage morphology, they should be fast, have short TE, and should yield images with high SNR, high CNR, high-spatial resolution, and no image artifacts. Although SPGR/FLASH sequences are the most common, emerging pulse sequences with higher cartilage to fluid contrast are in the process of validation. Segmentation plays a central role in quantitative imaging-based measures of cartilage morphology. The tomographic capability of MRI yielding 3D scans with aligned-contiguous slices, should be taken into consideration and as an advantage to compute 3D measures. Morphological analysis of cartilage based on small regions, may be more sensitive to change than global metrics. The technical accuracy and precision of quantitative measurements of cartilage morphology have been validated, and any new technique should be tested and validated. This process should be done in conditions that are similar to those encountered *in vivo*. The clinical utility of quantitative MRI cartilage morphology in knee OA is undergoing a strong validation process that looks promising. Cross-sectional and longitudinal studies have demonstrated the effectiveness of MRI at detecting cartilage loss over time, differentiating between patients with knee OA from those without it, establishing relationships with other tissues within the joint, as well as indicating relationships with several risk factors and an important clinical outcome, such as TKA. Studies mentioned in this chapter and many others omitted due to space constraints, as well as future results of the OAI, warrant further investigation to better understand and treat knee OA.

References

1. Hunziker EB, Quinn TM, Hauselmann HJ. Quantitative structural organization of normal adult human articular cartilage. *Osteoarthr Cartil* 2002;10(7):564–572.
2. Mow VC, Ateshian GA, Spilker RL. Biomechanics of diarthrodial joints: a review of twenty years of progress. *J Biomech Eng* 1993;115(4B):460–467.
3. Mow VC, Holmes MH, Lai WM. Fluid transport and mechanical properties of articular cartilage: a review. *J Biomech* 1984;17(5):377–394.
4. Felson DT, Zhang Y, Hannan MT, Naimark A, Weissman BN, Aliabadi P, Levy D. The incidence and natural history of knee osteoarthritis in the elderly. The Framingham Osteoarthritis Study. *Arthritis Rheum* 1995;38(10):1500–1505.
5. Vignon E, Conrozier T, Piperno M, Richard S, Carrillon Y, Fantino O. Radiographic assessment of hip and knee osteoarthritis. Recommendations: recommended guidelines. *Osteoarthr Cartil* 1999;7(4):434–436.
6. Brandt KD, Mazzuca SA, Conrozier T, Dacre JE, Peterfy CG, Provvedini D, Ravaud P, Taccoen A, Vignon E. Which is the best radiographic protocol for a clinical trial of a structure modifying drug in patients with knee osteoarthritis? *J Rheumatol* 2002;29(6):1308–1320.
7. Buckland-Wright C. Review of the anatomical and radiological differences between fluoroscopic and non-fluoroscopic positioning of osteoarthritic knees. *Osteoarthr Cartil* 2006;14(Suppl A):A19–31.
8. Le Graverand MP, Mazzuca S, Lassere M, Guermazi A, Pickering E, Brandt K, Peterfy C, Cline G, Nevitt M, Woodworth T, Conaghan P, Vignon E. Assessment of the radioanatomic positioning of the osteoarthritic knee in serial radiographs: comparison of three acquisition techniques. *Osteoarthr Cartil* 2006;14(Suppl A): A37–43.
9. Ding C, Cicuttini F, Jones G. How important is MRI for detecting early osteoarthritis? *Nat Clin Pract Rheumatol* 2008;4(1):4–5.
10. Brandt KD, Fife RS, Braunstein EM, Katz B. Radiographic grading of the severity of knee osteoarthritis: relation of the Kellgren and Lawrence grade to a grade based on joint space narrowing, and correlation with arthroscopic evidence of articular cartilage degeneration. *Arthritis Rheum* 1991;34(11):1381–1386.
11. Gale DR, Chaisson CE, Totterman SM, Schwartz RK, Gale ME, Felson D. Meniscal subluxation: association with osteoarthritis and joint space narrowing. *Osteoarthr Cartil* 1999;7(6):526–532.
12. Adams JG, McAlindon T, Dimasi M, Carey J, Eustace S. Contribution of meniscal extrusion and cartilage loss to joint space narrowing in osteoarthritis. *Clin Radiol* 1999;54(8):502–506.
13. Hunter DJ, Zhang YQ, Tu X, Lavalley M, Niu JB, Amin S, Guermazi A, Genant H, Gale D, Felson DT. Change in joint space width: hyaline articular cartilage loss or alteration in meniscus? *Arthritis Rheum* 2006;54(8):2488–2495.
14. Eckstein F, Hudelmaier M, Putz R. The effects of exercise on human articular cartilage. *J Anat* 2006;208(4):491–512.
15. Gold GE, Burstein D, Dardzinski B, Lang P, Boada F, Mosher T. MRI of articular cartilage in OA: novel pulse sequences and compositional/functional markers. *Osteoarthr Cartil* 2006;14(Suppl A):A76–86.

16. Eckstein F, Cicuttini F, Raynauld JP, Waterton JC, Peterfy C. Magnetic resonance imaging (MRI) of articular cartilage in knee osteoarthritis (OA): morphological assessment. *Osteoarthr Cartil* 2006;14(Suppl A):A46–75.

17. Hardy PA, Recht MP, Piraino DW. Fat suppressed MRI of articular cartilage with a spatial-spectral excitation pulse. *J Magn Reson Imaging* 1998;8(6):1279–1287.

18. Glaser C, Faber S, Eckstein F, Fischer H, Springer V, Heudorfer L, Stammberger T, Englmeier KH, Reiser M. Optimization and validation of a rapid high-resolution T1-w 3D FLASH water excitation MRI sequence for the quantitative assessment of articular cartilage volume and thickness. *Magn Reson Imaging* 2001;19(2): 177–185.

19. Mohr A, Priebe M, Taouli B, Grimm J, Heller M, Brossmann J. Selective water excitation for faster MR imaging of articular cartilage defects: initial clinical results. *Eur Radiol* 2003;13(4):686–689.

20. Hardya PA, Newmark R, Liu YM, Meier D, Norris S, Piraino DW, Shah A. The influence of the resolution and contrast on measuring the articular cartilage volume in magnetic resonance images. *Magn Reson Imaging* 2000;18(8):965–972.

21. Link TM, Majumdar S, Peterfy C, Daldrup HE, Uffmann M, Dowling C, Steinbach L, Genant HK. High resolution MRI of small joints: impact of spatial resolution on diagnostic performance and SNR. *Magn Reson Imaging* 1998;16(2): 147–155.

22. Marshall KW, Guthrie BT, Mikulis DJ. Quantitative cartilage imaging. *Br J Rheumatol* 1995;34(Suppl 1):29–31.

23. Cicuttini F, Morris KF, Glisson M, Wluka AE. Slice thickness in the assessment of medial and lateral tibial cartilage volume and accuracy for the measurement of change in a longitudinal study. *J Rheumatol* 2004;31(12):2444–2448.

24. Zhai G, Ding C, Cicuttini F, Jones G. Optimal sampling of MRI slices for the assessment of knee cartilage volume for cross-sectional and longitudinal studies. *BMC Musculoskelet Disord* 2005;6:10.

25. Eckstein F, Charles HC, Buck RJ, Kraus VB, Remmers AE, Hudelmaier M, Wirth W, Evelhoch JL. Accuracy and precision of quantitative assessment of cartilage morphology by magnetic resonance imaging at 3.0T. *Arthritis Rheum* 2005;52(10):3132–3136.

26. Tieschky M, Faber S, Haubner M, Kolem H, Schulte E, Englmeier KH, Reiser M, Eckstein F. Repeatability of patellar cartilage thickness patterns in the living, using a fat-suppressed magnetic resonance imaging sequence with short acquisition time and three-dimensional data processing. *J Orthop Res* 1997;15(6):808–813.

27. Eckstein F, Tieschky M, Faber SC, Haubner M, Kolem H, Englmeier KH, Reiser M. Effect of physical exercise on cartilage volume and thickness *in vivo*: MR imaging study. *Radiology* 1998;207(1):243–248.

28. Eckstein F, Tieschky M, Faber S, Englmeier KH, Reiser M. Functional analysis of articular cartilage deformation, recovery, and fluid flow following dynamic exercise *in vivo*. *Anat Embryol (Berl)* 1999;200(4):419–424.

29. Hohe J, Faber S, Muehlbauer R, Reiser M, Englmeier KH, Eckstein F. Three-dimensional analysis and visualization of regional MR signal intensity distribution of articular cartilage. *Med Eng Phys* 2002;24(3):219–227.

30. Stammberger T, Herberhold C, Faber S, Englmeier KH, Reiser M, Eckstein F. A method for quantifying time dependent changes in MR signal intensity of articular cartilage as a function of tissue deformation in intact joints. *Med Eng Phys* 1998;20(10):741–749.

31. Disler DG. Fat-suppressed three-dimensional spoiled gradient-recalled MR imaging: assessment of articular and physeal hyaline cartilage. *AJR Am J Roentgenol* 1997;169(4):1117–1123.

32. Recht MP, Piraino DW, Paletta GA, Schils JP, Belhobek GH. Accuracy of fat-suppressed three-dimensional spoiled gradient-echo FLASH MR imaging in the detection of patellofemoral articular cartilage abnormalities. *Radiology* 1996;198(1):209–212.

33. Wang SF, Cheng HC, Chang CY. Fat-suppressed three-dimensional fast spoiled gradient-recalled echo imaging: a modified FS 3D SPGR technique for assessment of patellofemoral joint chondromalacia. *Clin Imaging* 1999;23(3): 177–180.

34. Peterfy CG, van Dijke CF, Janzen DL, Gluer CC, Namba R, Majumdar S, Lang P, Genant HK. Quantification of articular cartilage in the knee with pulsed saturation transfer subtraction and fat-suppressed MR imaging: optimization and validation. *Radiology* 1994;192(2):485–491.

35. Eckstein F, Sittek H, Milz S, Putz R, Reiser M. The morphology of articular cartilage assessed by magnetic resonance imaging (MRI). Reproducibility and anatomical correlation. *Surg Radiol Anat* 1994;16(4):429–438.

36. Eckstein F, Gavazzeni A, Sittek H, Haubner M, Losch A, Milz S, Englmeier KH, Schulte E, Putz R, Reiser M. Determination of knee joint cartilage thickness using three-dimensional magnetic resonance chondro-crassometry (3D MR-CCM). *Magn Reson Med* 1996;36(2):256–265.

37. Eckstein F, Schnier M, Haubner M, Priebsch J, Glaser C, Englmeier KH, Reiser M. Accuracy of cartilage volume and thickness measurements with magnetic resonance imaging. *Clin Orthop Relat Res* 1998;352:137–148.

38. Burgkart R, Glaser C, Hyhlik-Durr A, Englmeier KH, Reiser M, Eckstein F. Magnetic resonance imaging — based assessment of cartilage loss in severe osteoarthritis: accuracy, precision, and diagnostic value. *Arthritis Rheum* 2001;44(9): 2072–2077.

39. Graichen H, von Eisenhart-Rothe R, Vogl T, Englmeier KH, Eckstein F. Quantitative assessment of cartilage status in osteoarthritis by quantitative magnetic resonance imaging: technical validation for use in analysis of cartilage volume and further morphologic parameters. *Arthritis Rheum* 2004;50(3):811–816.

40. Zuo J, Li X, Banerjee S, Han E, Majumdar S. Parallel imaging of knee cartilage at 3 Tesla. *J Magn Reson Imaging* 2007;26(4):1001–1009.

41. Banerjee S, Krug R, Carballido-Gamio J, Kelley DA, Xu D, Vigneron DB, Majumdar S. Rapid *in vivo* musculoskeletal MR with parallel imaging at 7T. *Magn Reson Med* 2008;59(3):655–660.

42. Hargreaves BA, Gold GE, Lang PK, Conolly SM, Pauly JM, Bergman G, Vandevenne J, Nishimura DG. MR imaging of articular cartilage using driven equilibrium. *Magn Reson Med* 1999;42(4):695–703.

43. Peterfy CG, Gold G, Eckstein F, Cicuttini F, Dardzinski B, Stevens R. MRI protocols for whole-organ assessment of the knee in osteoarthritis. *Osteoarthr Cartil* 2006;14(Suppl A):A95–111.

44. Peterfy CG, Schneider E, Nevitt M. The osteoarthritis initiative: report on the design rationale for the magnetic resonance imaging protocol for the knee. *Osteoarthr Cartil* 2008;16(12):1433–1441.

45. Gold GE, Hargreaves BA, Reeder SB, Vasanawala SS, Beaulieu CF. Controversies in protocol selection in the imaging of articular cartilage. *Semin Musculoskelet Radiol* 2005;9(2):161–172.

46. Eckstein F, Hudelmaier M, Wirth W, Kiefer B, Jackson R, Yu J, Eaton CB, Schneider E. Double echo steady state magnetic resonance imaging of knee articular cartilage at 3 Tesla: a pilot study for the Osteoarthritis Initiative. *Ann Rheum Dis* 2006;65(4):433–441.

47. Eckstein F, Kunz M, Hudelmaier M, Jackson R, Yu J, Eaton CB, Schneider E. Impact of coil design on the contrast-to-noise ratio, precision, and consistency of quantitative cartilage morphometry at 3 Tesla: a pilot study for the osteoarthritis initiative. *Magn Reson Med* 2007;57(2):448–454.

48. Eckstein F, Kunz M, Schutzer M, Hudelmaier M, Jackson RD, Yu J, Eaton CB, Schneider E. Two year longitudinal change and test-retest-precision of knee cartilage morphology in a pilot study for the osteoarthritis initiative. *Osteoarthr Cartil* 2007;15(11):1326–1332.

49. Hunter DJ, Niu J, Zhang Y, Totterman S, Tamez J, Dabrowski C, Davies R, Hellio Le Graverand MP, Luchi M, Tymofyeyev Y, Beals CR. Change in cartilage morphometry: a sample of the progression cohort of the Osteoarthritis Initiative. *Ann Rheum Dis* 2009;68:349–356.

50. Eckstein F, Maschek S, Wirth W, Hudelmaier M, Hitzl W, Wyman B, Nevitt M, Hellio Le Graverand MP. One year change of knee cartilage morphology in the first release of participants from the Osteoarthritis Initiative progression subcohort — association with sex, body mass index, symptoms, and radiographic osteoarthritis status. *Ann Rheum Dis* 2009;68:674–679.

51. Peterfy CG, Guermazi A, Zaim S, Tirman PF, Miaux Y, White D, Kothari M, Lu Y, Fye K, Zhao S, Genant HK. Whole-Organ Magnetic Resonance Imaging Score (WORMS) of the knee in osteoarthritis. *Osteoarthr Cartil* 2004;12(3):177–190.

52. Kornaat PR, Ceulemans RY, Kroon HM, Riyazi N, Kloppenburg M, Carter WO, Woodworth TG, Bloem JL. MRI assessment of knee osteoarthritis: Knee Osteoarthritis Scoring System (KOSS) — inter-observer and intra-observer reproducibility of a compartment-based scoring system. *Skeletal Radiol* 2005;34(2):95–102.

53. Hunter DJ, Lo GH, Gale D, Grainger AJ, Guermazi A, Conaghan PG. The reliability of a new scoring system for knee osteoarthritis MRI and the validity of bone marrow lesion assessment: BLOKS (Boston Leeds Osteoarthritis Knee Score). *Ann Rheum Dis* 2008;67(2):206–211.

54. Hunter DJ, Conaghan PG, Peterfy CG, Bloch D, Guermazi A, Woodworth T, Stevens R, Genant HK. Responsiveness, effect size, and smallest detectable

difference of Magnetic Resonance Imaging in knee osteoarthritis. *Osteoarthr Cartil* 2006;14(Suppl A):A112–115.

55. Eckstein F, Ateshian G, Burgkart R, Burstein D, Cicuttini F, Dardzinski B, Gray M, Link TM, Majumdar S, Mosher T, Peterfy C, Totterman S, Waterton J, Winalski CS, Felson D. Proposal for a nomenclature for magnetic resonance imaging based measures of articular cartilage in osteoarthritis. *Osteoarthr Cartil* 2006;14(10): 974–983.

56. Eckstein F, Reiser M, Englmeier KH, Putz R. *In vivo* morphometry and functional analysis of human articular cartilage with quantitative magnetic resonance imaging — from image to data, from data to theory. *Anat Embryol (Berl)* 2001;203(3): 147–173.

57. Eckstein F, Winzheimer M, Hohe J, Englmeier KH, Reiser M. Interindividual variability and correlation among morphological parameters of knee joint cartilage plates: analysis with three-dimensional MR imaging. *Osteoarthr Cartil* 2001;9(2):101–111.

58. Faber SC, Eckstein F, Lukasz S, Muhlbauer R, Hohe J, Englmeier KH, Reiser M. Gender differences in knee joint cartilage thickness, volume and articular surface areas: assessment with quantitative three-dimensional MR imaging. *Skeletal Radiol* 2001;30(3):144–150.

59. Otterness IG, Eckstein F. Women have thinner cartilage and smaller joint surfaces than men after adjustment for body height and weight. *Osteoarthr Cartil* 2007;15(6):666–672.

60. Cicuttini F, Forbes A, Morris K, Darling S, Bailey M, Stuckey S. Gender differences in knee cartilage volume as measured by magnetic resonance imaging. *Osteoarthr Cartil* 1999;7(3):265–271.

61. Otterness IG, Le Graverand MP, Eckstein F. Allometric relationships between knee cartilage volume, thickness, surface area and body dimensions. *Osteoarthr Cartil* 2008;16(1):34–40.

62. Burgkart R, Glaser C, Hinterwimmer S, Hudelmaier M, Englmeier KH, Reiser M, Eckstein F. Feasibility of T and Z scores from magnetic resonance imaging data for quantification of cartilage loss in osteoarthritis. *Arthritis Rheum* 2003;48(10): 2829–2835.

63. Lee KY, Dunn TC, Steinbach LS, Ozhinsky E, Ries MD, Majumdar S. Computer-aided quantification of focal cartilage lesions of osteoarthritic knee using MRI. *Magn Reson Imaging* 2004;22(8):1105–1115.

64. Lee KY, Masi JN, Sell CA, Schier R, Link TM, Steinbach LS, Safran M, Ma B, Majumdar S. Computer-aided quantification of focal cartilage lesions using MRI: accuracy and initial arthroscopic comparison. *Osteoarthr Cartil* 2005;13(8): 728–737.

65. Graichen H, Al-Shamari D, Hinterwimmer S, von Eisenhart-Rothe R, Vogl T, Eckstein F. Accuracy of quantitative magnetic resonance imaging in the detection of *ex vivo* focal cartilage defects. *Ann Rheum Dis* 2005;64(8):1120–1125.

66. Cohen ZA, McCarthy DM, Kwak SD, Legrand P, Fogarasi F, Ciaccio EJ, Ateshian GA. Knee cartilage topography, thickness, and contact areas from MRI: *in-vitro* calibration and *in-vivo* measurements. *Osteoarthr Cartil* 1999;7(1):95–109.

67. Cohen ZA, McCarthy DM, Ateshian GA, Kwak SD, Peterfy CG, Alderson P, et al. Knee joint cartilage topography, thickness, and contact areas: validation of measurements from MRI. *ASME Proc Bioeng Conf* 1997;BED 35:45–46 (Abstract).

68. Ahmad CS, Cohen ZA, Levine WN, Ateshian GA, Mow VC. Biomechanical and topographic considerations for autologous osteochondral grafting in the knee. *Am J Sports Med* 2001;29(2):201–206.

69. Stammberger T, Eckstein F, Michaelis M, Englmeier KH, Reiser M. Inter-observer reproducibility of quantitative cartilage measurements: comparison of B-spline snakes and manual segmentation. *Magn Reson Imaging* 1999;17(7): 1033–1042.

70. Lynch JA, Zaim S, Zhao J, Stork A, Peterfy CG, Genant HK. Cartilage segmentation of 3D MRI scans of the osteoarthritic knee combining user knowledge and active contours. *Proc. SPIE* Vol. 3979, pp. 925–935, Medical Imaging 2000: Image Processing, Kenneth M. Hanson; Ed.

71. Grau V, Mewes AU, Alcaniz M, Kikinis R, Warfield SK. Improved watershed transform for medical image segmentation using prior information. *IEEE Trans Med Imaging* 2004;23(4):447–458.

72. Pakin SK, Tamez-Pena JG, Totterman S, Parker KJ. Segmentation, surface extraction, and thickness computation of articular cartilage. *Proc SPIE* Vol. 4684, pp. 155–166, Medical Imaging 2002: Image Processing, Milan Sonka; J. Michael Fitzpatrick; Eds.

73. Warfield SK, Kaus M, Jolesz FA, Kikinis R. Adaptive, template moderated, spatially varying statistical classification. *Med Image Anal* 2000;4(1):43–55.

74. Stammberger T, Eckstein F, Englmeier KH, Reiser M. Determination of 3D cartilage thickness data from MR imaging: computational method and reproducibility in the living. *Magn Reson Med* 1999;41(3):529–536.

75. Hohe J, Ateshian G, Reiser M, Englmeier KH, Eckstein F. Surface size, curvature analysis, and assessment of knee joint incongruity with MRI *in vivo*. *Magn Reson Med* 2002;47(3):554–561.

76. Carballido-Gamio J, Bauer JS, Stahl R, Lee KY, Krause S, Link TM, Majumdar S. Inter-subject comparison of MRI knee cartilage thickness. *Med Image Anal* 2008;12(2):120–135.

77. Kauffmann C, Gravel P, Godbout B, Gravel A, Beaudoin G, Raynauld JP, Martel-Pelletier J, Pelletier JP, de Guise JA. Computer-aided method for quantification of cartilage thickness and volume changes using MRI: validation study using a synthetic model. *IEEE Trans Biomed Eng* 2003;50(8):978–988.

78. Ateshian GA, Soslowsky LJ, Mow VC. Quantitation of articular surface topography and cartilage thickness in knee joints using stereophotogrammetry. *J Biomech* 1991;24(8):761–776.

79. Kshirsagar AA, Watson PJ, Tyler JA, Hall LD. Measurement of localized cartilage volume and thickness of human knee joints by computer analysis of three-dimensional magnetic resonance images. *Invest Radiol* 1998;33(5):289–299.

80. Koo S, Gold GE, Andriacchi TP. Considerations in measuring cartilage thickness using MRI: factors influencing reproducibility and accuracy. *Osteoarthr Cartil* 2005;13(9):782–789.

81. Stammberger T, Hohe J, Englmeier KH, Reiser M, Eckstein F. Elastic registration of 3D cartilage surfaces from MR image data for detecting local changes in cartilage thickness. *Magn Reson Med* 2000;44(4):592–601.

82. Lynch JA, Zaim S, Zhao J, Peterfy CG, Genant HK. Automating measurement of subtle changes in articular cartilage from MRI of the knee by combining 3D image registration and segmentation. San Diego, CA, 2001.

83. Jaremko JL, Cheng RW, Lambert RG, Habib AF, Ronsky JL. Reliability of an efficient MRI-based method for estimation of knee cartilage volume using surface registration. *Osteoarthr Cartil* 2006;14(9):914–922.

84. Pelletier JP, Raynauld JP, Berthiaume MJ, Abram F, Choquette D, Haraoui B, Beary JF, Cline GA, Meyer JM, Martel-Pelletier J. Risk factors associated with the loss of cartilage volume on weight-bearing areas in knee osteoarthritis patients assessed by quantitative magnetic resonance imaging: a longitudinal study. *Arthritis Res Ther* 2007;9(4):R74.

85. Carballido-Gamio J, Link TM, Majumdar S. New techniques for cartilage magnetic resonance imaging relaxation time analysis: texture analysis of flattened cartilage and localized intra- and inter-subject comparisons. *Magn Reson Med* 2008;59(6):1472–1477.

86. Cohen ZA, Mow VC, Henry JH, Levine WN, Ateshian GA. Templates of the cartilage layers of the patellofemoral joint and their use in the assessment of osteoarthritic cartilage damage. *Osteoarthr Cartil* 2003;11(8):569–579.

87. Stahl R, Blumenkrantz G, Carballido-Gamio J, Zhao S, Munoz T, Hellio Le Graverand-Gastineau MP, Li X, Majumdar S, Link TM. MRI-derived T2 relaxation times and cartilage morphometry of the tibio-femoral joint in subjects with and without osteoarthritis during a 1-year follow-up. *Osteoarthr Cartil* 2007;15(11): 1225–1234.

88. Wirth W, Eckstein F. A technique for regional analysis of femorotibial cartilage thickness based on quantitative magnetic resonance imaging. *IEEE Trans Med Imaging* 2008;27(6):737–744.

89. Wirth W, Hellio Le Graverand MP, Wyman BT, Maschek S, Hudelmaier M, Hitzl W, Nevitt M, Eckstein F. Regional analysis of femorotibial cartilage loss in a subsample from the Osteoarthritis Initiative progression subcohort. *Osteoarthr Cartil* 2009;17(3):291–297.

90. Hellio Le Graverand MP, Buck RJ, Wyman BT, Vignon E, Mazzuca SA, Brandt KD, Piperno M, Charles HC, Hudelmaier M, Hunter DJ, Jackson C, Kraus VB, Link TM, Majumdar S, Prasad PV, Schnitzer TJ, Vaz A, Wirth W, Eckstein F. Change in regional cartilage morphology and joint space width in osteoarthritis participants versus healthy controls — a multicenter study using 3.0 Tesla MRI and Lyon Schuss radiography. *Ann Rheum Dis* (in press).

91. Eckstein F, Wirth W, Hudelmaier M, Stein V, Lengfelder V, Cahue S, Marshall M, Prasad P, Sharma L. Patterns of femorotibial cartilage loss in knees with neutral, varus, and valgus alignment. *Arthritis Rheum* 2008;59(11):1563–1570.

92. Sittek H, Eckstein F, Gavazzeni A, Milz S, Kiefer B, Schulte E, Reiser M. Assessment of normal patellar cartilage volume and thickness using MRI: an analysis of currently available pulse sequences. *Skeletal Radiol* 1996;25(1):55–62.

93. Eckstein F, Sittek H, Milz S, Schulte E, Kiefer B, Reiser M, Putz R. The potential of magnetic resonance imaging (MRI) for quantifying articular cartilage thickness — a methodological study. *Clin Biomech (Bristol, Avon)* 1995;10(8):434–440.

94. Eckstein F, Sittek H, Gavazzeni A, Schulte E, Milz S, Kiefer B, Reiser M, Putz R. Magnetic resonance chondro-crassometry (MR CCM): a method for accurate determination of articular cartilage thickness? *Magn Reson Med* 1996;35(1): 89–96.

95. Eckstein F, Adam C, Sittek H, Becker C, Milz S, Schulte E, Reiser M, Putz R. Non-invasive determination of cartilage thickness throughout joint surfaces using magnetic resonance imaging. *J Biomech* 1997;30(3):285–289.

96. Haubner M, Eckstein F, Schnier M, Losch A, Sittek H, Becker C, Kolem H, Reiser M, Englmeier KH. A non-invasive technique for 3-dimensional assessment of articular cartilage thickness based on MRI. Part 2: Validation using CT arthrography. *Magn Reson Imaging* 1997;15(7):805–813.

97. Glüer CC, Blake G, Blunt BA, Jergas M, Genant HK. Accurate assessment of precision errors: How to measure the reproducibility of bone densitometry techniques. *Osteoporosis Int* 1995;5:262–270.

98. Eckstein F, Burstein D, Link TM. Quantitative MRI of cartilage and bone: degenerative changes in osteoarthritis. *NMR Biomed* 2006;19(7):822–854.

99. Hyhlik-Durr A, Faber S, Burgkart R, Stammberger T, Maag KP, Englmeier KH, Reiser M, Eckstein F. Precision of tibial cartilage morphometry with a coronal water-excitation MR sequence. *Eur Radiol* 2000;10(2):297–303.

100. Eckstein F, Lemberger B, Gratzke C, Hudelmaier M, Glaser C, Englmeier KH, Reiser M. *In vivo* cartilage deformation after different types of activity and its dependence on physical training status. *Ann Rheum Dis* 2005;64(2):291–295.

101. Kornaat PR, Reeder SB, Koo S, Brittain JH, Yu H, Andriacchi TP, Gold GE. MR imaging of articular cartilage at 1.5T and 3.0T: comparison of SPGR and SSFP sequences. *Osteoarthr Cartil* 2005;13(4):338–344.

102. Kornaat PR, Koo S, Andriacchi TP, Bloem JL, Gold GE. Comparison of quantitative cartilage measurements acquired on two 3.0T MRI systems from different manufacturers. *J Magn Reson Imaging* 2006;23(5):770–773.

103. Eckstein F, Buck RJ, Burstein D, Charles HC, Crim J, Hudelmaier M, Hunter DJ, Hutchins G, Jackson C, Kraus VB, Lane NE, Link TM, Majumdar LS, Mazzuca S, Prasad PV, Schnitzer TJ, Taljanovic MS, Vaz A, Wyman B, Le Graverand MP. Precision of 3.0 Tesla quantitative magnetic resonance imaging of cartilage morphology in a multicentre clinical trial. *Ann Rheum Dis* 2008;67(12):1683–1688.

104. Hudelmaier M, Glaser C, Hohe J, Englmeier KH, Reiser M, Putz R, Eckstein F. Age-related changes in the morphology and deformational behavior of knee joint cartilage. *Arthritis Rheum* 2001;44(11):2556–2561.

105. Hudelmaier M, Glaser C, Englmeier KH, Reiser M, Putz R, Eckstein F. Correlation of knee-joint cartilage morphology with muscle cross-sectional areas vs. anthropometric variables. *Anat Rec A Discov Mol Cell Evol Biol* 2003;270(2):175–184.

106. Beattie KA, Duryea J, Pui M, O'Neill J, Boulos P, Webber CE, Eckstein F, Adachi JD. Minimum joint space width and tibial cartilage morphology in the knees of healthy individuals: a cross-sectional study. *BMC Musculoskelet Disord* 2008;9:119.

107. Jones G, Ding C, Scott F, Glisson M, Cicuttini F. Early radiographic osteoarthritis is associated with substantial changes in cartilage volume and tibial bone surface area in both males and females. *Osteoarthr Cartil* 2004;12(2):169–174.

108. Hellio Le Graverand MP, Buck RJ, Wyman BT, Vignon E, Mazzuca SA, Brandt KD, Piperno M, Charles HC, Hudelmaier M, Hunter DJ, Jackson C, Kraus VB, Link TM, Majumdar S, Prasad PV, Schnitzer TJ, Vaz A, Wirth W, Eckstein F. Subregional femorotibial cartilage morphology in women — comparison between healthy controls and participants with different grades of radiographic knee osteoarthritis. *Osteoarthr Cartil* 2009.

109. Hunter DJ, Niu J, Zhang YQ, McLennan C, LaValley M, Tu X, Hudelmaier M, Eckstein F, Felson DT. Cartilage volume must be normalized to bone surface area in order to provide satisfactory construct validity: The Framingham study. *Osteoarthr Cartil* 2004;12(Suppl B):S2.

110. von Eisenhart-Rothe R, Graichen H, Hudelmaier M, Vogl T, Sharma L, Eckstein F. Femorotibial and patellar cartilage loss in patients prior to total knee arthroplasty, heterogeneity, and correlation with alignment of the knee. *Ann Rheum Dis* 2006;65(1):69–73.

111. Reichenbach S, Yang M, Eckstein F, Niu J, Hunter DJ, McLennan CE, Guermazi A, Roemer FW, Hudelmaier M, Aliabadi P, Felson DT. Do cartilage volume or thickness distinguish knees with and without mild radiographic osteoarthritis? The Framingham Study. *Ann Rheum Dis* 2009.

112. Kellgren J, Lawrence J. Radiologic assessment of osteoarthritis. *Ann Rheum Dis* 1957;16:494–502.

113. Calvo E, Palacios I, Delgado E, Ruiz-Cabello J, Hernandez P, Sanchez-Pernaute O, Egido J, Herrero-Beaumont G. High-resolution MRI detects cartilage swelling at the early stages of experimental osteoarthritis. *Osteoarthr Cartil* 2001;9(5): 463–472.

114. Calvo E, Palacios I, Delgado E, Sanchez-Pernaute O, Largo R, Egido J, Herrero-Beaumont G. Histopathological correlation of cartilage swelling detected by magnetic resonance imaging in early experimental osteoarthritis. *Osteoarthr Cartil* 2004;12(11):878–886.

115. Watson PJ, Carpenter TA, Hall LD, Tyler JA. Cartilage swelling and loss in a spontaneous model of osteoarthritis visualized by magnetic resonance imaging. *Osteoarthr Cartil* 1996;4(3):197–207.

116. Vignon E, Arlot M, Hartmann D, Moyen B, Ville G. Hypertrophic repair of articular cartilage in experimental osteoarthrosis. *Ann Rheum Dis* 1983;42(1):82–88.

117. Adams ME, Brandt KD. Hypertrophic repair of canine articular cartilage in osteoarthritis after anterior cruciate ligament transection. *J Rheumatol* 1991;18(3):428–435.

118. Andreisek G, White LM, Sussman MS, Kunz M, Hurtig M, Weller I, Essue J, Marks P, Eckstein F. Quantitative MR imaging evaluation of the cartilage thickness and subchondral bone area in patients with ACL-reconstructions 7 years after surgery. *Osteoarthr Cartil* 2009;17(7):857–864.

119. Wluka AE, Wolfe R, Davis SR, Stuckey S, Cicuttini FM. Tibial cartilage volume change in healthy postmenopausal women: a longitudinal study. *Ann Rheum Dis* 2004;63(4):444–449.

120.   Hanna F, Ebeling PR, Wang Y, O'Sullivan R, Davis S, Wluka AE, Cicuttini FM. Factors influencing longitudinal change in knee cartilage volume measured from magnetic resonance imaging in healthy men. *Ann Rheum Dis* 2005;64(7): 1038–1042.

121.   Wluka AE, Stuckey S, Snaddon J, Cicuttini FM. The determinants of change in tibial cartilage volume in osteoarthritic knees. *Arthritis Rheum* 2002;46(8):2065–2072.

122.   Ding C, Cicuttini F, Blizzard L, Scott F, Jones G. A longitudinal study of the effect of sex and age on rate of change in knee cartilage volume in adults. *Rheumatology (Oxford)* 2007;46(2):273–279.

123.   Cicuttini F, Wluka A, Wang Y, Stuckey S. The determinants of change in patella cartilage volume in osteoarthritic knees. *J Rheumatol* 2002;29(12):2615–2619.

124.   Wang Y, Wluka AE, Cicuttini FM. The determinants of change in tibial plateau bone area in osteoarthritic knees: a cohort study. *Arthritis Res Ther* 2005;7(3):R687–693.

125.   Eckstein F, Hudelmaier M, Cahue S, Marshall M, Sharma L. Medial-to-lateral ratio of tibiofemoral subchondral bone area is adapted to alignment and mechanical load. *Calcif Tissue Int* 2009;84(3):186–194.

126.   Gandy SJ, Dieppe PA, Keen MC, Maciewicz RA, Watt I, Waterton JC. No loss of cartilage volume over three years in patients with knee osteoarthritis as assessed by magnetic resonance imaging. *Osteoarthr Cartil* 2002;10(12):929–937.

127.   Frobell RB, Le Graverand MP, Buck R, Roos EM, Roos HP, Tamez-Pena J, Totterman S, Lohmander LS. The acutely ACL injured knee assessed by MRI: changes in joint fluid, bone marrow lesions, and cartilage during the first year. *Osteoarthr Cartil* 2009;17(2):161–167.

128.   Cicuttini FM, Wluka AE, Forbes A, Wolfe R. Comparison of tibial cartilage volume and radiologic grade of the tibiofemoral joint. *Arthritis Rheum* 2003;48(3): 682–688.

129.   Cicuttini F, Hankin J, Jones G, Wluka A. Comparison of conventional standing knee radiographs and magnetic resonance imaging in assessing progression of tibiofemoral joint osteoarthritis. *Osteoarthr Cartil* 2005;13(8):722–727.

130.   Cicuttini FM, Wluka AE, Hankin J, Stuckey S. Comparison of patella cartilage volume and radiography in the assessment of longitudinal joint change at the patellofemoral joint. *J Rheumatol* 2004;31(7):1369–1372.

131.   Raynauld JP, Martel-Pelletier J, Berthiaume MJ, Labonte F, Beaudoin G, de Guise JA, Bloch DA, Choquette D, Haraoui B, Altman RD, Hochberg MC, Meyer JM, Cline GA, Pelletier JP. Quantitative magnetic resonance imaging evaluation of knee osteoarthritis progression over two years and correlation with clinical symptoms and radiologic changes. *Arthritis Rheum* 2004;50(2):476–487.

132.   Bruyere O, Genant H, Kothari M, Zaim S, White D, Peterfy C, Burlet N, Richy F, Ethgen D, Montague T, Dabrowski C, Reginster JY. Longitudinal study of magnetic resonance imaging and standard X-rays to assess disease progression in osteoarthritis. *Osteoarthr Cartil* 2007;15(1):98–103.

133.   Link TM, Steinbach LS, Ghosh S, Ries M, Lu Y, Lane N, Majumdar S. Osteoarthritis: MR imaging findings in different stages of disease and correlation with clinical findings. *Radiology* 2003;226(2):373–381.

134.   Hunter DJ, March L, Sambrook PN. The association of cartilage volume with knee pain. *Osteoarthr Cartil* 2003;11(10):725–729.

135. Bellamy N, Buchanan WW, Goldsmith CH, Campbell J, Stitt LW. Validation study of WOMAC: a health status instrument for measuring clinically important patient relevant outcomes to antirheumatic drug therapy in patients with osteoarthritis of the hip or knee. *J Rheumatol* 1988;15(12):1833–1840.

136. Wluka AE, Wolfe R, Stuckey S, Cicuttini FM. How does tibial cartilage volume relate to symptoms in subjects with knee osteoarthritis? *Ann Rheum Dis* 2004;63(3):264–268.

137. Phan CM, Link TM, Blumenkrantz G, Dunn TC, Ries MD, Steinbach LS, Majumdar S. MR imaging findings in the follow-up of patients with different stages of knee osteoarthritis and the correlation with clinical symptoms. *Eur Radiol* 2006;16(3):608–618.

138. Teichtahl AJ, Wluka AE, Davies-Tuck ML, Cicuttini FM. Imaging of knee osteoarthritis. *Best Pract Res Clin Rheumatol* 2008;22(6):1061–1074.

139. Cicuttini FM, Jones G, Forbes A, Wluka AE. Rate of cartilage loss at two years predicts subsequent total knee arthroplasty: a prospective study. *Ann Rheum Dis* 2004;63(9):1124–1127.

140. Berthiaume MJ, Raynauld JP, Martel-Pelletier J, Labonte F, Beaudoin G, Bloch DA, Choquette D, Haraoui B, Altman RD, Hochberg M, Meyer JM, Cline GA, Pelletier JP. Meniscal tear and extrusion are strongly associated with progression of symptomatic knee osteoarthritis as assessed by quantitative magnetic resonance imaging. *Ann Rheum Dis* 2005;64(4):556–563.

141. Raynauld JP, Martel-Pelletier J, Berthiaume MJ, Beaudoin G, Choquette D, Haraoui B, Tannenbaum H, Meyer JM, Beary JF, Cline GA, Pelletier JP. Long term evaluation of disease progression through the quantitative magnetic resonance imaging of symptomatic knee osteoarthritis patients: correlation with clinical symptoms and radiographic changes. *Arthritis Res Ther* 2006;8(1):R21.

142. Ding C, Martel-Pelletier J, Pelletier JP, Abram F, Raynauld JP, Cicuttini F, Jones G. Knee meniscal extrusion in a largely non-osteoarthritic cohort: association with greater loss of cartilage volume. *Arthritis Res Ther* 2007;9(2):R21.

143. Sharma L, Eckstein F, Song J, Guermazi A, Prasad P, Kapoor D, Cahue S, Marshall M, Hudelmaier M, Dunlop D. Relationship of meniscal damage, meniscal extrusion, malalignment, and joint laxity to subsequent cartilage loss in osteoarthritic knees. *Arthritis Rheum* 2008;58(6):1716–1726.

144. Lindsey CT, Narasimhan A, Adolfo JM, Jin H, Steinbach LS, Link T, Ries M, Majumdar S. Magnetic resonance evaluation of the interrelationship between articular cartilage and trabecular bone of the osteoarthritic knee(1). *Osteoarthr Cartil* 2004;12(2):86–96.

145. Blumenkrantz G, Lindsey CT, Dunn TC, Jin H, Ries MD, Link TM, Steinbach LS, Majumdar S. A pilot, two-year longitudinal study of the interrelationship between trabecular bone and articular cartilage in the osteoarthritic knee. *Osteoarthr Cartil* 2004;12(12):997–1005.

146. Cicuttini F, Wluka A, Hankin J, Wang Y. Longitudinal study of the relationship between knee angle and tibiofemoral cartilage volume in subjects with knee osteoarthritis. *Rheumatology (Oxford)* 2004;43(3):321–324.

147.   Teichtahl AJ, Davies-Tuck ML, Wluka AE, Jones G, Cicuttini FM. Change in knee angle influences the rate of medial tibial cartilage volume loss in knee osteoarthritis. *Osteoarthr Cartil* 2009;17(1):8–11.

148.   Hunter DJ, Zhang Y, Niu J, Goggins J, Amin S, LaValley MP, Guermazi A, Genant H, Gale D, Felson DT. Increase in bone marrow lesions associated with cartilage loss: a longitudinal magnetic resonance imaging study of knee osteoarthritis. *Arthritis Rheum* 2006;54(5):1529–1535.

149.   Raynauld JP, Martel-Pelletier J, Berthiaume MJ, Abram F, Choquette D, Haraoui B, Beary JF, Cline GA, Meyer JM, Pelletier JP. Correlation between bone lesion changes and cartilage volume loss in patients with osteoarthritis of the knee as assessed by quantitative magnetic resonance imaging over a 24-month period. *Ann Rheum Dis* 2008;67(5):683–688.

150.   Wluka AE, Wang Y, Davies-Tuck M, English DR, Giles GG, Cicuttini FM. Bone marrow lesions predict progression of cartilage defects and loss of cartilage volume in healthy middle-aged adults without knee pain over 2 years. *Rheumatology (Oxford)* 2008;47(9):1392–1396.

151.   Cicuttini F, Ding C, Wluka A, Davis S, Ebeling PR, Jones G. Association of cartilage defects with loss of knee cartilage in healthy, middle-age adults: a prospective study. *Arthritis Rheum* 2005;52(7):2033–2039.

152.   Ding C, Cicuttini F, Scott F, Boon C, Jones G. Association of prevalent and incident knee cartilage defects with loss of tibial and patellar cartilage: a longitudinal study. *Arthritis Rheum* 2005;52(12):3918–3927.

153.   Ding C, Cicuttini F, Scott F, Cooley H, Jones G. Knee structural alteration and BMI: a cross-sectional study. *Obes Res* 2005;13(2):350–361.

154.   Ding C, Garnero P, Cicuttini F, Scott F, Cooley H, Jones G. Knee cartilage defects: association with early radiographic osteoarthritis, decreased cartilage volume, increased joint surface area and type II collagen breakdown. *Osteoarthr Cartil* 2005;13(3):198–205.

7

Functional Imaging of the Knee Joint

by Gabrielle Blumenkrantz, Xiaojuan Li,
Ravinder R. Regatte, Alexej Jerschow
and Sharmila Majumdar

Preview

Osteoarthritis (OA) is one of the most common forms of musculoskeletal degenerative disease. The integrity of cartilage tissue is a significant factor in the initiation and progression of OA. Cartilage has a well-defined biochemical structure.[1] Integrity is provided by the collagen 3D mesh-like framework into which proteoglycans (PGs) are entrapped. The major PGs are glycosaminoglycans (GAGs), a highly negatively-charged, long branch polysaccharide. The negatively-charged GAG attracts ^{23}Na ions in its vicinity. In turn, the high concentration of ^{23}Na produces osmotic pressure, which absorbs large amounts of water into the extracellular matrix. This effect leads to high swelling pressure, providing the favorable load-bearing properties of the cartilage.[2] Cartilage also contains a small population of chondrocytes ($<1\%$ of volume) to maintain the macromolecular moiety.[3]

Although MRI is widely used for the clinical diagnosis of OA, conventional imaging protocols assess degeneration primarily based on morphological changes (late stage in the disease process). Quantitative MR methods for measuring the relaxation properties in cartilage may aid in the diagnosis of early OA prior to irreversible morphologic changes. Such methods, which characterize changes in the molecular composition of the extracellular matrix, include $T_{1\rho}$ relaxometry, ^{23}Na MRI, and gagCEST, T_2 relaxometry, and T_{1Gd} relaxometry (delayed gadolinium enhanced MRI contrast, dGEMRIC). This chapter will review the above MR imaging quantification techniques for cartilage assessment and their applications in OA imaging.

$T_{1\rho}$ Relaxation Time

$T_{1\rho}$ relaxation time describes the spin-lattice relaxation in the rotating frame.[4] It probes the slow motion interactions between motion-restricted water molecules and their local macromolecular environment, and therefore provides unique biochemical information in the low-frequency regime, typically from a few hundred hertz (Hz) to a few kilohertz (kHz). Spin-lock (SL) techniques, first described by Redfield in solid materials,[5] enable the study of $T_{1\rho}$ relaxation at very low field without sacrificing the signal-to-noise ratio (SNR) afforded by higher field strengths. In a SL experiment, spins are flipped into the transverse plane along one axis, immediately after which a long-duration, low energy SL radio-frequency (RF) pulse is applied along the same axis. Since the magnetization and RF field are along the same direction, the magnetization is said to be "spin-locked" provided the locking condition is satisfied, i.e. the magnetic field B_1 of locking pulses is much stronger than the local magnetic fields generated by, for example, magnetic moments of nuclei. Thus, neither the normal transverse relaxation (characterized by the relaxation time T_2) will take place, nor the longitudinal relaxation (characterized by the relaxation time T_1) along B_0 will occur because of the effect of the locking pulse. The spins will relax with a time constant $T_{1\rho}$ along the B_1 of locking pulses in the transverse plane.[4] The amplitude of the SL pulse is commonly referenced in terms of the nutation frequency ($f = \gamma B_1$), where γ is the gyromagnetic ratio of a nuclear species. $T_{1\rho}$ relaxation phenomena are sensitive to physicochemical processes with inverse correlation times on the order of the nutation frequency of the SL pulse. By setting the amplitude of the SL pulse to coincide with the frequency of the molecular processes of interest, the signal from the SL-MRI sequence becomes heavily $T_{1\rho}$-weighted. $T_{1\rho}$ can be computed by acquiring a series of $T_{1\rho}$-weighted images at various SL pulse durations called times of SL (TSLs). $T_{1\rho}$ increases as the strength of the SL field increases, a phenomenon termed $T_{1\rho}$ dispersion. $T_{1\rho}$ dispersions may also have tissue specificity.[4]

As discussed previously in Chapter 1, hyaline articular cartilage is composed by few chondrocytes surrounded by a large extracellular matrix (ECM). The ECM is composed primarily by water and two groups of macromolecules: proteoglycan (PG) and collagen fibers. These macromolecules in the ECM restrict the motion of water protons. Changes to the ECM, such as PG loss, therefore, may be reflected in measurements of $T_{1\rho}$ of water protons. Since the loss of PG has been shown to be an initiating event in early stages of OA, $T_{1\rho}$ mapping may be a promising diagnostic tool for early OA evaluation.[6] *In-vivo* $T_{1\rho}$ quantification techniques have been developed in the past decade for imaging biochemical changes in cartilage matrix. The major applications have been in osteoarthritis (OA) and acutely injured knees that have a high risk of developing OA. We will discuss the details on acquiring $T_{1\rho}$-weighted images, concerns that need to be taken care of during sequence implementation, clinical applications of $T_{1\rho}$ quantifications as well as comparison with T_2 quantifications in the following sections.

Sequence Implementation

The $T_{1\rho}$-weighted imaging sequences are composed of two parts: $T_{1\rho}$ pre-encoding with SL pulse cluster, followed by either two-dimensional (2D) or three-dimensional (3D) data acquisition, as shown in (Fig. 1). The SL pulse cluster consists of a hard 90° pulse followed by a SL pulse and a hard −90° pulse. The first 90° pulse is applied along the x-axis and flips the longitudinal magnetization into the transverse plane along the y-axis. Then, a long low power pulse is applied along the y-axis to spin-lock the magnetization. The second 90° pulse flips this spin-locked magnetization back to the z-axis. The phase of the second half of the SL pulse is shifted 180° from the first half to reduce artifacts caused by $B1$ inhomogeneity.[7] Residual transverse magnetization is dephased by a

G. Blumenkrantz et al.

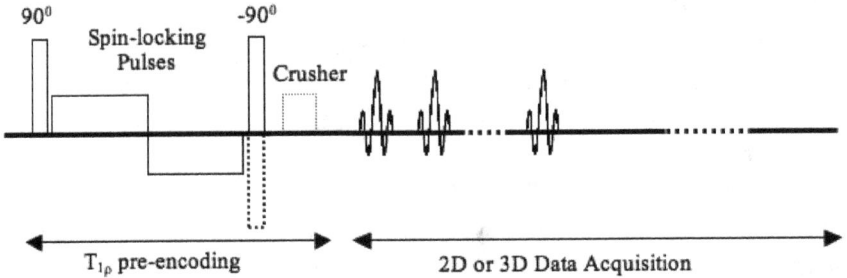

Fig. 1. Diagram of a $T_{1\rho}$-weighted imaging sequence. The sequence is composed of two parts: $T_{1\rho}$ pre-encoding with spin-lock pulse cluster, followed by a 2D or 3D data acquisition.

crusher gradient. Magnetization stored along the z-axis is read out by the following sequences.

Current $T_{1\rho}$ quantification techniques are based on either 2D spin echo (SE), fast spin echo (FSE),[8] spiral imaging,[9] echo planar imaging (EPI)[10] or 3D gradient echo sequences.[11–13] These sequences have been implemented at both 1.5T and 3T on scanners from different manufacturers.

The initial development of $T_{1\rho}$-weighted imaging was based on single-slice 2D spin echo (SE) or fast spin echo (FSE)[8] sequences. $T_{1\rho}$-weighted images with varying TSLs are acquired and the $T_{1\rho}$ maps can be reconstructed pixel-by-pixel using the equation below:

$$S(\text{TSL}) \propto e^{(-\text{TSL}/T_{1\rho})}. \tag{1}$$

The nonselective pulses (hard pulses) used in spin-lock experiments will saturate the longitudinal magnetization from non-excited regions, thus making the implementation of the $T_{1\rho}$ sequence in multi-slice mode not straightforward. Wheaton *et al.* experimentally measured and theoretically modeled this longitudinal saturation as $T_{2\rho}$ decay.[8] The saturation data was used to correct the image data as a function of the TSL to enable quantitative measurements of $T_{1\rho}$ using a multi-slice FSE sequence. The $T_{1\rho}$ quantification using this saturation-corrected multi-slice data was reported to be identical to that measured using single-slice spin-lock sequence.

Li *et al.* developed a multi-slice $T_{1\rho}$-weighted imaging based on spiral acquisition.[9] A spiral interleave from each prescribed slice is acquired in rapid succession, followed by a period of RF and gradient dead-time for T_1

recovery. A RF cycling technique was used to eliminate T_1 contamination in the $T_{1\rho}$-weighted images.[14] In this technique, as first described by Wright *et al.*[14] longitudinal magnetization is inverted immediately after alternate $T_{1\rho}$ preparation. The longitudinal magnetization at the time of acquisition after $T_{1\rho}$ preparation (T_a) can then be described as follows:

$$M_z(T_a) = M_z^{\text{prep}} e^{-T_a/T_1} + M_0(1 - e^{-T_a/T_1}) \quad \text{without inversion} \quad (2)$$

$$M_z(T_a) = -M_z^{\text{prep}} e^{-T_a/T_1} + M_0(1 - e^{-T_a/T_1}) \quad \text{with inversion} \quad (3)$$

where M_z^{prep} is the longitudinal magnetization immediately after $T_{1\rho}$ preparation. The second term of the equation describes the amount of longitudinal recovery between the end of $T_{1\rho}$ preparation and T_a. Subtracting Equation (3) from Equation (2) yields:

$$M_z(T_a) = 2M_z^{\text{prep}} e^{-T_a/T_1} \quad (4)$$

where M_z^{prep} is proportional to $\exp(-\text{TSL}/T_{1\rho})$. By using this RF cycling technique, the T_1 term, as indicated in Equation (4), is constant for a fixed T_a, and therefore does not contaminate the acquired $T_{1\rho}$-weighted images. Instead, the net effect of T_1 is the exponential reduction of SNR with increased T_a. Multiple $T_{1\rho}$-weighted images are acquired with different TSL to reconstruct the $T_{1\rho}$ map. This technique needs no correction and modeling for longitudinal saturation. The $T_{1\rho}$ measurement has been validated using MR spectroscopy method and single-slice acquisition.[9] Reproducibility was assessed using the average coefficient of variation (CV) of median $T_{1\rho}$ that was 0.68% in phantoms and 4.8% in healthy volunteers.[9]

Compared with 2D methods, 3D imaging is free from artifacts caused by slice crosstalk. Therefore 3D sequences can generally have a thinner slice thickness, and consequently may provide a more accurate assessment of cartilage degeneration. High-spatial resolution MRI is particularly attractive in the context of OA where cartilage becomes very thin — on the order of or less than 1 mm. Furthermore, a 3D acquisition is desired due to the non-slice-selective nature of the $T_{1\rho}$ preparation pulses (spin-lock pulses).

Borthakur *et al.* have developed a 3D $T_{1\rho}$ mapping technique based on a steady-state spoiled gradient echo (SPGR) imaging sequence.[11,12,15] This method showed clinical promise at both 1.5 T and 3 T. However, using this method, the energy deposited by the sequence (as estimated by the specific absorption rate, SAR) is high because $T_{1\rho}$ preparation pulses are applied every repetition time (TR). Relatively long TRs (140 ms at 1.5 T and 175 ms at 3 T) are used in order to comply with the maximum SAR mandated by the Food and Drug Administration (FDA). This long TR results in long acquisition times. In addition, this technique requires a prior knowledge of T_1 (or an assumption) for $T_{1\rho}$ quantification as T_1-dependent steady state signals are used.

Very recently, novel 3D acquisitions have been developed for *in vivo* knee $T_{1\rho}$ mapping based on SPGR.[16] (referred as Magnetization-prepared Angle-modulated Partitioned-k-space Spoiled Gradient-Echo Snapshots, MAPSS) and balanced gradient echo (b-GRE).[13] In both methods, transient signal evolving towards the steady-state were acquired, which allows multiple TR acquisitions per spin-lock pre-encoding. Thus, these sequences are less SAR intensive than the previous 3D SPGR $T_{1\rho}$-weighted imaging using the steady-state signals. In MAPSS, the acquisition was an interleaved segmented elliptical centric phase encoding order immediately after a $T_{1\rho}$ magnetization preparation sequence. RF cycling was applied to eliminate the adverse impact of longitudinal relaxation on quantitative accuracy. This RF cycling scheme also yields a transient signal evolution that is independent of the prepared magnetization M_{prep}. A variable flip angle train was designed to provide a flat signal response to eliminate the filtering effect in k-space caused by transient signal evolution. Experiments in phantoms agreed well with results from simulation. Measurements *in vivo* using MAPSS agree well with previously developed 2D methods. The $T_{1\rho}$ values were 42.4 ± 5.2 ms in overall cartilage of healthy volunteers. The average CV of mean $T_{1\rho}$ values for overall cartilage from healthy volunteers was 1.6%, with regional CV ranging from 1.7% to 8.7%.[16]

In the method using b-GRE sequence, the transient signal decay during b-GRE image acquisition was corrected using a k-space filter. However, because the transient signal decay depended on the initial $T_{1\rho}$-preparation, the corresponding $T_{1\rho}$ map was altered by variations in the point spread function with TSL. Measurement of $T_{1\rho}$ using the $T_{1\rho}$-prepared b-GRE sequence matches standard $T_{1\rho}$-prepared SE in the medial patellar and lateral patellar cartilage compartments.

$T_{1\rho}$ sequences have also been implemented using parallel imaging techniques.[17,18] In these studies, no significant differences were found between parallel versus non-parallel $T_{1\rho}$ quantification.

Applications

In vitro studies have evaluated the relationship between $T_{1\rho}$ relaxation time and the biochemical composition of cartilage. Akella *et al.* have demonstrated that over 50% depletion of PG from bovine articular cartilage resulted in average $T_{1\rho}$ increases from 110–170 ms.[19] Regression analysis of the data showed a strong correlation ($R^2 = 0.987$) between changes in PG and $T_{1\rho}$. In another study on bovine cartilage at 4 T, $T_{1\rho}$ has been proposed as a more specific indicator of PG content than T_2 relaxation in trypsinized cartilage.[20] The authors reported that there was an excellent correlation ($R^2 = 0.89$) between $1/T_{1\rho}$ and GAG concentration while the correlation between $1/T_2$ and GAG concentration was rather poor ($R^2 = 0.01$). Wheaton *et al.* found correlations between $T_{1\rho}$ relaxation time, proteoglycan, and mechanical properties of bovine cartilage explants including aggregate modulus and hydraulic permeability.[21] In human OA cartilage obtained from patients who underwent total knee arthroplasty, a significant but moderate correlation was reported between $T_{1\rho}$ relaxation times and GAG concentration ($R = 0.55$, $P = 0.04$).[22] These studies form the experimental basis for using the $T_{1\rho}$ mapping techniques in studying cartilage pathology in OA.

In vivo studies showed increased cartilage $T_{1\rho}$ values in OA subjects compared to controls.[6,9,12,23] Figure 2 shows color-coded $T_{1\rho}$ maps overlaid on SPGR images for a healthy volunteer (a, male, age = 30) and an OA patient (b, female, age = 27, post-traumatic OA).[9] Significant elevated $T_{1\rho}$ values in different regions of cartilage were observed in the patient although there were no obvious changes in cartilage morphology yet. In a recent cohort study using 3 T MRI,[23] the average $T_{1\rho}$ and T_2 values were significantly increased in OA patients compared with controls (52.04 ± 2.97 ms versus 45.53 ± 3.28 ms with $P = 0.0002$ for $T_{1\rho}$, and 39.63 ± 2.69 versus 34.74 ± 2.48 with $P = 0.001$ for T_2). Increased $T_{1\rho}$ and T_2 values were also correlated with increased severity in radiographic and MR grading of OA. $T_{1\rho}$ had a larger range and higher effect size than

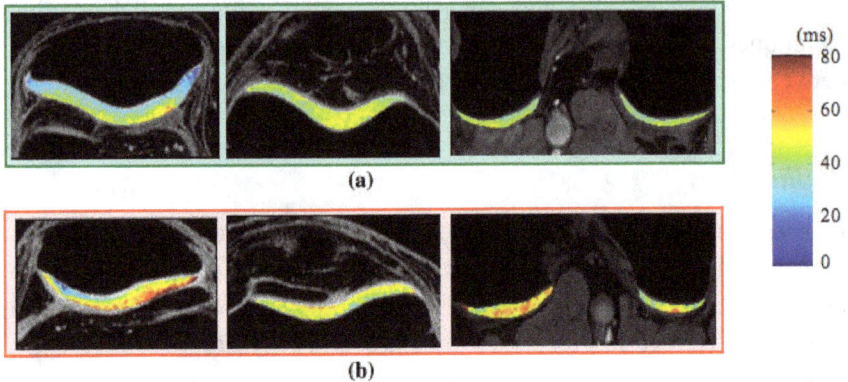

Fig. 2. Color-coded $T_{1\rho}$ maps overlaid on SPGR images. Left: patellar cartilage; middle: anterior femoral (trochlea) cartilage; right: posterior femoral cartilage. **(a)** A healthy volunteer, male, 30 years old and **(b)** a patient with early OA, female, 27 years old. The $T_{1\rho}$ values were 40.05 ± 11.43 ms in the volunteer and 50.56 ± 19.26 ms in the patient, respectively.

T_2, 3.7 versus 3.0. These studies reflect the potential for $T_{1\rho}$ imaging for non-invasive evaluation of diseased cartilage.

Another *in vivo* study applied T_2 and $T_{1\rho}$ measurements in physically active and sedentary healthy subjects as well as in patients with early OA.[24] Nine out of 13 active healthy subjects had focal cartilage abnormalities. $T_{1\rho}$ and T_2 values in active subjects with and without focal cartilage abnormalities differed significantly ($P < 0.05$). $T_{1\rho}$ and T_2 values were significantly higher ($P < 0.05$) in early OA patients compared to healthy subjects. $T_{1\rho}$ measurements were superior to T_2 in differentiating OA patients from healthy subjects, yet $T_{1\rho}$ was moderately age-dependent. The authors suggested that $T_{1\rho}$ and T_2 could be parameters suited to identify active healthy subjects at higher risk for developing cartilage pathology.

Studies have also used $T_{1\rho}$ imaging to evaluate cartilage overlying bone marrow edema-like lesions (BMEL) in OA knees.[25] In a one-year longitudinal study with 23 OA patients,[26] Zhao *et al.* found that patients with BMEL showed overall higher $T_{1\rho}$ values in cartilage compared with those who had no BMEL (42.0 ± 3.7 ms versus 39.8 ± 1.4 ms, $P = 0.032$), suggesting BMEL may be correlated with disease severity of OA. Furthermore, in patients with BMEL, both $T_{1\rho}$ values and clinical Whole-Organ MRI Score (WORMS) grading were elevated significantly

(P < 0.05) in cartilage overlying BMEL compared to the surrounding cartilage, suggesting a local spatial correlation between BMEL and more advanced cartilage degeneration. At one-year follow up, cartilage overlying BMEL showed a significantly higher $T_{1\rho}$ value increase compared with surrounding cartilage, suggesting BMEL is indicative of accelerated cartilage degeneration. Interestingly, no such difference was found using WORMS scoring. This result suggests that quantitative cartilage imaging, such as $T_{1\rho}$, may be a more sensitive indicator of cartilage degeneration than semi-quantitative scoring systems.

In addition to evaluating cartilage in patients with OA, $T_{1\rho}$ quantification techniques have been applied to cartilage in patients with acutely injured knees, who have a high risk of developing OA. In patients with acute anterior cruciate ligament (ACL) tears, significantly increased $T_{1\rho}$ values were found in cartilage overlying BMEL when compared with surrounding cartilage at the lateral tibia (LT, P < 0.05), but no significant difference was found in the lateral femoral condyle.[25,27] Two patients were confirmed to have cartilage damage in regions with elevated $T_{1\rho}$ values using arthroscopic images, as shown in (Fig. 3).[28] Preliminary longitudinal follow-up on these ACL injured knees showed that (1) in lateral sides,

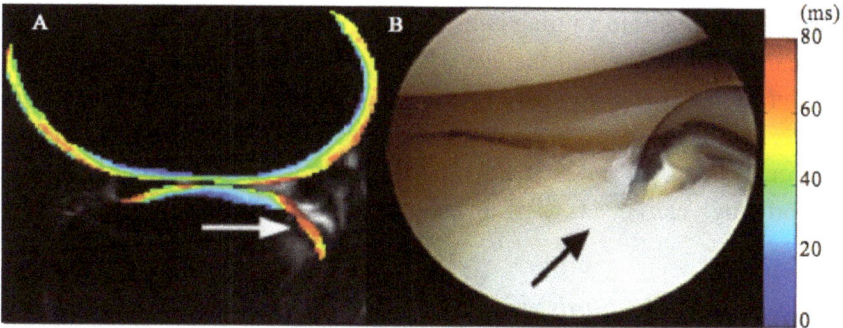

Fig. 3. A patient with ACL tear showed BMEL in lateral tibia. **(A)** Color coded $T_{1\rho}$ relaxation time map. $T_{1\rho}$ values were significantly elevated in BMEL-overlying cartilage in posterolateral tibia plateau (white arrow) versus surrounding cartilage in the same compartment (60.2 ± 13.7 versus 37.5 ± 14.3 ms). **(B)** Arthroscopic picture demonstrating grade I softening of the postero-lateral tibial plateau with linear partial fissures along the articular cartilage overlying the region of the BMEL (black arrow). Reproduced from Ref. 43 with permission.

despite the resolution of BMEL, cartilage overlying the baseline BMEL still show significantly higher $T_{1\rho}$ compared to the surrounding cartilage, suggesting potential irreversible damage of cartilage in these regions and (2) in medial sides, $T_{1\rho}$ values in medical tibial and medial femoral condyles show significant elevation at one- and two-year follow-up compared to healthy controls.[29] These results suggest cartilage damage after acute knee injuries that can be the risk factors for predisposing OA to these knees. Quantitative $T_{1\rho}$ may probe these degenerations at earlier time points than radiographs or conventional MRI.

Furthermore, $T_{1\rho}$ quantification has been evaluated in meniscus in OA and ACL-injured knees.[30,31] *In vivo* $T_{1\rho}$ measurements in the meniscus showed excellent reproducibility (CV < 5%). Significant differences between three subject groups (controls $n = 27$; mild OA patient $n = 23$; severe OA patient $n = 10$) were found: Mean $T_{1\rho}$ values were 14.7 ± 5.5 ms for healthy controls ($n = 27$), 16.1 ± 6.6 ms for mild OA patients ($n = 23$), and 19.3 ± 7.6 ms for severe OA patients ($n = 10$), respectively. In acutely ACL-injured knees, significantly elevated $T_{1\rho}$ values were found in the lateral meniscus in patients compared with controls ($P < 0.01$). A significant correlation ($R^2 = 0.47$, $P = 0.007$) was found between $T_{1\rho}$ values of posterior horn of lateral meniscus and $T_{1\rho}$ values of posterior sub-compartment of lateral tibia cartilage in patients. This correlation suggested a strong injury-related relationship between meniscus and cartilage biochemical changes. However, because menisci have a much shorter $T_{1\rho}$ ($\sim$20 ms) compared to cartilage, acquisition sequences need to be optimized to quantify such a short relaxation time. The relationship between $T_{1\rho}$ values and biochemical composition (collagen, mainly type I, and proteoglycan) needs to be investigated.

$T_{1\rho}$ *Imaging Mechanism*

Previous studies showed that collagen structure and orientation are dominating factors that affect T_2 relaxation in cartilage. This results in the "magic angle" effect and commonly seen laminar appearance in cartilage imaging.[32,33] Similar to T_2, studies have demonstrated regional variations of cartilage $T_{1\rho}$. $T_{1\rho}$ values were highest at the superficial zone, decreased gradually in the middle zone, and increased in the region near the subchondral bone in bovine cartilage,[19] human cartilage specimens,[34] and human *in vivo* cartilage.[35] Although the trend of $T_{1\rho}$ and T_2 values are similar, $T_{1\rho}$ shows a larger dynamic range from the bone/cartilage interface to the cartilage surface,[34] and a larger difference between controls and patients,[35] particularly, in the superficial layer, indicating that it may be more sensitive to degenerative changes occurring in cartilage OA. Furthermore, less laminar appearance was observed in $T_{1\rho}$-weighted images compared to T_2-weighted images due to reduced dipolar interaction during $T_{1\rho}$ relaxation.[36]

During cartilage degeneration, T_2 has been found to correlate poorly with PG content in controlled *in vitro* studies.[20,37] In $T_{1\rho}$ quantification experiments, the spin-lock techniques reduce dipolar interactions and therefore reduce the dependence of the relaxation time constant on collagen fiber orientation.[36] This may enable more accurate diagnoses of early degenerative changes in cartilage. $T_{1\rho}$ relaxation rate $(1/T_{1\rho})$ has been shown to decrease linearly with decreasing PG content in *ex vivo* bovine patellae[38] and has been proposed as a more specific indicator of PG content than T_2 relaxation in trypsinized cartilage.[20]

The mechanism of $T_{1\rho}$ relaxation time in biological tissues, particularly in cartilage, is not yet fully understood. Using native and immobilized protein solution, Makela *et al.* suggested that proton exchange between the protein side chain groups and bulk water contribute significantly to the $T_{1\rho}$ relaxation.[39] Based on spectroscopy experiments with peptide solutions, GAG solutions and bovine cartilage samples before and after PG degradation, Duvvuri *et al.* further suggested that in cartilage hydrogen exchange from NH and OH groups to water may dominate the low-frequency (0–1.5 KHz) water $T_{1\rho}$ dispersion.[40] They speculated that increase of the low-frequency correlation rate with PG loss could be the result of increased proton exchange rates. Other evidence of a proton exchange pathway is the PH dependency of $T_{1\rho}$ values in the ischemic rat brain tissues.[41] Mlynarik *et al.*, on the other hand, have suggested that the dominant relaxation mechanism in the rotating frame in cartilage at $B_0 \leq 3\,T$ seems to be dipolar interaction.[42] The contribution of scalar relaxation caused by proton exchange is only relevant at high fields such as 7 T. Clearly, further investigations are needed to better understand this relaxation mechanism.

The correlation and differences between T_2 and $T_{1\rho}$ in cartilage have been explored both *in vitro* and *in vivo*. Mlyranik *et al.*[43] showed that the $T_{1\rho}$ relaxation times obtained were slightly longer than the corresponding T_2 values, but both parameters showed almost identical spatial distributions. Menezes *et al.*[44] have shown that $T_{1\rho}$ and T_2 changes in articular cartilage do not necessarily coincide, and might provide complementary information. These investigators showed that $T_{1\rho}$ and T_2 reflect changes that may be associated with proteoglycan, collagen content and hydration and the true mechanism of $T_{1\rho}$ may arise from a weighted-average of multiple biochemical changes occurring in cartilage in OA.

A recent *in vivo* study quantified the pixel-by-pixel correlation of $T_{1\rho}$ and T_2 values in OA patients ($n = 10$) and healthy controls ($n = 10$). The investigators showed that, although the average $T_{1\rho}$ and T_2 values correlated significantly, the pixel-by-pixel correlation between $T_{1\rho}$ and T_2 showed a large range in both controls and OA patients ($R = 0.522 \pm 0.183$, ranging from 0.221 to 0.763 in OA patients versus $R = 0.624 \pm 0.060$, ranging from 0.547 to 0.726 in controls).[35] Figure 4 shows $T_{1\rho}$ and T_2 maps from a control subject, a subject with mild OA, and a subject with severe OA. The differences between the $T_{1\rho}$ and T_2 maps are evident. These results suggested $T_{1\rho}$ and T_2 show different spatial distribution and may provide complementary information regarding cartilage degeneration in OA. Combining these two parameters may further improve our capability to diagnose early cartilage degeneration and injury.

As spatial variation was observed in a number of $T_{1\rho}$ and T_2 studies, texture analysis[45] has been applied to examine the spatial distribution of pixel values and quantify the heterogeneity in $T_{1\rho}$ and T_2 maps. The most commonly used texture analysis parameters are those extracted from the grey-level co-occurrence matrix (GLCM) as proposed by Haralick *et al.*[46] The GLCM determines the frequency that neighboring grey-level values occur in an image. Parameters derived from GLCM provide information on the variation between neighboring pixels and directly quantify the distribution of the image signal. Blumenkrantz *et al.* demonstrated that mild OA patients ($n = 8$) had significantly elevated GLCM entropy and reduced angular second moment (ASM) of cartilage T_2 values than controls ($n = 14$). Similarly, Li *et al.* reported that overall elevated GLCM contrast and entropy measurements, and lower ASM and GLCM mean

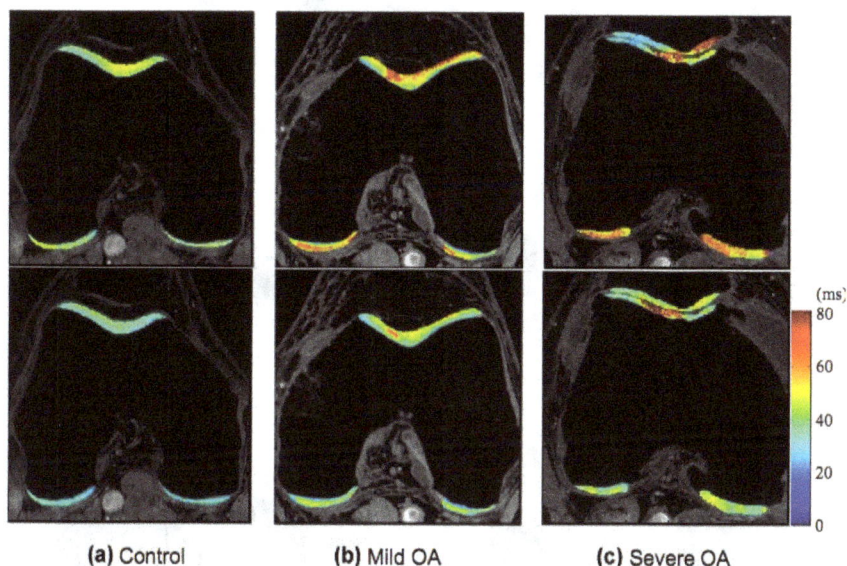

(a) Control   **(b)** Mild OA   **(c)** Severe OA

Fig. 4. $T_{1\rho}$ maps (first row) and T_2 maps (second row) for a healthy control **(a)**, a patient with mild OA **(b)**, and a patient with severe OA **(c)**. (a) Control: The average $T_{1\rho}$ value was 40.1 ± 11.4 ms and T_2 values was 33.3 ± 10.5 ms in cartilage. (b) A patient with early OA (male, 66 years old). The average $T_{1\rho}$ value was 45.5 ± 14.5 ms and T_2 values was 35.0 ± 10.9 ms in cartilage. (c) A patient with advanced OA (male, 46 years old). The average $T_{1\rho}$ value was 55.4 ± 26.0 ms and T_2 values was 43.8 ± 11.1 ms in cartilage. The maps illustrate the differences in $T_{1\rho}$ and T_2 between OA severity, and demonstrate potential different spatial distribution between T_2 and $T_{1\rho}$ elevation in osteoarthritic cartilage (patient C).

measurements of both $T_{1\rho}$ and T_2 values were observed in patients with OA ($n = 10$) when compared to controls ($n = 10$).[35] These differences, however, appear more prevalent in $T_{1\rho}$ measurements, as shown in (Fig. 5). The results indicate that these relaxation time constants are not only increased but are also more heterogeneous in osteoarthritic cartilage.

Sodium MRI

Sodium plays an important role in cellular function, synaptic transmission, osmotic balance, and solute transport in biological tissues.[47–51] The ^{23}Na nucleus is the only naturally occurring nucleus of sodium and has a spin quantum number $I = 3/2$. This implies that there are four possible orientations of the sodium nucleus with respect to the static external magnetic

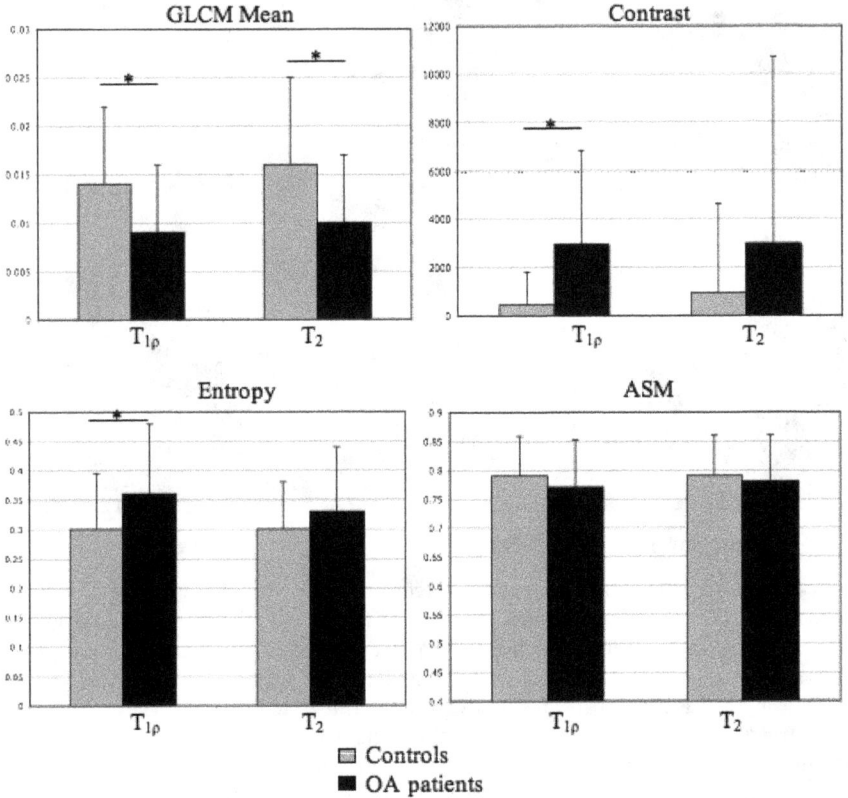

Fig. 5. Texture parameters of $T_{1\rho}$ and T_2 values in overall cartilage in controls and OA patients in $0°$ and 1 pixel offset. OA subjects had greater overall contrast and entropy, but lower overall GLCM mean and ASM of cartilage $T_{1\rho}$ and T_2 than of controls at $0°$ and $90°$ in all pixel offsets. These differences were significant ($P < 0.05$) in the GLCM mean, contrast, and entropy of cartilage $T_{1\rho}$ and in the GLCM mean of cartilage T_2, as indicated by $*$ in the figure.

field (B_0). ^{23}Na has a low gyromagnetic ratio [11.3 MHz/Tesla (T)] when compared to protons (42.6 MHz/T). Average *in-vivo* sodium concentrations lie in the range between 250 and 350 mM/L in connective tissues (e.g. articular cartilage, intervertebral disc). In general, the sensitivity of the nucleus is directly proportional to $\gamma^{11/4}I(I + 1)$ for a given B_0 field. The MR sensitivity of ^{23}Na is only 9.2% of the one of ^{1}H-MR and the *in vivo* concentration is $\sim$366 times lower than the *in vivo* water proton concentration. The combination of these factors results in a ^{23}Na signal which is approximately 3978 (2.52×10^{-4}) times smaller than the ^{1}H signal.

The Quadrupolar Interaction

The ^{23}Na nucleus exhibits a quadrupolar interaction when located in an anisotropic environment.[52-54] This effect originates from the interaction between the non-spherically symmetric nucleus and the surrounding electric field gradients, which forms usually the strongest NMR-active interaction for a ^{23}Na nucleus. Hence, the appearance of a quadrupolar interaction is diagnostic of the presence of an asymmetry in the electronic environment of the ^{23}Na nucleus. The interaction may be averaged out partly or completely by molecular tumbling. For tissue samples, the residual interaction is relatively weak and can be described to a good approximation by the Hamiltonian

$$H_Q = A_Q \frac{1}{2}[I_Z^2 - I(I+1)/3] \tag{5}$$

where the time averaged quadrupolar coupling is:

$$A_Q = \langle 3\omega_Q[P_2(\cos\beta) + (\eta/2)\cos 2\alpha \sin^2\beta]\rangle \tag{6}$$

with η being the asymmetry parameter given by the tensor components as $\eta = (q_{xx} - q_{yy})/q_{zz}$, and α, β, γ describing the rotation from the principal frame of the interaction to the laboratory frame. For axial symmetry $\eta = 0$. The strength of the interaction is further determined by the electric field gradient, typically written as eq and the nuclear quadrupole moment via the relationship

$$\omega_Q = e^2 q Q/2I(2I-1). \tag{7}$$

The angular brackets in Equation (6) denote spatial and temporal averaging on a time scale faster than the time it takes to perform a MR measurement.

A nonzero quadrupolar interaction as described by Equation (5) leads to shifts in energy levels and the appearance of three inequivalent transitions at the frequencies $\omega_o + A_q/2\pi$, ω_o and $\omega_o - A_q/2\pi$. This effect is readily seen in liquid crystalline solutions, but is also well known in cartilage samples. In the latter case, the sodium ions are associated with the type-II collagen/proteoglycan framework with the electric field gradient from the fixed charges causing the relatively large quadrupolar splitting.

Quadrupolar Relaxation

In addition to a line splitting, the instantaneous quadrupolar coupling fluctuates due to tumbling [the part inside the angled brackets in Equation (6)], and leads to accelerated relaxation of the magnetization. Even in phosphate buffered saline (PBS) solutions T_1 is typically as short as 30–40 ms, which represents the longest T_1 times observable for ^{23}Na in the context of MRI. As motion becomes slower (lower temperature, or higher viscosity), the relaxation time drops further until it bifurcates and leads to the appearance of two different T_1 times, a fast one and a slow one. In cartilage the slow relaxation time is typically on the order of 15 ms, while the fast one may be on the order of 5 ms. The same happens for T_2, but the constants are slightly shorter than the corresponding T_1 times. Typical transverse relaxation times in cartilage, for example, are between 1–3 ms for the fast component and 8–15 ms for the slow component.[55,56] Motional restriction in cartilage can be assumed to arise due to the association with the type-II collagen/proteoglycan framework. The charges hold the ions in place, and the whole complex moves very slowly.

The fast relaxing outer transitions (+3/2 to +1/2 and from −3/2 to −1/2) account for 60% of the signal, while the inner transition relaxes more slowly. This process is indeed typically seen in NMR spectra of cartilage samples. The fast component of T_2 is frequently invisible in conventional MR pulse sequences because of echo time limitations.

It was first reported by Hubbard[55] that the interaction between the nuclear electric quadrupole moment and the fluctuating EFG can produce multiexponential relaxation. The satellite and central transitions of sodium transverse relaxation rates differ in the following way

$$R_{2f} = -C(J_0 + J_1), \quad R_{2s} = -C(J_1 + J_2), \tag{8}$$

where the spectral density function, J_n is defined as

$$J_n = \frac{2\tau_c}{1 + (n\omega_0\tau_c)^2} \tag{9}$$

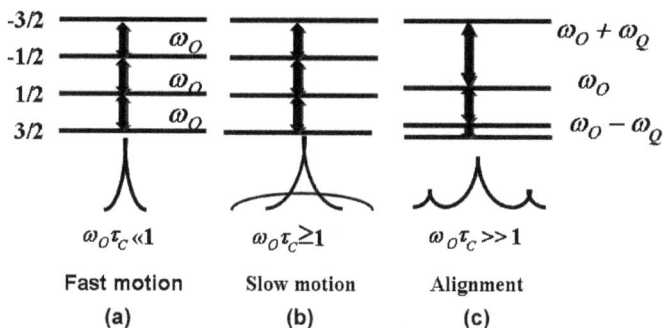

Fig. 6. ^{23}Na ($I = 3/2$) energy levels with different motional regimes (fast, slow and oriented environments).

with τ_c being the rotational correlation time. The constant C is

$$C = \frac{1}{40} \left(\frac{e^2 q Q}{h} \right)^2 \left(1 + \frac{\eta^2}{3} \right). \tag{10}$$

Under the extreme narrowing condition ($\omega_o \tau_c \ll 1$), one has $J_0 = J_1 = J_2 = 2\tau_c$ (i.e. both satellite and central transitions decay at the same rate). However, if the motion is slowed down sufficiently, such as in the case of cartilage, biexponential transverse relaxation results. Figure 6 shows representative ^{23}Na ($I = 3/2$) energy levels and schematic spectra with different motional characteristics.

Measuring Sodium Concentration in Cartilage

Sodium concentrations monitored by ^{23}Na-MRI show a strong linear correlation with fixed charge densities (FCD),[57] which has been demonstrated by several investigators in *ex vivo* model systems as well as *in vivo*.[58–60]

Distinguishing Sodium Based on Motion

Many MR investigations have dealt with the distinction between sodium ions based on the time scales of their motion. The regime of slow motion is assumed to be fulfilled for intracellular sodium, for which the biexponential regime is obeyed. By contrast, extracellular sodium moves quickly and hence has monoexponential relaxation. In the biexponential regime, it is further possible to create triple-quantum coherences, and a so-called triple-quantum filtered (TQF) experiment can be used to select the slow component. Although sodium in cartilage is primarily extracellular, its motion is sufficiently slowed down so that TQF signals can also be seen.[57,61,62]

Isotropic and Anisotropic ^{23}Na Pools

The assessment of free and bound sodium can hold strong diagnostic power for cartilage and other tissue pathologies.[62,63] The bound or ordered sodium signal overlaps frequently with the signal arising from free sodium. In the literature bound and ordered sodium is sometimes used to refer to intracellular sodium, although this kind of sodium is not necessarily bound to any molecules. Even in cartilage, where most of the sodium is extracellular, when one refers to bound sodium, there is no strong bonding, but rather sodium can be thought of as twirling around the macromolecules in clouds held loosely by electrostatic forces. Nonetheless, significant quadrupolar splittings are routinely observed for cartilage sodium. Bound sodium can be detected by using a double-quantum filtered (DQF) experiment. As mentioned above, a TQF will also lead to detectable signal because motion of sodium in cartilage is sufficiently restricted. The least ambiguous experiment, however is the DQF experiment with magic angle pulses, in which slow motion sodium does not contribute to the signal (unless it also shows a nonvanishing residual quadrupolar coupling).[64,65] A typical pulse sequence for multiple quantum filtering is shown in (Fig. 7). The main disadvantages of the DQF or TQF experiments are large phase cycle, a large number of RF pulses, and low sensitivity which makes them challenging to implement in routine clinical MRI. It has been reported that omitting the π-pulse enhances the sensitivity.[57,59,62,65] These sequences are usually difficult to implement in imaging, because the application of several pulses may lead to SAR complications. Furthermore, the RF pulses are usually fairly long, leading to sizable relaxation interferences during the pulses.

Recently several other methods have been developed, such as central peak suppression (CPS)[66] and the quadrupolar filter by nutation (QFN),[62] which may more directly sample the presence of a quadrupolar coupling and

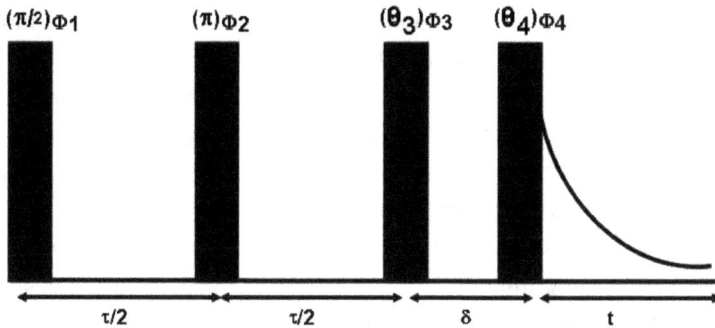

Fig. 7. A typical pulse sequence for multiple quantum filtered experiment.

thereby select bound sodium. Inversion recovery (IR)[67] has also been shown recently to select cartilage sodium by exploiting simply the difference in T_1 values between cartilage sodium and synovial fluid sodium. Recent results also showed that the numerical optimization of a RF waveform may also provide improved SNR of bound sodium.[68]

There is indication that the quadrupolar coupling of sodium in cartilage significantly correlates with early degenerative changes[61,67] thus lending motivation to the development of novel pulse sequences which would highlight this anisotropic interaction as contrast in the images, but these have not been clinically tested yet.

Technical Challenges for Sodium Imaging at Clinical Scanners

The lower physiological sodium concentration (110 M versus 300 mM), 3.8-fold smaller gyromagnetic ratio, in biological tissues, and shorter T_2 relaxation time make sodium MRI less attractive in many respects compared to conventional proton MRI. Therefore, one has to compromise image quality in order to gain sensitivity. The short T_1 of sodium ($\sim$20 ms) allows for rapid signal averaging, which partially offsets the loss in signal/unit time. Sodium MRI is advantageous in investigating pathology where the change in sodium MR properties of the tissue of interest is more pronounced than the changes in relaxation times and water content. The negatively charged

GAG plays an important role in determining tissue integrity by maintaining a fixed charge density (FCD) in cartilage. Positively charged sodium ions are attracted by the FCD. There is a strong linear correlation between FCD and GAG.[58,69,70] Previous studies have already shown that sodium MRI has a potential advantage over conventional proton MRI in investigating biochemical markers in cartilage during the early stages of OA.[56,63,70,71] To avoid signal loss due to the fast T_2 component, sodium MRI requires both innovative three-dimensional ultra short echo pulse sequences such as 3D radial sequences[72] or twisted projection imaging (3D-TPI)[57,73] that achieve short echo times as well as high field systems (3T and above) for adequate signal-to-noise ratio (SNR). Even at 3T the sodium imaging time of the whole knee joint would be approximately 30 to 45 minutes in order to achieve adequate SNR. Recent advances in magnet technology, improved gradient performance, multi coil RF technology (parallel receive as well as transmit) may make sodium MRI clinically feasible on high fields systems. There is strong evidence that an ultra-high field 7T-MRI system will further improve SNR, sensitivity, specificity, and spatial and temporal resolution. Although sodium MRI has high specificity and does not require any exogenous contrast agent, it does require special hardware capabilities (multinuclear), specialized RF coils (transmit/receive) and novel 3D-UTE pulse sequences. These challenges currently limit the clinical use of sodium MRI at standard clinical scanners. A representative volumetric sodium image of the knee joint acquired in less than 15 minutes at 7T is shown in Fig. 8.

gagCEST

A new method for GAG mapping in cartilage based on chemical exchange saturation transfer (gagCEST) has been proposed recently.[74-76] In this section, we outline the potential applications for GAG mapping in OA or in repair treatment. Being an endogenous method, gagCEST avoids some of the limitations that contrast-agent-based methods may face. In contrast to $T_{1\rho}$ relaxometry, it may allow measurements to be performed with lower rf powers, and may be more specific to GAG. One limitation of gagCEST, however, is that artifacts may be pronounced in the presence of large B_0 inhomogeneities. Such a drawback could be offset by performing

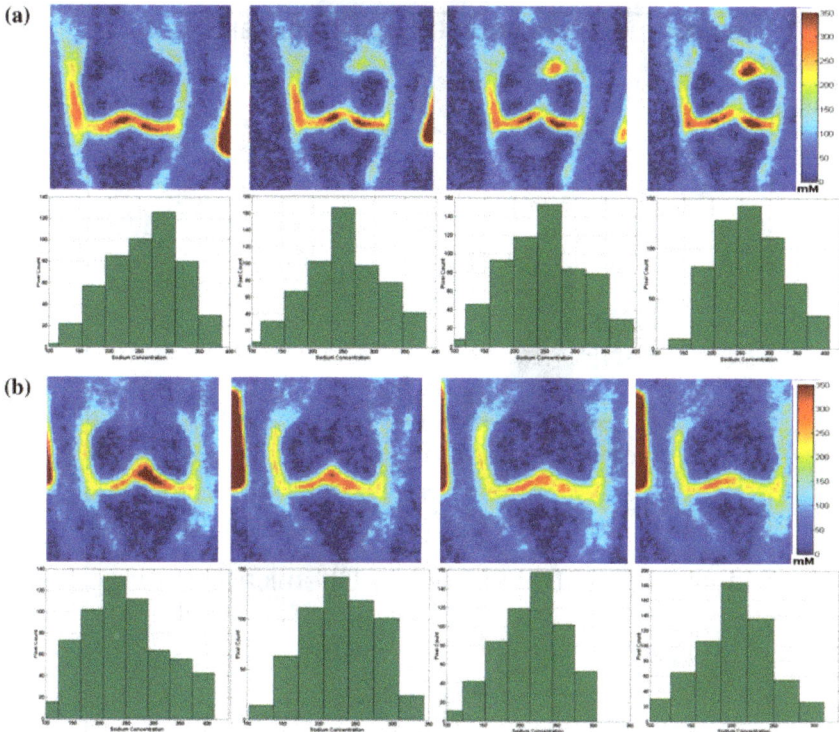

Fig. 8. 3D-Isotropic volumetric sodium mapping of knee joint acquired at 7T in less than 15 minutes **(a)** Healthy volunteer (top) and the corresponding histograms and **(b)** OA patient (bottom) and corresponding histograms.

B_0 correction schemes based on water saturation shift referencing (WASSR).[77]

Chemical Exchange Saturation Transfer (CEST) Mechanism

Chemical exchange saturation transfer (CEST) contrast exploits the fact that some protons from a small fraction of molecules (metabolites, macromolecules, etc.) can interchange with those of bulk water, which in turn is the major contributor to the observed MRI signal. The small pool of exchangeable protons is first saturated by a radio frequency (RF) pulse, and upon chemical exchange with bulk water, the degree of saturation is

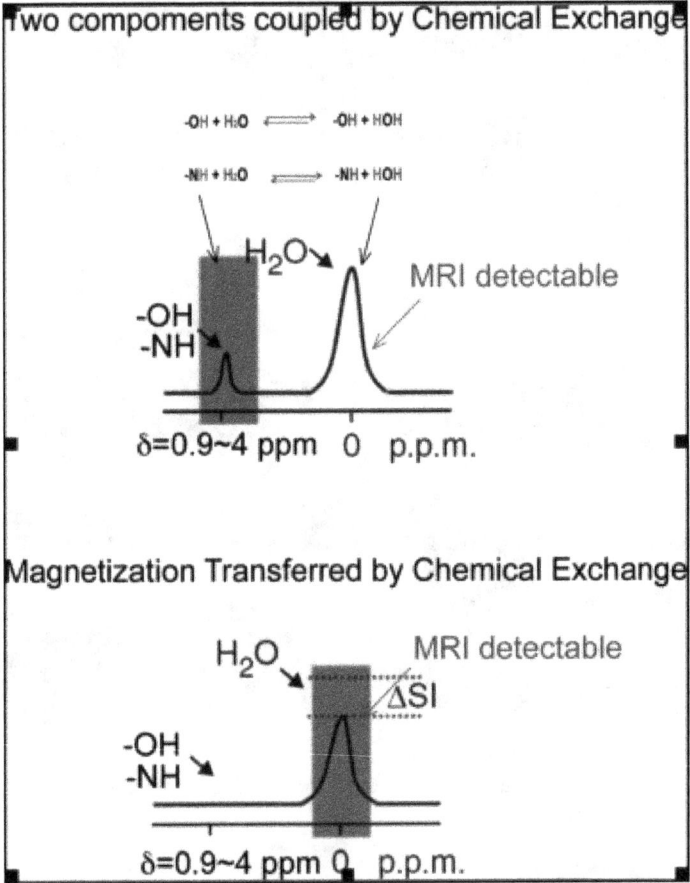

Fig. 9. Schematic diagram illustrating the CEST mechanism.

perceptible as a decrease in the bulk water signal (Fig. 9). As a result, the water pool acts as a detector of the concentration of a small portion of the molecules.[78,79] As a result, the CEST method can achieve larger contrast enhancement when compared with the directly-detected signal arising from these molecules.[80] The CEST approach has already been employed to image tissue pH,[80] to map brain proteins,[80] to monitor glycogen concentration in liver,[81] and to map specific gene expressions *in vivo*.[82]

The existence of endogenous exchangeable protons within GAG molecules leads to the logical next step of exploiting them as possible

CEST agents. In cartilage, every GAG unit has one −NH, and three −OHs. −NH has an intermediate exchange rate ($k_{sw} \approx 10 \, \text{s}^{-1}$, where k_{sw} is the exchange rate of the labile proton with bulk water) and a large chemical shift relative to the water signal ($\Delta\delta \geq 3 \, \text{ppm}$), which makes it ideal for many CEST applications.[80] Although the chemical exchange rate of −OH is in the fast regime ($k_{sw} \approx 10^3) \, \text{s}^{-1}$ and its chemical shift relative to the water signal is usually small ($\Delta\delta \leq 2 \, \text{ppm}$),[80,83] it has already been demonstrated suitable for various CEST applications.[79,82] We refer to the acronym gagCEST.

Assessing GAG with CEST

In cartilage, the collagen framework is relatively solid, which gives rise to an MR signal broadened to up to 15–20 kHz, due to the strong residual dipolar interactions. Hence it is typically invisible in NMR spectra unless solid-state techniques such as magic-angle spinning and dipolar decoupling are used.[84] GAG, instead, is a flexible molecule, and as a result, GAG, as well as some small metabolites, contribute to the major signals visible in the 1D-^{1}H spectra of cartilage.[74,84,85] A comparison between Figs. 10a and 10b illustrates that most of the resonances arise from GAG, except in the aliphatic region between −5 ppm and −2 ppm, where metabolites contribute significantly to the signals. z-Spectroscopy, in which the bulk water intensity is plotted as a function of the pre-saturation frequency with respect to the center of the main water resonance, is a convenient way to visualize the CEST effect and to select potential exchangeable groups for providing contrast.[86] Such spectra are displayed in Figs. 10c and 10d. As is customary in z-spectroscopy, 0 ppm here refers to the center of the water resonance.[86] Among the GAG signals, the amide proton (−NH) at +3.2 ppm, the hydroxyl protons (−OH) at +0.9 to +1.9 ppm (only visible in Fig. 10a at lower temperature), the non-exchangeable protons from the carbohydrate ring between −2.5 and −0.5 ppm, and the N-acetyl group at −2.7 ppm are of interest for the exploration of GAG quantification and characterization.[74,75] Moreover, it appears likely that the PG core protein also contributes to the +2.7 ppm signal (Fig. 10b), which probably is either an amine or amide proton.

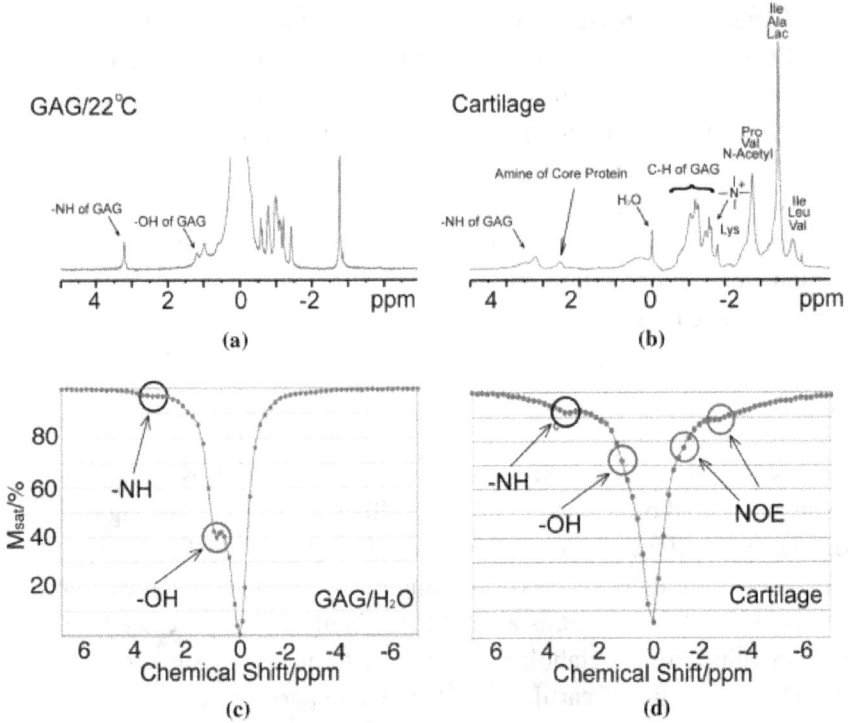

Fig. 10. (a) 1D proton NMR spectrum of GAG at 22°C. (b) 1D proton NMR spectrum of cartilage. (c) z-spectrum of GAG. (d) z-spectrum of cartilage.

In the z-spectra (Figs. 10c and 10d), the exchangeable protons demonstrate dips at $+3.2$ ppm and $+1.0$ ppm. Under the assumption of complete saturation of the irradiated group, the reduction of the water magnetization is given by[80]

$$\text{CEST} = k_{sw} \times T_{1w}/[(M_{0w}/M_{0s}) + k_{sw} \times T_{1w}], \qquad (11)$$

where T_{1w} is the water longitudinal relaxation time and M_{0s}, M_{0w} are the equilibrium magnetizations of the labile protons and water protons, respectively. Although this assumption is often violated, Equation (11) gives a useful account of the factors that contribute to an enhanced appearance of the CEST effect. Another magnetization transfer mechanism, the Nuclear Overhauser Effect (NOE), also introduces dips at $\delta = -2.6$ ppm and -1.0 ppm in the z-spectra as in Fig. 10d, which correspond to the magnetization transfer from the CH and N-acetyl residues in GAG, respectively.[75] Other aliphatic groups may contribute to this effect as well. The NOE enhancement factor of the water signal can be expressed as[87]

$$NOE_{water} = T_{1w} \times \sigma, \tag{12}$$

where σ is the cross-relaxation constant between water and GAG. σ is negative when the rotational motion of GAG is slow, which is a reasonable assumption since GAGs are entrapped within the collagen framework. It is common practice to quantify the CEST effect as[79]

$$\%CEST(\delta) = [S(-\delta) - S(+\delta)]/S(-\delta) \times 100, \tag{13}$$

where δ is the offset of the irradiation relative to the water signal and $S(\delta)$ is the water intensity acquired after a long saturation pulse at offset δ. In addition to the specific exchange effects, magnetization transfer (MT) effects may contribute to the measured signals, which arise from a nonspecific exchange of protons on water molecules that are bound to macromolecules.[88,89] The subtraction of the signal obtained after irradiation on the opposite side of the water resonance avoids some artifacts due to MT effects from bound water, and some of the direct water saturation effects. It is recognized, however, that MT effects may also be asymmetric with respect to the water resonance center,[90] and may hence contribute to the value determined by Equation (13).

The normalization should also cancel out proton density variations. On the other hand, this subtraction is not useful in the case of −NH groups, since the NOE transfer effects according to Equation (12) partially mask the CEST effect. Therefore, in practice the −OH CEST effect has been found to be more useful for characterizing cartilage GAGs.[74,75]

Figure 11 shows an *in-vivo* CEST measurement on a patellofemoral human knee joint performed on a clinical 3T scanner. In this image, the patellar cartilage region is clearly demarcated (Fig. 11). The accumulation of joint effusion (fluid) in the knee is almost entirely subtracted in the difference image. A loss of GAG concentration is also shown on the medial side of the patellofemoral knee joint. The regional variation of the GAG concentration in the knee joint is comparable to previously published data extracted from [23]Na MRI:[56] across the cartilage (~33%), the lateral side of

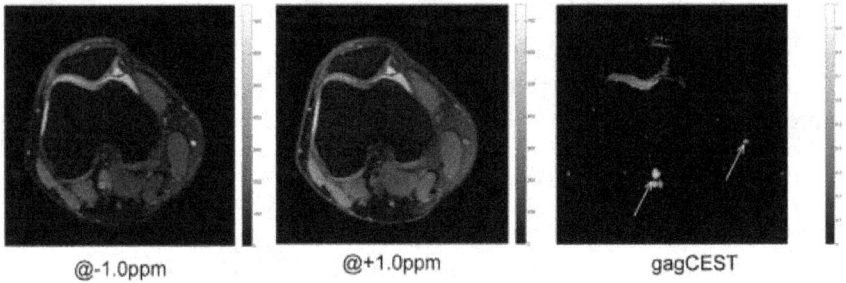

@-1.0ppm   @+1.0ppm   gagCEST

Fig. 11. *In-vivo* images of a human patellofemoral knee with irradiation at $\delta = -1.0$ ppm, $\delta = +1.0$ ppm, and the corresponding gagCEST map. The blood vessels (white arrows) also give rise to substantial CEST effects most likely due to proteins and saccharides in the blood.

the patella (~22%), and the medial side of the patella (~18%). Figure 12 shows routine clinical ^{1}H, non-spectroscopic images obtained from the same volunteer at 3T. Weak morphologic signs of chondramalacia and joint effusion are seen on the clinically acquired proton density (PD), T_1- and T_2-weighted images, although at this point it is unclear how these abnormalities would be reflected in the gagCEST images. Figure 11 also illustrates that other areas, in this case blood vessels light up in the image (arrows), due to the presence of saccharides and proteins in blood. The fact that most other areas of the knee are suppressed in the image points to the relative robustness of this particular implementation and can serve as an internal standard for assessing the variability of B_0 across the tissue of interest. Large B_0 inhomogeneities would lead to "false positives," in rarer cases to "false negatives," but could be corrected using a water shift referencing method.[77]

Extension of gagCEST to Intervertebral Disc

Intervertebral discs (IVDs) represent the largest avascular, aneural structures in the body, each unit consisting of two anatomical regions: the annulus fibrosus and the nucleus pulposus.[3,91] It has a similar biochemical makeup as cartilage. Loss of GAG in the nucleus is the most marked change in degenerative disc diseases (DDD), which also costs hundreds of billions of dollars annually in developed countries.[92] Work is in progress showing that gagCEST can be used to measure the GAG concentration changes in

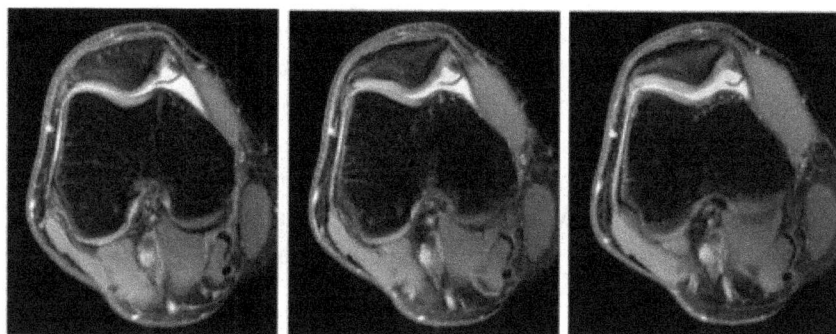

(a) Axial Proton Image with Fat Saturation

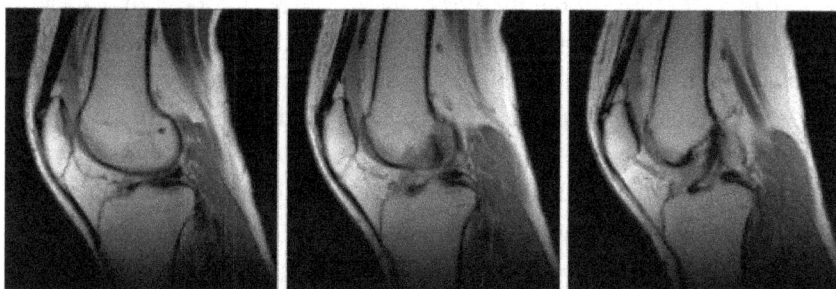

(b) Sagittal Proton Image without Fat Saturation

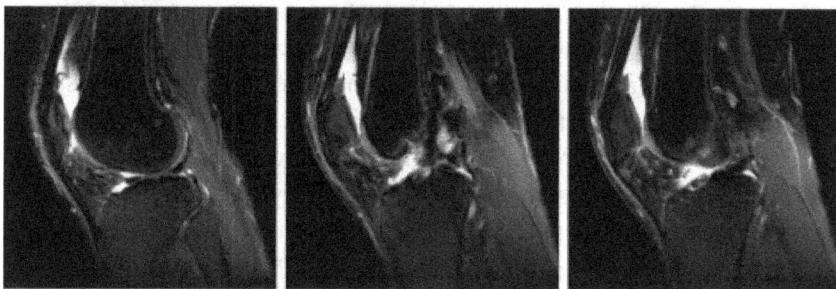

(c) Sagittal T2 Image with Fat Saturation

Fig. 12. Representative conventional clinical images [proton density (PD) and T_2-weighted] obtained at 3T with the following imaging parameters: Fast spin echo (FSE) sequence with FOV $= 150 \times 150$ mm, slice thickness $= 3$ mm, matrix $= 256 \times 256$, **(a)** TR/TE $= 2500$ ms/28 ms (axial PD with fat saturation), **(b)** TR/TE $= 2500$ ms/30 ms (sagittal PD without fat saturation) and **(c)** TR/TE $= 3040$ ms/78 ms (sagittal T_2-weighted with fat saturation).

induced disc degeneration *in vitro*.[93] Since the nucleus pulposus does not take up contrast agents in significant concentrations, dGEMRIC is not a good option for studying this tissue. The nucleus pulposus can be regarded as the most "isolated" tissue in the human body. As a result, its metabolism is easily perturbed. Since the amide proton concentration is relatively high in the nucleus (~350 mM), one could also use amide-proton based pH imaging (based on CEST) for assessing cell metabolism.[76,91]

T_2 Relaxation Time

Quantitative T_2 relaxation time is a non-invasive marker of cartilage degeneration because it is sensitive to tissue hydration and biochemical composition. Immobilization of water protons in cartilage by the collagen-proteoglycan matrix promotes T_2 decay and renders the cartilage low in signal intensity on long-TE (T_2-weighted) images, while mobile water protons in synovial fluid retain their high signal. Loss of collagen and proteoglycan in degenerating cartilage increases the mobility of water, thus increasing its signal intensity on T_2-weighted images.[94] Signal intensity is further augmented in degenerative disease by the elevation of cartilage water content (i.e. proton density) that accompanies matrix loss.[95] Consistent with this, foci of high signal intensity are often seen within the cartilage of knees with OA on T_2-weighted images and have been shown to correspond to arthroscopically demonstrable abnormalities.[96,97]

Cartilage T_2 maps are created using the following process: Typically, T_2-weighted multi-echo, spin echo images with varying echo times (TE) and identical repetition times (TR) are acquired. Second, T_2 maps are computed (Fig. 13) assuming exponential signal decay. T_2 is defined as the time at which the signal decays to 37% of the maximum signal.

In Vitro Imaging

In vitro imaging studies have evaluated the relationship between biochemistry of cartilage and T_2 measurements. Cartilage T_2 is affected by hydration and the integrity of the collagen matrix; however, the relationship between T_2 and proteoglycan content remains controversial in literature. Proteoglycan loss in rat patellar cartilage induced by hyaluronidase degradation (which does not alter the collagen network) was associated with

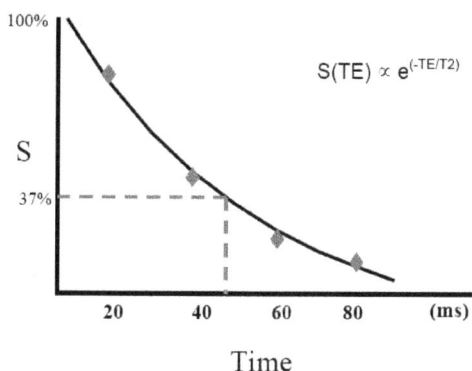

$$S(TE) \propto e^{(-TE/T2)}$$

Time

Fig. 13. An example of T_2 calculation using four T_2-weighted images acquired with different echo-times (TE). The graph shows signal (S) as a function of time. T_2 is calculated for each pixel in an image using the above equation, and is defined as the time at which the signal decays to 37% of the maximum signal.

significantly increased global T_2.[98] However, other studies[43,73,99] found that the depletion of proteoglycan had minimal effects on T_2. A positive relationship between water content and T_2 has been reported.[100,101] These studies demonstrate that the biochemical changes associated with cartilage degeneration are related to elevated T_2; however the effects of proteoglycan concentration on T_2 must be further evaluated.

The relationship between T_2 relaxation time and the mechanical properties of cartilage is under investigation. A recent *in vitro* study[102] has reported that T_2 relaxation time in human patellar cartilage is significantly correlated to Young's Modulus, suggesting that T_2 quantification may predict the mechanical properties of cartilage.

The signal intensity of cartilage in an MR image is dependent on its orientation to the main magnetic field. An *in vitro* study using high-field (8.6T) microscopic MRI (μMRI) suggested that the angular dependency of T_2 with respect to the main magnetic field (*B*0) can provide specific information about the collagen ultra-structure.[103] However, the requirement for the specific orientation of cartilage to the main magnetic field and the required ultra-high resolution (at 13.7 μm) preclude it from *in vivo* applications with current techniques. Goodwin *et al.*[104] have described how T_2 varies with depth from the articular surface due to collagen fibril orientation to *B*0. Imaging of the femoral condyles can be challenging due to the bulk curvature of the cartilage altering the depth-dependent fibril orientation. However, a comprehensive *in vivo* study has shown that the "magic-angle effect" may not be the major determinant of T_2 heterogeneity in high-curvature articular cartilage.[105]

In Vivo Imaging

In vivo MR T_2 mapping has primarily been performed at 1.5 and 3.0 Tesla; however recent studies have demonstrated the feasibility of measuring relaxation properties in cartilage at 7.0 Tesla,[106-108] thus providing increased SNR. The acquisition time for each sequence is an important consideration in study design — minimal acquisition time (while retaining accurate quantification of relaxation properties) is desirable, such that the chances of motion during scans are minimized and the number of scans per study is maximized. Generally, the T_2 mapping acquisition time ranges from about 10–20 minutes,[109] however various techniques have been recently developed to reduce acquisition time: Fast T_2 imaging using gradient and spin echo (GRASE) MR imaging has been recently developed and validated at 1.5 Tesla, yielding an acquisition time of 1 minute and 51 seconds.[110] Parallel imaging sequences with an acceleration factor of 2 (AF = 2) have been developed at 3.0 Tesla for the measurement of cartilage relaxation times ($T_{1\rho}$, T_2) and morphologic measures (volume and thickness), demonstrating comparable results to the conventional method.[18] These studies highlight the novel technical advancements in MR sequence development for T_2 mapping.

In vivo imaging studies have evaluated the affects of gender,[111] age,[112,113] disease,[112,114–117] activity level,[118–120] and treatment (e.g. chondrocyte transplantation on T_2 relaxation time[121]). Studies have demonstrated that cartilage T_2 values are related to age, and vary from the subchondral bone to the cartilage surface.[112,122] Dunn et al. have shown that the cartilage T_2 values are associated with the severity of OA, and variations exist between tibial and femoral cartilage T_2.[123] The precision errors of T_2 measurements in patellar cartilage have been evaluated.[124,125] The precision errors of T_2 were markedly smaller than the differences in T_2 between healthy and diseased cartilage, suggesting that T_2 may be a discriminatory biomarker for disease. Dunn et al. used Z-score maps to compare cartilage T_2 values of OA subjects to those in control subjects.[123] Voxel based Z-scores were generated in each compartment of the articular cartilage for the T_2 images. A voxel in a Z–image was calculated by $(Voxel_I - Mean_{normal,compartment})/SD_{normal,compartment}$, where $Voxel_I$ is the T_2 in the voxel of interest, $Mean_{normal,compartment}$ is the mean T_2 for all voxels of the normal knees in that compartment, and the $SD_{normal,compartment}$ is the standard deviation of the same normal T_2 distribution. The Z-score maps normalize the T_2 results for each subject to the mean value of the control subjects. Figure 14 illustrates Z-score maps of a control, a mild OA subject, and a severe OA subject, respectively. These maps demonstrate the heterogeneity of cartilage T_2 values. Studies have evaluated the spatial distribution of cartilage T_2: Dray *et al.*[126] found no difference between mean T_2 values in OA cartilage; however, they showed visual differences in the spatial distribution of the T_2 values. These results demonstrate the necessity to characterize and quantify the spatial distribution of cartilage T_2 values. A recent study employed grey level o-occurrence matrix (GLCM) texture analysis to quantify the differences in spatial distribution of cartilage T_2 values in OA patients and controls. The mean, standard deviation, and GLCM entropy of cartilage T_2 was significantly greater in OA patients than in controls,[127] demonstrating that T_2 values in osteoarthritic cartilage are not only elevated, but also more heterogeneous than those in healthy cartilage. Moreover, Carballido-Gamio *et al.* have demonstrated the feasibility of flattening cartilage for texture analysis, thus obtaining measurements both

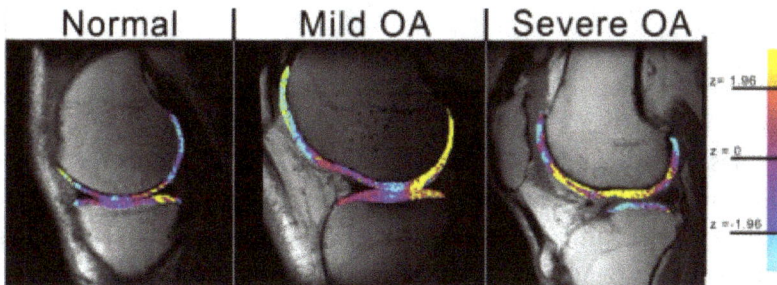

Fig. 14. Representative Z-score maps of a control, a mild OA subject, and a severe OA subject. The maps show an increase in area of regions of high Z-scores in the OA subjects. The regional variations in femoral and tibial cartilage compared to control subjects are also evident. Adapted from Dunn *et al.*[123]

parallel and perpendicular to the natural cartilage layers.[128] By non-invasively evaluating cartilage integrity, T_2 relaxation time may provide insight on both global (mean T_2) and focal (local spatial distribution of T_2) changes in cartilage degeneration in OA.

The evaluation of cartilage repair tissue using quantitative MRI is an emerging avenue of research. In addition to morphologic imaging techniques, T_2 relaxation time has been used to quantitatively assess the biochemical composition of cartilage repair tissue, thus providing insight on the tissue integrity. Previous studies have measured T_2 relaxation time to assess cartilage following cartilage repair procedures including chondrocyte transplantation[121,129–133] and microfracture.[130,132,134] A recent longitudinal study by Welsch *et al.* performed MRI examinations on patients one year after they had undergone matrix-associated autologous chondrocyte transplantation.[129] While there were no significant changes to cartilage morphology at one-year follow-up, changes to zonal T_2 values were evident. This study demonstrates the T_2 mapping may be an emerging tool to non-invasively and assess the longitudinal outcome of cartilage repair, and may supplement standard morphological cartilage assessment.

T_2 relaxation time has primarily been evaluated in cartilage in both healthy subjects and those with OA, however recent studies have measured T_2 in the meniscus.[135] Rauscher *et al.* demonstrated differences in T_2 between OA patients and controls, as well as correlations with clinical findings.[135] This study highlights that relaxation times measurements in both the cartilage and meniscus may be sensitive to degenerative changes in OA.

The relationship between T_2 and cartilage morphology has been evaluated cross-sectionally and longitudinally. Studies have shown an inverse relationship between cartilage T_2 and cartilage thickness.[116,123] Another study has shown that higher medial cartilage T_2 results in greater loss of medial cartilage volume at 12 months, demonstrating a relationship between cartilage T_2 and cartilage volume.[136] The relationship between cartilage T_2 and the underlying bone structure has been investigated.[137,138] Bolbos *et al.* reported a negative relationship between T_2 relaxation time, and bone structural parameters including bone volume fraction (BV/TV), and trabecular number (Tb.N),[137] highlighting the interplay between cartilage and bone structure.

Table 1. Inclusion criteria for the three subject groups in the OAI.

Progression cohort	Incidence cohort	Control cohort
Those who have frequent knee symptoms defined as "pain aching or stiffness in or around the knee on most days" for at least one month during the past 12 months and radiographic finding relating to the presence of OA corresponding to Kellgren-Lawrence grade ≥ 2.	Those who have characteristics that place them at increased risk for developing OA during the course of the study. These include being overweight, having previous knee injury, having previous knee surgery, having family history, and/or repetitive knee bending occupations.	Those who have no pain aching or stiffness in either knee in the past year, no radiographic findings of OA (Kellgren-Lawrence grade = 0), and no eligibility risk factors from the incidence cohort.

The Osteoarthritis Initiative (OAI) is a national and multi-center, ~5000-patient natural history and prevalence database of OA images. This study aims to evaluate the pathogenesis of OA and to classify biomarkers that can predict the development and progression of the disease. The OAI is a cross-sectional and longitudinal dataset that includes both MRI and radiographic images of subjects scanned annually over five years. MR images of cartilage to assess cartilage morphology and T_2 are available. Three subject groups (ages 45–79 years) will participate in the study: (1) the progression cohort: those with symptomatic knee OA at baseline, (2) the incidence cohort: those with an elevated risk of developing symptomatic OA during the course of the study, and (3) a control cohort. The inclusion criteria for each group are shown in Table 1. This database will provide a means to study and evaluate MRI biomarkers including T_2 relaxation time, in the development and progression of OA, thus providing a wealth of information for the scientific and medical community.

dGEMRIC Imaging

The change in glycosaminoglycan (GAG) concentration evident in early OA is associated with a change in tissue fixed charge density (FCD). This change in FCD (arising due to the loss of proteoglycans), can be detected by differences in the uptake of a charged contrast agent such as Gd-DTPA^{2-}.[139] Delayed gadolinium-enhanced MRI of cartilage (dGEMRIC) can be used to study cartilage GAG content and distribution in the knee[140–149] and the hip.[106,150–152] In dGEMRIC imaging, negatively-charged, intra-venous Gd-DTPA^{2-} is absorbed in articular cartilage. The negatively charged GAG in articular cartilage repels the negatively charged contrast agent. In diseased cartilage, the contrast agent is easily absorbed due to the lack of GAG. However, in healthy cartilage, the contrast agent is less likely to be absorbed due to the abundance of GAG. The distribution of Gd-DTPA^{2-} is calculated based on the T_1 relaxation time of the tissue.

dGEMRIC Imaging Protocol

In the dGEMRIC imaging protocol, the contrast agent is injected intra-venously, the subject exercises for approximately 10 minutes, and imaging is performed after about 1.5 hours for the knee and 20–30 minutes for the hip.[144] The reproducibility of this technique is 10%–15% for images taken several weeks apart.[144] The inter-observer variability (six investigators) for calculating T_1 values using a large region of interest (ROI) in both the lateral and medial femoral weight-bearing cartilage was 1.3%–2.3%. The intra-observer reproducibility for T_1 measurements was 2.6% for the lateral femoral cartilage and 1.5% for the medial femoral cartilage.[153] A recent study investigated the effects of intra-articular injection of contrast in dGEMRIC imaging in a canine model.[154] The results showed that the SNR was not significantly different between intravenous and intra-articular injection; however intra-articular injection provided superior visualization of GAG distribution. The low inter- and intra-observer variability for the intravenous dGEMRIC technique demonstrates the potential role of *in vivo* contrast-enhanced MR imaging in quantifying articular cartilage changes in OA.

Bashir *et al.* found that regions of cartilage degeneration (from trypsin or interleukin) showed histological differences, as well as differences in the post-contrast (Gd-DTPA^{2-}) signal intensity and T_1 relaxation time. When injected in subjects, intra-venous Gd-DTPA^{2-} is absorbed in articular cartilage two to eight hours post-injection, and this uptake is manifested as a signal intensity and T_1 change.[139]

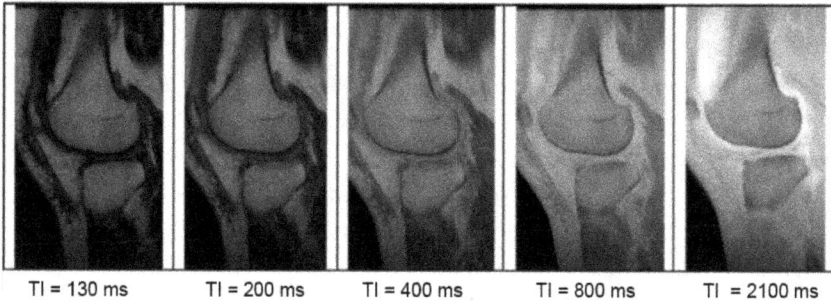

| TI = 130 ms | TI = 200 ms | TI = 400 ms | TI = 800 ms | TI = 2100 ms |

Fig. 15. An example of sagittal images of the knee (identical window and level) used to measure $T1$ relaxation time and determine the distribution of Gd-DTPA^{2-} in cartilage. A fast gradient echo sequence is used with the following scanning parameters: TI1/TI2/TI3/TI4/TI5 = 130/200/400/800/2100 ms, TR = 6.2 ms, resolution = 0.625 × 0.625×3 mm^3, FOV = 16 cm. The images reflect an uptake of Gd-DTPA^{2-} as demonstrated by the increases image signal intensity, particularly in the cartilage.

Three-dimensional dGEMRIC sequences have been implemented at 1.5 T and 3.0 T for use in clinical studies.[142] Recently, the feasibility of dGEMRIC scanning at 7.0 Tesla has been reported.[106] Figure 15 illustrates sagittal images of the knee (identical window and level) that can be used to measure T_1 relaxation time and determine the distribution of Gd-DTPA^{2-} in cartilage. The sensitivity of dGEMRIC is affected by various factors: For example, the amount of contrast agent absorbed in cartilage is dependent on the dose. A study by Burstein *et al.* showed that T_1 in patellar cartilage was 636 ± 70 msec after one dose and was 506 ± 38 msec after a double dose. With an increase in dose, there was a less noticeable difference in the contrast absorbed in cartilage, demonstrating that a greater dose provides increased sensitivity.[144] Body mass index (BMI) also affects contrast concentration and, must be carefully considered when designing cross-sectional studies.[145]

dGEMRIC has been used to evaluate osteoarthritic cartilage, since one of the initiating characteristics of OA is loss of cartilage proteogly-cans. dGEMRIC has been used to distinguish symptomatic from non-symptomatic OA patients.[141] In OA, the dGEMRIC index is associated with joint space width, Kellgren Lawrence (KL) grading scale and malalignment. Varus malaligment is associated with a lower dGEMRIC index on the medial side, while the opposite trend is evident in valgus malalignment.[141]

Knee cartilage in a given KL score has a wide range of dGEMRIC values, demonstrating that dGEMRIC may provide additional information to the radiographic classification of OA.[141] A recent longitudinal study reported that a low dGEMRIC index at baseline was significantly associated with the development of radiographic OA at six years follow-up.[146] These studies demonstrate the utility of dGEMRIC in evaluating cartilage integrity in patients with malalignment and symptomatic disease. Both cross-sectional and longitudinal assessments using dGEMRIC show promise in the assessment of cartilage integrity OA.

In Vitro Studies

Studies have demonstrated a relationship between dGEMRIC and mechanical properties of cartilage.[102,155,156] Kurkijarvi *et al.* found that dGEMRIC is correlated with compressive stiffness in non-arthritic human knee cartilage specimens.[157] In another study, tibial plateaus from patients undergoing total knee arthroplasty were indented to determine the relationship between compressive stiffness and GAG content. The strength of the correlation between GAG and local stiffness was dependent on the depth of the region in which the average GAG content was calculated. The highest correlations were found when GAG content was averaged in a region similar in depth to the indentation,[158] reflecting the heterogeneity of GAG distribution in cartilage. A study by Nieminen *et al.* indicated that the combination of T_2 quantification and $Gd\text{-}DTPA^{2-}$ enhanced imaging best characterized the mechanical properties of cartilage.[159] These results suggest that the combination of quantitative MR imaging techniques may predict the mechanical properties of cartilage.

In Vivo Studies

dGEMRIC studies have evaluated potential therapies in OA, demonstrated that moderate exercise can improve knee cartilage GAG content in patients with high risk of OA,[140] and showed that dGEMRIC can be used to monitor GAG content in autologous chondrocyte transplantation[121,149,160–162] and microfracture.[149] A study by Trattnig *et al.* performed dGEMRIC scans on patients who had undergone matrix associated autologous chondrocyte transplantation (MACT) ($n = 10$) and microfracture (MFX) ($n = 10$).

The study reported a higher cartilage GAG content, as measured by dGEMRIC, in the MACT group as compared to the MFX group.[149] These studies demonstrate that dGEMRIC is not only useful in evaluating diseased cartilage, but is also valuable in assessing the integrity of cartilage following cartilage repair.

Although dGEMRIC has been used primarily to evaluate cartilage, recent studies have used this method to evaluate the meniscus. A recent study has established the feasibility of evaluating the meniscus using dGEMRIC in both symptomatic and asymptomatic subjects.[148] The results demonstrate a relationship between dGEMRIC values in cartilage and the meniscus. The authors suggest that dGEMRIC is a potential method to evaluate the meniscus in arthritis. Since OA is a multi-factorial disease that affects the various tissues in the joint, it is interesting to assess various tissues with degeneration in OA. These studies suggest that dGEMRIC may have potential to assess various joint tissues in the course of osteoarthritis.

dGEMRIC is valuable in assessing early OA as it provides specific information on the distribution and content of GAG in cartilage. When implementing dGEMRIC, factors such as the concentration of contrast agent and the delay-time for imaging post-injection must be carefully considered. Research studies have shown that dGEMRIC can be used to assess the integrity of cartilage in the evolution of OA and to monitor the efficacy of cartilage repair techniques. Research studies on contrast-enhanced MRI establish the utility for using dGEMRIC to evaluate diseased cartilage and warrant further studies to evaluate the therapeutic efficacy of treatments for OA.

Summary

This chapter has discussed various MR imaging methods that probe early degenerative changes in cartilage biochemistry associated with OA. Quantitative MR imaging techniques including T_2 mapping, $T_{1\rho}$ mapping gagCEST, sodium imaging, and dGEMRIC have been used to evaluate the extracellular matrix of cartilage non-invasively. Each of these techniques is unique in its inherent mechanism for cartilage assessment, and each offers a distinctive perspective in the assessment of various components to the extracellular matrix.

One of the fundamental goals of MR imaging in OA is to diagnose OA at an early stage, such that treatment may be implemented before irreversible morphologic degeneration occurs. Since $T_{1\rho}$, T_2, dGEMRIC, gagCEST, and sodium imaging techniques are sensitive to different aspects of cartilage degeneration, future research on the combination of these techniques may be useful in the characterization of early OA. Quantitative MR imaging that is sensitive to biochemical changes appears promising and may potentially provide information beyond morphological changes in articular cartilage, with regards to early cartilage degeneration and biochemistry. The techniques discussed in this chapter hold promise for the evaluation of early cartilage disease, and the relationships between MR parameters, biochemistry, loading, gene and protein expression, disease progression and pain are clearly warranted.

Abbreviations

−NH: Amide proton
−OH: Hydroxyl proton
CEST: Chemical exchange dependent saturation transfer
DDD: Degenerative disc disease
GAG: Glycosaminogycan
IVD: Intervertebral disc
NMR: Nuclear magnetic resonance
NOE: Nuclear Overhauser effect
OA: Osteoarthritis
PG: Proteoglycan
SAR: Specific absorption rate
dGEMRIC: Delayed gadolinium-enhanced MRI contrast
gagCEST: CEST approach specialized in detecting GAG
k_{sw}: Chemical exchange rate from solute proton to water proton.

Acknowledgments

We would like to thank Wen Ling, Mark E. Schweitzer, and Gil Navon for their contributions to the gagCEST section of this chapter. We also thank Dr. Robert E. LaPrade for contributing Fig. 13.

References

1. Moskowitz RW, Altman RD, Hochberg MC, Buckwalter JA, Goldberg VM. *Osteoarthritis: Diagnosis and Medical / Surgical Management.* Philadelphia, PA: Lippincott Williams & Wilkins, 2007, p. 470.
2. Roughley PJ. The structure and function of cartilage proteoglycans. *Eur Cells Mater* 2006;12:92–101.
3. Kurtz SM, Edidin AA, editors. *Spine Technology Handbook.* London: Elsevier Academic Press, 2006.
4. Sepponen R. Rotating frame and magnetization transfer. In: Stark DD, Bradley WGJ, editors. *Magnetic Resonance Imaging,* Vol. 1. St. Louis: Mosby-Year Book, 1992, pp. 204–218.
5. Redfield AG. Nuclear spin thermodynamics in the rotating frame. *Science* 1969;164:1015–1023.
6. Duvvuri U, Charagundla SR, Kudchodkar SB, Kaufman JH, Kneeland JB, Rizi R, Leigh JS, Reddy R. Human knee: *in vivo* T1(rho)-weighted MR imaging at 1.5 T — preliminary experience. *Radiology* 2001;220(3):822–826.
7. Charagundla SR, Borthakur A, Leigh JS, Reddy R. Artifacts in T(1rho)-weighted imaging: correction with a self-compensating spin-locking pulse. *J Magn Reson* 2003;162(1):113–121.
8. Wheaton AJ, Borthakur A, Kneeland JB, Regatte RR, Akella SV, Reddy R. *In vivo* quantification of T1rho using a multislice spin-lock pulse sequence. *Magn Reson Med* 2004;52(6):1453–1458.
9. Li X, Han E, Ma C, Link T, Newitt D, Majumdar S. *In vivo* 3T spiral imaging based multi-slice T(1rho) mapping of knee cartilage in osteoarthritis. *Magn Reson Med* 2005;54(4):929–936.
10. Borthakur A, Hulvershorn J, Gualtieri E, Wheaton A, Charagundla S, Elliott M, Reddy R. A pulse sequence for rapid *in vivo* spin-locked MRI. *J Magn Reson Imaging* 2006;23(4):591–596.
11. Borthakur A, Wheaton A, Charagundla SR, Shapiro EM, Regatte RR, Akella SV, Kneeland JB, Reddy R. Three-dimensional T1rho-weighted MRI at 1.5 Tesla. *J Magn Reson Imaging* 2003;17(6):730–736.
12. Regatte RR, Akella SV, Wheaton AJ, Lech G, Borthakur A, Kneeland JB, Reddy R. 3D-T1rho-relaxation mapping of articular cartilage: *in vivo* assessment of early degenerative changes in symptomatic osteoarthritic subjects. *Acad Radiol* 2004;11(7):741–749.
13. Witschey W, Borthakur A, Elliott M, Fenty M, Sochor M, Wang C, Reddy R. T1rho-prepared balanced gradient echo for rapid 3D T1rho MRI. *J Magn Reson Imaging* 2008;28(3):744–754.
14. Wright GA, Brittain JH, Stainsby JA. Preserving T1 or T2 contrast in magnetization preparation sequences. In: *Proc Soc Magn Reson, 4th scientific Meeting.* New York, 1996, p. 1474.
15. Pakin S, Schweitzer M, Regatte R. 3D-T1rho quantitation of patellar cartilage at 3.0T. *J Magn Reson Imaging* 2006;24(6):1357–1363.

16. Li X, Han E, Busse R, Majumdar S. *In vivo* T1rho mapping in cartilage using 3D magnetization-prepared angle-modulated partitioned k-space spoiled gradient echo snapshots (3D MAPSS). *Magn Reson Med* 2008;59(2):298–307.

17. Pakin S, Schweitzer M, Regatte R. Rapid 3D-T1rho mapping of the knee joint at 3.0T with parallel imaging. *Magn Reson Med* 2006;56(3):563–571.

18. Zuo J, Li X, Banerjee S, Han E, Majumdar S. Parallel imaging of knee cartilage at 3 Tesla. *J Magn Reson Imaging* 2007;26(4):1001–1009.

19. Akella SV, Regatte RR, Gougoutas AJ, Borthakur A, Shapiro EM, Kneeland JB, Leigh JS, Reddy R. Proteoglycan-induced changes in T1rho-relaxation of articular cartilage at 4T. *Magn Reson Med* 2001;46(3):419–423.

20. Regatte RR, Akella SV, Borthakur A, Kneeland JB, Reddy R. Proteoglycan depletion-induced changes in transverse relaxation maps of cartilage: comparison of T2 and T1rho. *Acad Radiol* 2002;9(12):1388–1394.

21. Wheaton A, Dodge G, Elliott D, Nicoll S, Reddy R. Quantification of cartilage biomechanical and biochemical properties via T1rho magnetic resonance imaging. *Magn Reson Med* 2005;54(5):1087–1093.

22. Cheng J, Saadat E, Bolbos R, Jobke B, Siddiqui S, Ries M, Link T, Li X, Majumdar S. *Detection of Proteoglycan Content in Human Osteoarthritic Cartilage Samples with Magnetic Resonance T1rho Imaging.* 2008 May 5–9, Toronto, CA.

23. Li X, Ma C, Link T, Castillo D, Blumenkrantz G, Lozano J, Carballido-Gamio J, Ries M, Majumdar S. *In vivo* T1rho and T2 mapping of articular cartilage in osteoarthritis of the knee using 3 Tesla MRI. *Osteoarthr Cartil* 2007;15(7): 789–797.

24. Stahl R, Luke A, Li X, Carballido-Gamio J, Ma C, Majumdar S, Link T. T1rho, T(2) and focal knee cartilage abnormalities in physically active and sedentary healthy subjects versus early OA patients-a 3.0-Tesla MRI study. *Eur Radiol* 2009;19(1): 132–143.

25. Li X, Ma C, Bolbos R, Stahl R, Lozano J, Zuo J, Lin K, Link T, Safran M, Majumdar S. Quantitative assessment of bone marrow edema pattern and overlying cartilage in knees with osteoarthritis and anterior cruciate ligament tear using MR imaging and spectroscopic imaging. *J Magn Reson Imaging* 2008;28(2):453–461.

26. Zhao J, Bolbos R, Majumdar S, Link T, Li X. *Bone Marrow Edema-Like Lesions and Cartilage Degeneration in Osteoarthirits Using 3T MR T1rho Quantification: Longitudinal Assessment.* 2009 Apr 20–24, Honolulu, USA.

27. Bolbos R, Ma C, Link T, Majumdar S, Li X. *In vivo* T1rho quantitative assessment of knee cartilage after anterior cruciate ligament injury using 3 Tesla magnetic resonance imaging. *Invest Radiol* 2008;43(11):782–788.

28. Lozano J, Li X, Link T, Safran M, Majumdar S, Ma C. Detection of posttraumatic cartilage injury using quantitative T1rho magnetic resonance imaging. A report of two cases with arthroscopic findings. *J Bone Joint Surg Am* 2006;88(6): 1349–1352.

29. Kuo D, Theologis A, Bolbos R, Ma C, Li X. *Longitudinal Quantitative Evaluation of Cartilage Damage in ACL-Injured Knees Using MR T1ρ at 3T.* 2009 April 20–24, Honolulu, USA.

30. Rauscher I, Stahl R, Cheng J, Li X, Huber M, Luke A, Majumdar S, Link T. Meniscal measurements of T1rho and T2 at MR imaging in healthy subjects and patients with osteoarthritis. *Radiology* 2008;249(2):591–600.

31. Bolbos R, Link T, Ma C, Majumdar S, Li X. T1rho relaxation time of the meniscus and its relationship with T1rho of adjacent cartilage in knees with acute ACL injuries at 3T. *Osteoarthr Cartil* 2009;17(1):12–18.

32. Xia Y, Farquhar T, Burton-Wuster N, Ray E, Jelinski L. Difiusion and relaxation mapping of cartilage-bone plugs and excised disks using microscopic magnetic resonance imaging. *Magn Reson Med* 1994;31:273–282.

33. David-Vaudey E, Ghosh S, Ries M, Majumdar S. T2 relaxation time measurements in osteoarthritis. *Magn Reson Imaging* 2004;22(5):673–682.

34. Regatte R, Akella S, Lonner J, Kneeland J, Reddy R. T1rho relaxation mapping in human osteoarthritis (OA) cartilage: comparison of T1rho with T2. *J Magn Reson Imaging* 2006;23(4):547–553.

35. Li X, Pai A, Blumenkrantz G, Carballido-Gamio J, Link T, Ma C, Ries M, Majumdar S. Spatial distribution and relationship of T1rho and T2 relaxation times in knee cartilage with osteoarthritis. *Magn Reson Med* 2009;61(6):1310–1318.

36. Akella SV, Regatte RR, Wheaton AJ, Borthakur A, Reddy R. Reduction of residual dipolar interaction in cartilage by spin-lock technique. *Magn Reson Med* 2004;52(5):1103–1109.

37. Nieminen MT, Toyras J, Rieppo J, Hakumaki JM, Silvennoinen J, Helminen HJ, Jurvelin JS. Quantitative MR microscopy of enzymatically degraded articular cartilage. *Magn Reson Med* 2000;43(5):676–681.

38. Duvvuri U, Reddy R, Patel SD, Kaufman JH, Kneeland JB, Leigh JS. T1rho-relaxation in articular cartilage: effects of enzymatic degradation. *Magn Reson Med* 1997;38(6):863–867.

39. Makela HI, Grohn OH, Kettunen MI, Kauppinen RA. Proton exchange as a relaxation mechanism for T1 in the rotating frame in native and immobilized protein solutions. *Biochem Biophys Res Commun* 2001;289(4):813–818.

40. Duvvuri U, Goldberg AD, Kranz JK, Hoang L, Reddy R, Wehrli FW, Wand AJ, Englander SW, Leigh JS. Water magnetic relaxation dispersion in biological systems: the contribution of proton exchange and implications for the noninvasive detection of cartilage degradation. *Proc Natl Acad Sci USA* 2001;98(22): 12479–12484.

41. Kettunen M, Gröhn O, Silvennoinen M, Penttonen M, Kauppinen R. Effects of intracellular pH, blood, and tissue oxygen tension on T1rho relaxation in rat brain. *Magn Reson Med* 2002;48(3):470–477.

42. Mlynarik V, Szomolanyi P, Toffanin R, Vittur F, Trattnig S. Transverse relaxation mechanisms in articular cartilage. *J Magn Reson* 2004;169(2):300–307.

43. Mlynarik V, Trattnig S, Huber M, Zembsch A, Imhof H. The role of relaxation times in monitoring proteoglycan depletion in articular cartilage. *J Magn Reson Imaging* 1999;10(4):497–502.

44. Menezes NM, Gray ML, Hartke JR, Burstein D. T2 and T1rho MRI in articular cartilage systems. *Magn Reson Med* 2004;51(3):503–509.

45. Petrou M, Sevilla PG. *Dealing with Texture*. England: John Wiley & Sons, 2006.

46. Haralick R, Shanmugam K, Dinstein I. Textural features for image classification. *IEEE Trans Syst Man Cybern* 1973;3(6):610–618.

47. Hilal SK, Maudsley AA, Ra JB, Simon HE, Roschmann P, Wittekoek S, Cho ZH, Mun SK. *In vivo* NMR imaging of sodium-23 in the human head. *J Comput Assist Tomogr* 1985;9(1):1–7.

48. Maudsley AA, Hilal SK. Biological aspects of sodium-23 imaging. *Br Med Bull* 1984;40(2):165–166.

49. Garner WH, Hilal SK, Lee SW, Spector A. Sodium-23 magnetic resonance imaging of the eye and lens. *Proc Natl Acad Sci USA* 1986;83(6):1901–1905.

50. Ra JB, Hilal SK, Oh CH, Mun IK. *In vivo* magnetic resonance imaging of sodium in the human body. *Magn Reson Med* 1988;7(1):11–22.

51. Springer C. Biological systems: spin-3/2 nuclei. In: Grant DM Harris RK, editors. *Encyclopedia of Nuclear Magnetic Resonance*. New York: John Wiley and Sons, 1996, pp. 940–951.

52. Abragam A. *The Principles of Nuclear Magnetism*. London: Oxford University Press, 1961, p. 60.

53. Slichter C. *Principles of Magnetic Resonance*. Berlin: Springer, 1990.

54. Slichter C. *Principles of Magnetic Resonance*. Berlin: Springer, 1996.

55. Hubbard P. Nonexponential relaxation of rotating three-spin systems in molecules of a liquid. *J Chem Phys* 1970;52(2):563–568.

56. Shapiro EM, Borthakur A, Gougoutas A, Reddy R. 23Na MRI accurately measures fixed charge density in articular cartilage. *Mag Reson Med* 2002;47(2): 284–291.

57. Borthakur A, Hancu I, Boada FE, Shen GX, Shapiro EM, Reddy R. *In vivo* triple quantum filtered twisted projection sodium MRI of human articular cartilage. *J Magn Reson* 1999;141(2):286–290.

58. Shapiro EM, Borthakur A, Dandora R, Kriss A, Leigh JS, Reddy R. Sodium visibility and quantitation in intact bovine articular cartilage using high field (23)Na MRI and MRS. *J Magn Reson* 2000;142(1):24–31.

59. Reddy R, Insko EK, Leigh JS. Triple quantum sodium imaging of articular cartilage. *Magn Reson Med* 1997;38(2):279–284.

60. Duvvuri U, Kaufman JH, Patel SD, Bolinger L, Kneeland JB, Leigh JS, Reddy R. Sodium multiple quantum spectroscopy of articular cartilage: effects of mechanical compression. *Magn Reson Med* 1998;40(3):370–375.

61. Ling W, Regatte RR, Schweitzer ME, Jerschow A. Behavior of ordered sodium in enzymatically depleted cartilage tissue. *Magn Reson Med* 2006;56(5):1151–1155.

62. Choy J, Ling W, Jerschow A. Selective detection of ordered sodium signals via the central transition. *J Magn Reson* 2006;180(1):105–109.

63. Borthakur A, Mellon E, Niyogi S, Witschey W, Kneeland JB, Reddy R. Sodium and T1rho MRI for molecular and diagnostic imaging of articular cartilage. *NMR Biomed* 2006;19(7):781–821.

64. Navon G, Shinar H, Eliav U, Seo Y. Multiquantum filters and order in tissues. *NMR Biomed* 2001;14(2):112–132.

65. Reddy R, Shinnar M, Wang Z, Leigh JS. Multiple-quantum filters of spin-3/2 with pulses of arbitrary flip angle. *J Magn Reson B* 1994;104(2):148–152.

66. Eliav U, Keinan-Adamsky K, Navon G. A new method for suppressing the central transition in $I = 3/2$ NMR spectra with a demonstration for ^{23}Na in bovine articular cartilage. *J Magn Reson* 2003;165:276–281.

67. Rong P, Regatte RR, Jerschow A. Clean demarcation of cartilage tissue 23Na by inversion recovery. *J Magn Reson* 2008;193(2):207–209.

68. Lee JS, Regatte R, Jerschow A. Optimal nuclear magnetic resonance schemes for the central transition of a spin 3/2 in the presence of residual quadrupolar coupling. *J Chem Phys* 2008;129(22):224510–224515.

69. Wheaton AJ, Casey FL, Gougoutas AJ, Dodge GR, Borthakur A, Lonner JH, Schumacher HR, Reddy R. Correlation of T1rho with fixed charge density in cartilage. *J Magn Reson Imaging* 2004;20(3):519–525.

70. Reddy R, Insko EK, Noyszewski EA, Dandora R, Kneeland JB, Leigh JS. Sodium MRI of human articular cartilage *in vivo*. *Magn Reson Med* 1998;39(5):697–701.

71. Borthakur A, Shapiro EM, Beers J, Kudchodkar S, Kneeland JB, Reddy R. Sensitivity of MRI to proteoglycan depletion in cartilage: comparison of sodium and proton MRI. *Osteoarthr Cartil* 2000;8(4):288–293.

72. Wang L, Wu Y, Chang G, Oesingmann N, Schweitzer ME, Jerschow A, Regatte R. Rapid isotropic 3D-sodium MRI of the knee joint *in-vivo* at 7T. *J Magn Res Imag* 2009;30:606–614.

73. Boada FE, Shen GX, Chang SY, Thulborn KR. Spectrally weighted twisted projection imaging: reducing T2 signal attenuation effects in fast three-dimensional sodium imaging. *Magn Reson Med* 1997;38:1022–1028.

74. Ling W, Regatte RR, Schweitzer ME, Jerschow A. Characterization of bovine patellar cartilage by NMR. *NMR Biomed* 2008;21(3):289–295.

75. Ling W, Regatte RR, Navon G, Jerschow A. Assessment of glycosaminoglycan concentration *in vivo* by chemical exchange-dependent saturation transfer (gagCEST). *Proc Natl Acad Sci USA* 2008;105(7):2266–2270.

76. Ling W, Regatte RR, Schweitzer ME, Navon G, Jerschow A. gagCEST: a novel non-invasive MRI strategy to evaluate pathophysiology of musculoskeletal disorders. *US Musculoskel Rev* 2008;3(2):13–16.

77. Kim M, Gillen J, Landman BA, Zhou J, van Zijl PCM. Water saturation shift referencing (WASSR) for chemical exchange saturation transfer (CEST) experiments. *Mag Reson Med* 2009;61(6):1441–1450.

78. Guivel-Scharen V, Sinnwell T, Wolff SD, Balaban RS. Detection of proton chemical exchange between metabolites and water in biological tissues. *J Magn Reson* 1998;133(1):36–45.

79. Ward KM, Aletras AH, Balaban RS. A new class of contrast agents for MRI based on proton chemical exchange dependent saturation transfer (CEST). *J Magn Reson* 2000;143(1):79–87.

80. Zhou J, van Zijl PCM. Chemical exchange saturation transfer imaging and spectroscopy. *Prog NMR Spectr* 2006;48(2–3):109–136.

81. van Zijl PCM, Jones CK, Ren J, Malloy CR, Sherry AD. MRI detection of glycogen *in vivo* by using chemical exchange saturation transfer imaging (glycoCEST). *Proc Natl Acad Sci USA* 2007;104(11):4359–4364.

82. Gilad AA, Winnard PT Jr, van Zijl PCM, Bulte JWM. Developing MR reporter genes: promises and pitfalls. *NMR Biomed* 2007;20(3):275–290.

83. Hills BP, Cano C, Belton PS. Proton NMR relaxation studies of aqueous polysaccharide systems. *Macromolecules* 1991;24(10):2944–2950.

84.   Huster D, Schiller J, Naji L, Kaufmann J, Arnold K. NMR Studies of Cartilage —
       Dynamics, Diffusion, Degradation. *Lect Notes Phys* 2004;634:465–503.
85.   Schiller J, Naji L, Huster D, Kaufmann J, Arnold K. 1H and 13C HR-MAS NMR
       investigations on native and enzymatically digested bovine nasal cartilage. *MAGMA*
       2001;13(1):19–27.
86.   Grad J, Bryant RG. Nuclear magnetic cross-relaxation spectroscopy. *J Magn Reson*
       1990;90(1):1–8.
87.   Noggle JH, Schirmer RE. *The Nuclear Overhauser Effect, Chemical Application.*
       New York, NY: Academic Press, 1971.
88.   Balaban RS, Ceckler TL. Magnetization transfer contrast in magnetic resonance
       imaging. *Magn Reson Q* 1992;8:116–137.
89.   Wolff SD, Balaban RS. Magnetization transfer contrast (MTC) and tissue water
       proton relaxation *in vivo*. *Magn Reson Med* 1989;10:135–144.
90.   Hua J, Jones CK, Blakeley J, Smith SA, van Zijl PC, Zhou J. Quantitative description
       of the asymmetry in magnetization transfer effects around the water resonance in
       the human brain. *Magn Reson Med* 2007;58(4):786–793.
91.   Urban JPG, Winlove CP. Pathophysiology of the intervertebral disc and the
       challenges for MRI. *J Magn Reson Imaging* 2007;25(2):419–432.
92.   Katz JN. Lumbar disc disorders and low-back pain: socioeconomic factors and
       consequences. *J Bone Joint Surg Am* 2006;88(Suppl 2):21–24.
93.   Ling W, Saar G, Regatte RR, Jerschow A, Navon G. *Assessing the Intervertebral
       Disc via gagCEST*. ISMRM Conference, Honolulu, Hawaii, 2009.
94.   Konig H, Sauter R, Delmling M, Vogt M. Cartilage disorders: a comparison
       of spin-echo, CHESS, and FLASH sequence MR images. *Radiology* 1987;164:
       753–758.
95.   Lehner K, Rechl H, Gmeinwieser J, Heuck A, Lukas H, Kohl H. Structure, function,
       degeneration of bovine hyaline cartilage: assessment with MR imaging *in vitro*.
       Radiology 1989;170:495–499.
96.   Broderick L, Turner D, Renfrew D, Schnitzer T, Huff J, Harris C. Severity of articular
       cartilage abnormality in patients with osteoarthritis: evaluation with fast spin-echo
       MR vs arthroscopy. *AJR* 1994;162:99–103.
97.   Peterfy CG. Imaging of the disease process. *Curr Opin Rheumatol* 2002;14(5):
       590–596.
98.   Watrin-Pinzano A, Ruaud JP, Olivier P, Grossin L, Gonord P, Blum A, Netter P,
       Guillot G, Gillet P, Loeuille D. Effect of proteoglycan depletion on T2 mapping in
       rat patellar cartilage. *Radiology* 2005;234(1):162–170.
99.   Toffanin R, Mlynarik V, Russo S, Szomolanyi P, Piras A, Vittur F. Proteoglycan
       depletion and magnetic resonance parameters of articular cartilage. *Arch Biochem
       Biophys* 2001;390(2):235–242.
100.   Lusse S, Claassen H, Gehrke T, Hassenpflug J, Schunke M, Heller M, Gluer CC.
       Evaluation of water content by spatially resolved transverse relaxation times of
       human articular cartilage. *Magn Reson Imaging* 2000;18(4):423–430.
101.   Chou MC, Tsai PH, Huang GS, Lee HS, Lee CH, Lin MH, Lin CY, Chung HW.
       Correlation between the MR T2 value at 4.7 T and relative water content in articular
       cartilage in experimental osteoarthritis induced by ACL transection. *Osteoarthr
       Cartil* 2009;17(4):441–447.

102. Lammentausta E, Kiviranta P, Nissi MJ, Laasanen MS, Kiviranta I, Nieminen MT, Jurvelin JS. T2 relaxation time and delayed gadolinium-enhanced MRI of cartilage (dGEMRIC) of human patellar cartilage at 1.5 T and 9.4 T: relationships with tissue mechanical properties. *J Orthop Res* 2006;24(3):366–374.

103. Xia Y. Relaxation anisotropy in cartilage by NMR microscopy (muMRI) at 14-microm resolution. *Magn Reson Med* 1998;39(6):941–949.

104. Goodwin DW, Wadghiri YZ, Dunn JF. Micro-imaging of articular cartilage: T2, proton density, and the magic angle effect. *Acad Radiol* 1998;5(11):790–798.

105. Mosher TJ, Smith H, Dardzinski BJ, Schmithorst VJ, Smith MB. MR imaging and T2 mapping of femoral cartilage: *in vivo* determination of the magic angle effect. *AJR Am J Roentgenol* 2001;177(3):665–669.

106. Welsch GH, Mamisch TC, Hughes T, Zilkens C, Quirbach S, Scheffler K, Kraff O, Schweitzer ME, Szomolanyi P, Trattnig S. *In vivo* biochemical 7.0 Tesla magnetic resonance: preliminary results of dGEMRIC, zonal T2, and T2* mapping of articular cartilage. *Invest Radiol* 2008;43(9):619–626.

107. Krug R, Carballido-Gamio J, Banerjee S, Stahl R, Carvajal L, Xu D, Vigneron D, Kelley DA, Link TM, Majumdar S. *In vivo* bone and cartilage MRI using fully-balanced steady-state free-precession at 7 Tesla. *Magn Reson Med* 2007;58(6):1294–1298.

108. Pakin SK, Cavalcanti C, La Rocca R, Schweitzer ME, Regatte RR. Ultra-high-field MRI of knee joint at 7.0T: preliminary experience. *Acad Radiol* 2006;13(9):1135–1142.

109. Regatte RR, Schweitzer ME. Novel contrast mechanisms at 3 Tesla and 7 Tesla. *Semin Musculoskelet Radiol* 2008;12(3):266–280.

110. Quaia E, Toffanin R, Guglielmi G, Ukmar M, Rossi A, Martinelli B, Cova MA. Fast T2 mapping of the patellar articular cartilage with gradient and spin-echo magnetic resonance imaging at 1.5 T: validation and initial clinical experience in patients with osteoarthritis. *Skeletal Radiol* 2008;37(6):511–517.

111. Mosher TJ, Collins CM, Smith HE, Moser LE, Sivarajah RT, Dardzinski BJ, Smith MB. Effect of gender on *in vivo* cartilage magnetic resonance imaging T2 mapping. *J Magn Reson Imaging* 2004;19(3):323–328.

112. Mosher TJ, Dardzinski BJ, Smith MB. Human articular cartilage: influence of aging and early symptomatic degeneration on the spatial variation of T2–preliminary findings at 3T. *Radiology* 2000;214(1):259–266.

113. Mosher TJ, Liu Y, Yang QX, Yao J, Smith R, Dardzinski BJ, Smith MB. Age dependency of cartilage magnetic resonance imaging T2 relaxation times in asymptomatic women. *Arthritis Rheum* 2004;50(9):2820–2828.

114. Li X, Ma C, Link TM, Castillo DD, Blumenkrantz G, Lozano J, Carballido-Gamio J, Ries M, Majumdar S. *In vivo* T(1rho) and T(2) mapping of articular cartilage in osteoarthritis of the knee using 3T MRI. *Osteoarthr Cartil* 2007;15(7):789–797.

115. Stahl R, Blumenkrantz G, Carballido-Gamio J, Zhao S, Munoz T, Hellio Le Graverand-Gastineau MP, Li X, Majumdar S, Link TM. MRI-derived T2 relaxation times and cartilage morphometry of the tibio-femoral joint in subjects with and without osteoarthritis during a 1-year follow-up. *Osteoarthr Cartil* 2007;15(11):1225–1234.

116. Blumenkrantz G, Lindsey CT, Dunn TC, Jin H, Ries MD, Link TM, Steinbach LS, Majumdar S. A pilot, two-year longitudinal study of the interrelationship between trabecular bone and articular cartilage in the osteoarthritic knee. *Osteoarthr Cartil* 2004;12(12):997–1005.

117. Koff MF, Amrami KK, Kaufman KR. Clinical evaluation of T2 values of patellar cartilage in patients with osteoarthritis. *Osteoarthr Cartil* 2007;15(2): 198–204.

118. Mosher TJ, Smith HE, Collins C, Liu Y, Hancy J, Dardzinski BJ, Smith MB. Change in knee cartilage T2 at MR imaging after running: a feasibility study. *Radiology* 2005;234(1):245–249.

119. Stahl R, Luke A, Li X, Carballido-Gamio J, Ma CB, Majumdar S, Link TM. T1rho, T(2) and focal knee cartilage abnormalities in physically active and sedentary healthy subjects versus early OA patients — a 3.0-Tesla MRI study. *Eur Radiol* 2009;19(1):132–143.

120. Liess C, Lusse S, Karger N, Heller M, Gluer CC. Detection of changes in cartilage water content using MRI T2-mapping *in vivo*. *Osteoarthr Cartil* 2002;10(12): 907–913.

121. Kurkijarvi JE, Mattila L, Ojala RO, Vasara AI, Jurvelin JS, Kiviranta I, Nieminen MT. Evaluation of cartilage repair in the distal femur after autologous chondrocyte transplantation using T2 relaxation time and dGEMRIC. *Osteoarthr Cartil* 2007;15(4):372–378.

122. Dardzinski BJ, Laor T, Schmithorst VJ, Klosterman L, Graham TB. Mapping T2 relaxation time in the pediatric knee: feasibility with a clinical 1.5-T MR imaging system. *Radiology* 2002;225(1):233–239.

123. Dunn TC, Lu Y, Jin H, Ries MD, Majumdar S. T2 Relaxation time of cartilage at MR imaging: comparison with severity of knee osteoarthritis. *Radiology* 2004;232(2):592–598.

124. Glaser C, Mendlik T, Dinges J, Weber J, Stahl R, Trumm C, Reiser M. Global and regional reproducibility of T2 relaxation time measurements in human patellar cartilage. *Magn Reson Med* 2006;56(3):527–534.

125. Welsch GH, Mamisch TC, Weber M, Horger W, Bohndorf K, Trattnig S. High-resolution morphological and biochemical imaging of articular cartilage of the ankle joint at 3.0T using a new dedicated phased array coil: *in vivo* reproducibility study. *Skeletal Radiol* 2008;37(6):519–526.

126. Dray N, Williams A, Prasad PV, Sharma L, Burstein D. T2 in an OA population: metrics for reporting data? Miami, Florida, 2005, p 1995.

127. Blumenkrantz G, Stahl R, Carballido-Gamio J, Zhao S, Lu Y, Munoz T, Hellio Le Graverand-Gastineau MP, Jain SK, Link TM, Majumdar S. The feasibility of characterizing the spatial distribution of cartilage T(2) using texture analysis. *Osteoarthr Cartil* 2008;16(5):584–590.

128. Carballido-Gamio J, Link TM, Majumdar S. New techniques for cartilage magnetic resonance imaging relaxation time analysis: texture analysis of flattened cartilage and localized intra- and inter-subject comparisons. *Magn Reson Med* 2008;59(6):1472–1477.

129. Welsch GH, Mamisch TC, Marlovits S, Glaser C, Friedrich K, Hennig FF, Salomonowitz E, Trattnig S. Quantitative T2 mapping during follow-up after matrix-associated autologous chondrocyte transplantation (MACT): Full-thickness and zonal evaluation to visualize the maturation of cartilage repair tissue. *J Orthop Res* 2009;27(7):957–963.

130. Welsch GH, Trattnig S, Scheffler K, Szomonanyi P, Quirbach S, Marlovits S, Domayer S, Bieri O, Mamisch TC. Magnetization transfer contrast and T2 mapping in the evaluation of cartilage repair tissue with 3T MRI. *J Magn Reson Imaging* 2008;28(4):979–986.

131. Welsch GH, Mamisch TC, Quirbach S, Zak L, Marlovits S, Trattnig S. Evaluation and comparison of cartilage repair tissue of the patella and medial femoral condyle by using morphological MRI and biochemical zonal T2 mapping. *Eur Radiol* 2009;19(5):1253–1262.

132. Welsch GH, Mamisch TC, Domayer SE, Dorotka R, Kutscha-Lissberg F, Marlovits S, White LM, Trattnig S. Cartilage T2 assessment at 3-T MR imaging: *in vivo* differentiation of normal hyaline cartilage from reparative tissue after two cartilage repair procedures — initial experience. *Radiology* 2008;247(1): 154–161.

133. Trattnig S, Mamisch TC, Welsch GH, Glaser C, Szomolanyi P, Gebetsroither S, Stastny O, Horger W, Millington S, Marlovits S. Quantitative T2 mapping of matrix-associated autologous chondrocyte transplantation at 3 Tesla: an *in vivo* cross-sectional study. *Invest Radiol* 2007;42(6):442–448.

134. Domayer SE, Kutscha-Lissberg F, Welsch G, Dorotka R, Nehrer S, Gabler C, Mamisch TC, Trattnig S. T2 mapping in the knee after microfracture at 3.0 T: correlation of global T2 values and clinical outcome — preliminary results. *Osteoarthr Cartil* 2008;16(8):903–908.

135. Rauscher I, Stahl R, Cheng J, Li X, Huber MB, Luke A, Majumdar S, Link TM. Meniscal measurements of T1rho and T2 at MR imaging in healthy subjects and patients with osteoarthritis. *Radiology* 2008;249(2):591–600.

136. Blumenkrantz G, Dunn TC, Lindsey C, Ries MD, Link TM, Steinbach LS, Newitt DC, Majumdar S. *Cartilage T2 as a Marker of Progression of Osteoarthritis.* San Antonio, TX, 2004, p. 234.

137. Bolbos RI, Zuo J, Banerjee S, Link TM, Ma CB, Li X, Majumdar S. Relationship between trabecular bone structure and articular cartilage morphology and relaxation times in early OA of the knee joint using parallel MRI at 3T. *Osteoarthr Cartil* 2008;16(10):1150–1159.

138. Lammentausta E, Kiviranta P, Toyras J, Hyttinen MM, Kiviranta I, Nieminen MT, Jurvelin JS. Quantitative MRI of parallel changes of articular cartilage and underlying trabecular bone in degeneration. *Osteoarthr Cartil* 2007;15(10):1149–1157.

139. Bashir A, Gray M, Burstein D. Gd-DTPA2- as a measure of cartilage degradation. *Magn Reson Med* 1996;36:665–673.

140. Roos EM, Dahlberg L. Positive effects of moderate exercise on glycosaminoglycan content in knee cartilage: a four-month, randomized, controlled trial in patients at risk of osteoarthritis. *Arthritis Rheum* 2005;52(11):3507–3514.

141. Williams A, Sharma L, McKenzie CA, Prasad PV, Burstein D. Delayed gadolinium-enhanced magnetic resonance imaging of cartilage in knee osteoarthritis: findings at different radiographic stages of disease and relationship to malalignment. *Arthritis Rheum* 2005;52(11):3528–3535.

142. McKenzie CA, Williams A, Prasad PV, Burstein D. Three-dimensional delayed gadolinium-enhanced MRI of cartilage (dGEMRIC) at 1.5T and 3.0T. *J Magn Reson Imaging* 2006;24(4):928–933.

143. Tiderius CJ, Olsson LE, Leander P, Ekberg O, Dahlberg L. Delayed gadolinium-enhanced MRI of cartilage (dGEMRIC) in early knee osteoarthritis. *Magn Reson Med* 2003;49(3):488–492.

144. Burstein D, Velyvis J, Scott KT, Stock KW, Kim YJ, Jaramillo D, Boutin RD, Gray ML. Protocol issues for delayed Gd(DTPA)(2-)-enhanced MRI (dGEMRIC) for clinical evaluation of articular cartilage. *Magn Reson Med* 2001;45(1):36–41.

145. Tiderius C, Hori M, Williams A, Sharma L, Prasad PV, Finnell M, McKenzie C, Burstein D. dGEMRIC as a function of BMI. *Osteoarthr Cartil* 2006;14(11): 1091–1097.

146. Owman H, Tiderius CJ, Neuman P, Nyquist F, Dahlberg LE. Association between findings on delayed gadolinium-enhanced magnetic resonance imaging of cartilage and future knee osteoarthritis. *Arthritis Rheum* 2008;58(6):1727–1730.

147. Eckstein F, Buck RJ, Wyman BT, Kotyk JJ, Le Graverand MP, Remmers AE, Evelhoch JL, Hudelmaier M, Charles HC. Quantitative imaging of cartilage morphology at 3.0 Tesla in the presence of gadopentate dimeglumine (Gd-DTPA). *Magn Reson Med* 2007;58(2):402–406.

148. Krishnan N, Shetty SK, Williams A, Mikulis B, McKenzie C, Burstein D. Delayed gadolinium-enhanced magnetic resonance imaging of the meniscus: an index of meniscal tissue degeneration? *Arthritis Rheum* 2007;56(5):1507–1511.

149. Trattnig S, Mamisch TC, Pinker K, Domayer S, Szomolanyi P, Marlovits S, Kutscha-Lissberg F, Welsch GH. Differentiating normal hyaline cartilage from post-surgical repair tissue using fast gradient echo imaging in delayed gadolinium-enhanced MRI (dGEMRIC) at 3 Tesla. *Eur Radiol* 2008;18(6):1251–1259.

150. Boesen M, Jensen KE, Qvistgaard E, Danneskiold-Samsoe B, Thomsen C, Oster-gaard M, Bliddal H. Delayed gadolinium-enhanced magnetic resonance imaging (dGEMRIC) of hip joint cartilage: better cartilage delineation after intra-articular than intravenous gadolinium injection. *Acta Radiol* 2006;47(4):391–396.

151. Cunningham T, Jessel R, Zurakowski D, Millis MB, Kim YJ. Delayed gadolinium-enhanced magnetic resonance imaging of cartilage to predict early failure of Bernese periacetabular osteotomy for hip dysplasia. *J Bone Joint Surg Am* 2006;88(7): 1540–1548.

152. Tiderius CJ, Jessel R, Kim YJ, Burstein D. Hip dGEMRIC in asymptomatic volunteers and patients with early osteoarthritis: the influence of timing after contrast injection. *Magn Reson Med* 2007;57(4):803–805.

153. Tiderius CJ, Tjornstrand J, Akeson P, Sodersten K, Dahlberg L, Leander P. Delayed gadolinium-enhanced MRI of cartilage (dGEMRIC): intra- and interobserver variability in standardized drawing of regions of interest. *Acta Radiol* 2004;45(6): 628–634.

154. Kwack KS, Cho JH, Kim MM, Yoon CS, Yoon YS, Choi JW, Kwon JW, Min BH, Sun JS, Kim SY. Comparison study of intraarticular and intravenous gadolinium-enhanced magnetic resonance imaging of cartilage in a canine model. *Acta Radiol* 2008;49(1):65–74.

155. Nissi MJ, Toyras J, Laasanen MS, Rieppo J, Saarakkala S, Lappalainen R, Jurvelin JS, Nieminen MT. Proteoglycan and collagen sensitive MRI evaluation of normal and degenerated articular cartilage. *J Orthop Res* 2004;22(3):557–564.

156. Nissi MJ, Rieppo J, Toyras J, Laasanen MS, Kiviranta I, Nieminen MT, Jurvelin JS. Estimation of mechanical properties of articular cartilage with MRI - dGEMRIC, T2 and T1 imaging in different species with variable stages of maturation. *Osteoarthr Cartil* 2007;15(10):1141–1148.

157. Kurkijarvi JE, Nissi MJ, Kiviranta I, Jurvelin JS, Nieminen MT. Delayed gadolinium-enhanced MRI of cartilage (dGEMRIC) and T2 characteristics of human knee articular cartilage: topographical variation and relationships to mechanical properties. *Magn Reson Med* 2004;52(1):41–46.

158. Samosky JT, Burstein D, Eric Grimson W, Howe R, Martin S, Gray ML. Spatially-localized correlation of dGEMRIC-measured GAG distribution and mechanical stiffness in the human tibial plateau. *J Orthop Res* 2005;23(1):93–101.

159. Nieminen MT, Toyras J, Laasanen MS, Silvennoinen J, Helminen HJ, Jurvelin JS. Prediction of biomechanical properties of articular cartilage with quantitative magnetic resonance imaging. *J Biomech* 2004;37(3):321–328.

160. Gillis A, Bashir A, McKeon B, Scheller A, Gray ML, Burstein D. magnetic resonance imaging of relative glycosaminoglycan distribution in patients with autologous chondrocyte transplants. *Invest Radiol* 2001;36(12):743–748.

161. Trattnig S, Marlovits S, Gebetsroither S, Szomolanyi P, Welsch GH, Salomonowitz E, Watanabe A, Deimling M, Mamisch TC. Three-dimensional delayed gadolinium-enhanced MRI of cartilage (dGEMRIC) for *in vivo* evaluation of reparative cartilage after matrix-associated autologous chondrocyte transplantation at 3.0T: Preliminary results. *J Magn Reson Imaging* 2007;26(4):974–982.

162. Pinker K, Szomolanyi P, Welsch GC, Mamisch TC, Marlovits S, Stadlbauer A, Trattnig S. Longitudinal evaluation of cartilage composition of matrix-associated autologous chondrocyte transplants with 3-T delayed gadolinium-enhanced MRI of cartilage. *AJR Am J Roentgenol* 2008;191(5):1391–1396.

8

Bone and Osteoarthritis

by Janet Goldenstein, Gabrielle Blumenkrantz, Radu I. Bolbos and Xiaojuan Li

Preview

Although OA has been considered a disease primarily characterized by cartilage degeneration, the accompanying bone changes are critical in the pathogenesis of OA. The pathologic bone changes in OA include joint space narrowing, osteophytes, increased turnover in subchondral bone, thinning of the trabecular structure, bone marrow lesions, subchondral bone sclerosis, and bony cysts. This chapter will review the role of bone quantity and quality in the natural history of OA as well as the significant impact MRI had on these discoveries. The changes in bone remodeling, trabecular microstructure, mechanical properties, and bone mineral density in OA will be discussed in this chapter.

MR Imaging Bone for OA

Magnetic Resonance Imaging (MRI) has the unique ability to visualize both cartilage and bone non-invasively and without ionizing radiation. Clinically available pulse sequences such as $T1$-weighted Spoiled Gradient Echo (SPGR) provide visible distinction between cartilage and subchondral bone. Additionally fat-suppressed SPGR images show good contrast between bright cartilage and relatively dark bone. Specialized sequences can be implemented to visualize trabecular bone.

MR Imaging of Trabecular Bone

MRI is the only imaging method without ionizing radiation to visualize and quantify *in-vivo*, non-invasively, three-dimensional trabecular bone structure. Hydrogen, a proton present in water, is the most frequently studied atom in MR imaging. Bone tissue is a composite biomaterial made up mainly (~85%) of collagen (type I) and calcium hydroxyapatite, and a very low water content (~15%). Additionally, the protons within bone tissue water have a very short $T2$ relaxation time (250 microseconds).[1] As a result, bone has a relatively low MR-detectable magnetization and gives no signal in standard MR images. Bone is instead revealed indirectly through bone marrow visualization, which has a high water and fat content. In high-resolution MR images bone tissue appears black while bone marrow, due to its sufficient amounts of water and fat, produces a high signal. Figure 1 shows an MR image of the trabecular bone structure of the distal femur where the dark intensity areas represent the trabecular bone network and the areas of high intensity represent bone marrow in the trabecular spaces.

The ability to visualize and quantify trabecular bone structure depends on the pulse sequence implemented. The pulse sequence needs to allow for high-resolution, which ensures the voxel size is on the order of the

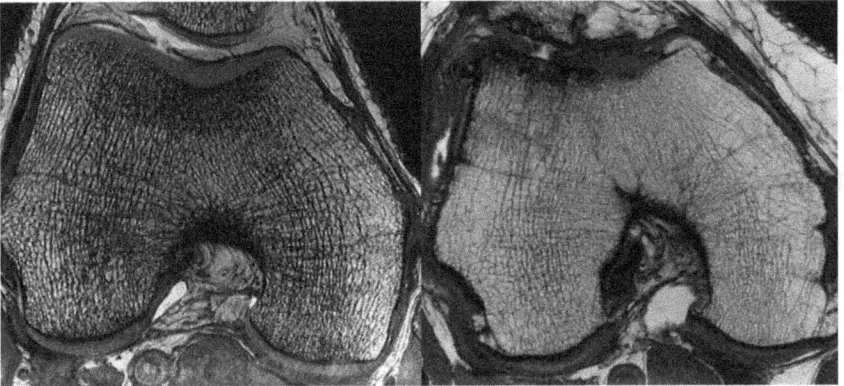

Fig. 1. MRI of the distal femur (knee) in a normal subject (left) and an OA subject (right). The trabecular bone network is represented by dark intensity while bone marrow appears bright in the image. While bone changes in response to OA vary due to location, the images below show decreased trabecular density in the OA patient.

trabecular structure (80–150 μm) and allow for an artifact free image with high signal-to-noise ratio (SNR). Additionally, it needs to allow for scanning of a large volume while ensuring that the scan time is within the limits of the patient's tolerance (10 to 15 minutes). Pulse sequences which meet these needs and are used for imaging trabecular bone of the knee can be classified as steady state gradient-echo type sequences[2] or steady state spin-echo type sequences.[3] There are trade-offs with all of these pulse sequences in terms of imaging time, SNR, and signal distortions which may effect the quantification of trabecular bone.[2–4]

In order to quantify trabecular bone structure, first each pixel pertaining to bone or to bone marrow needs to be identified. This binarization step becomes problematic in the presence of partial volume blurring. The spatial resolution of the image, especially in the slice direction, is greater than the dimension of the trabecular bone. Each pixel in a volume of interest (VOI) may contain a varying mixture of bone and marrow, not just one type of tissue (partial volume effects). Initially, a histogram of the distribution of signal intensities in the VOI is plotted. Due to the partial volume effects, the histogram does not have two distinct peaks corresponding to bone and marrow, but rather a single peak and an asymmetric tail. Therefore it is difficult to select an intensity to binarize the VOI into trabecular bone and marrow. The two main methods developed to address the complex binarization of bone are a histogram deconvolution algorithm (HDA)[5] and standardized histogram intensity based method.[6]

Many techniques have been developed to evaluate and quantify trabecular bone structure using MRI once the binarization step is complete. Most studies investigating the relationship between trabecular bone structure and OA have used MR-derived trabecular bone parameters analogous to those traditionally used in bone histomorphometry. Majumdar *et al.*[7] successfully adapted bone histomorphometric methods to MRI. For each slice in the VOI the total number of pixels contributing to the bone phase, Pp, are normalized to the total number of pixels. The total number of trabecular bone marrow boundaries that cross a set of parallel rays at a given angle, θ, through the image are counted to obtain $PL(\theta)$. The mean intercept length (MIL), an index of trabecular width, at a given angle, θ, is then computed as the ratio between the total area of trabecular bone and half the number of edges between bone and bone marrow that intersect the set of parallel rays passing through the image at that angle.

$$\text{MIL}(\theta) = 2P_p/P_L(\theta) \tag{1}$$

The mean value of the MIL for all angles provides a measurement of trabecular thickness, *Tb.Th*, such that *Tb.Th* $= 1/2$ average value of MIL(θ). From the measurements of P_p and *Tb.Th*, other histomorphometry measurements such as trabecular number, *Tb.N* $=$ area fraction of bone/*Tb.Th* and trabecular spacing, *Tb.Sp* $= (1/Tb.N) - Tb.Th$ can be calculated. High spatial resolution MR images of trabecular bone have voxel sizes on the order of trabecular thickness, thus partial volume effects, when each voxel in the image could represent more than one tissue type, influences MR-based trabecular structure assessment. MR images may not depict very thin trabeculae or may represent an average or projection of a few trabeculae. For this reason, MR-derived trabecular bone parameters are commonly termed "apparent" measures. A study conducted by Majumdar et al.[7] demonstrated the feasibility of using this technique to MR images to quantify trabecular structure. Studies which use Majumdar's technique to evaluate the relationship between trabecular bone structure and OA will be further discussed in subsequent sections of this chapter.

MR Imaging of Bone Marrow Edema Lesions (BMEL)

In addition to visualizing trabecular bone, MRI is also used to visualize bone marrow edema lesions (BMEL). BMEL do not show up in radiographs or other X-ray based images, but can be visualized using a MRI fat-suppressed SPGR sequence. Figure 4 shows a MR image of OA knee where the BMEL appears as a bright signal. The water-fat content of the bone marrow edema can also be determined using MR Spectroscopy.

OA and Bone

In OA, bone changes are evident on both the matrix and apparent levels. The "matrix level" refers to bone changes on the scale of 10 to 100's of microns. In OA, bone changes on this level include changes to the bone tissue such as altered remodeling and mineralization. The "apparent level" refers to bone changes on a scale of millimeters to centimeters. The bone changes on the apparent level are larger scale and include changes such as altered trabecular architecture. The mechanical properties of the "apparent level" include the effects from matrix level properties combined with the effects of bone mass and trabecular structure. The pathogenesis of osteoarthritic bone includes changes on both the matrix and apparent levels.

Bone Matrix Level

OA bone on the matrix level, on the scale of 10 to 100's of microns, has been evaluated and characterized. Reduced matrix mechanical properties may be due to decreased bone mineral density (BMD) of the bone matrix due to increase remodeling activity in osteoarthritic joints and due to an alteration in the college structure and network. Most OA bone research focuses on subchondral bone, the bone located directly below the cartilage.

Bone Mineral Density

Bone mineral density (BMD) is a measure of the amount of mineralized tissue in an area and has units of (g/cm^2). BMD is positively correlated with bone strength, and is often used as a predictor for risk of bone fracture. Studies evaluating the relationship between BMD in OA have mixed results: some finding positive correlation and others finding a negative correlation between BMD and OA.

Numerous cross-sectional studies indicated that OA is associated with increased BMD.[8–12] In a study of 1154 cohort subjects, mean femoral BMD of proximal femur was 5%–9% higher in patients with either Kellgren and Lawrence (KL) grade 1, grade 2, or grade 3 knee OA, compared with those with no knee OA.[8] Similarly a study of 979 women showed a small but significant increase in BMD in middle-aged women with OA defined on the basis of osteophytes of the hand, knee and lumbar spine.[9] The findings of a study by Newitt *et al.*[10] showed the same positive relationship between OA and increased BMD in hip OA. The study found that in 4855 elderly Caucasian women with moderate to severe radiographic hip OA had higher BMD in the hip, spine, and appendicular skeleton than did women without hip OA. Burger *et al.*[11] found that hip and knee radiographic OA of 2745 elderly subjects is associated with a higher BMD (3%–8%) and increased rate of bone loss. In a study of 485 premenopausal women aged 20–40 years found that women with radiographically defined knee OA have greater BMD (z-scores 0.3–0.8 higher) than do women without knee OA and are less likely to lose that higher level of BMD.[12] All of these studies agree that BMD is greater in bones of osteoarthritic patients bone compared to normal.

Several studies have not only evaluated the relationship between BMD and the incidence of OA but have also assessed the relationship between BMD and the progression of OA.[13–16] Bergink et al.[13] reported that high baseline femoral neck and lumbar spine BMD (the BMD at the beginning of a study which is used for comparison with later data) was positively correlated to the incidence and progression of knee OA, demonstrating a positive relationship between BMD and OA. A study of 473 women (ages 63 to 91 years) similarly found that high BMD and BMD gain was associated with an increased risk of incident knee OA, however it found different results in the association between BMD and progression of knee OA.[14] It found that high BMD and BMD gain decreased the risk of progression of radiographic knee OA and lowered the risk of joint space loss. Hart et al.[15] also confirmed that higher BMD in lumbar spine and hip is found in women who develop incident knee OA. However, they did not find a strong relationship between BMD and knee OA disease progression. A study examining 298 Caucasian men and 139 Caucasian women aged 20 and above found similar results by finding higher BMD at the lumbar spine but not at the femoral neck was associated with an increased risk of developing incident radiographic knee OA after adjustment for age, gender, and body mass index.[16] The study did not find a relationship between changes in bone mass and progression of OA. Differences in study results may be due to differences in bone remodeling in weight-bearing and non-weight-bearing joints, differences in the site and technique of bone mass measurement, and the relative location of the site of bone mass measurement.

Matrix Level Collagen Metabolism and Remodeling

Collagen is the major structural component of bone and provides tensile strength through cross-linking. In addition to its important structural role, collagen also provides a means for cellular communication. Changes in the nature of collagen structure, cross-linking, and metabolism, as well as bone remodeling in subchondral bone have been linked to osteoarthritic bone.[17-23] One study found increases in bone collagen metabolism in OA femoral heads compared to normal controls, with the greatest increase occurring in the subchondral bone.[19] However, the cross-linking in this study was similar in OA and healthy bone. The authors hypothesize that the changes in collagen synthesis in the bone matrix produces altered mechanical properties, thus exacerbating the degeneration of the other parts of the joint. Similarly another study found evidence of heightened collagen turnover in the subchondral trabecular bone in OA subjects when compared to age matched normal bone tissue.[20] Bailey *et al.* showed a 20-fold increase in subchondral bone turnover compared to normal in femoral head specimens.[21] They found narrow immature collagen fibers, a reduction in the collagen cross-linking, and decreased bone mineralization and suggested that these findings all contribute to a weakening of the mechanical properties of subchondral bone. Collagen structure was also shown to be altered in a follow-up study[22] which led the authors to suggest that this collagen structure alteration depends on the rate of turnover and hence the severity of OA. They also proposed that the change in collagen structure and decrease in cross-linking is due to increased water content of the fiber rather than a distortion of the molecular structure.[24]

Several studies have investigated the changes in bone cells[25-28] of OA patients, and results suggest that these changes may directly impact the surrounding cartilage. *Ex vivo* and *in vitro* results indicated altered activities of osteoblasts, bone formation cells, in OA.[25] The response of the osteoblasts from the bone of OA subjects to growth factors and cytokines, signaling molecules used in cellular communication, were altered compared to normal. A study by Bakker *et al.*[26] found that the cellular response to mechanical stress in bone cells is altered in OA femoral head specimens. Osteoblasts isolated from the bone of hip and knee explants from OA subjects were found to be capable of degrading cartilage proteoglycans in contrast to osteoblasts from normal bone.[27]

Microcracks in the subchondral bone or calcified cartilage stimulate focal remodeling and account for the increased vascularity in OA joints. Microcracks are found routinely in calcified cartilage from femoral heads of middle-aged nonarthritic humans and are associated with remodeling foci in OA cartilage.[29] Single or repetitive high-impact loads have been shown to cause microcracks,[30] which are followed by remodeling of the subchondral bone and degeneration of the overlying cartilage. Thus, microdamage in the calcified cartilage caused by mechanical stress, and the ensuing endochondral ossification, may play a vital role in the pathogenesis of OA.

Matrix Level Mechanical Properties

The mechanical properties of OA bone have been evaluated on the matrix level, on the scale of 10 to 100's of microns using *in vitro* mechanical testing and computer modeling. On the matrix level, osteoarthritic bone has a lower elastic modulus which corresponds to a lower stiffness. Using a combination of mechanical compression and ultrasound testing, Li and Aspden[31–33] tested the matrix level stiffness and composition of specimens from patients having hip arthroplasty, total hip replacement surgery. They found that OA has an altered subchondral bone plate composition in which the mass fraction of mineral is 12% less than normal and the matrix modulus, a measure of the matrix stiffness, is 15% less than normal. Using compression testing and finite element modeling of human osteoarthritic proximal tibia specimens, Day *et al.*[34] found the bone tissue modulus, the bone stiffness at the matrix level, was reduced by 60% in the medial condyle of the cases with cartilage damage compared to normal specimens. These studies both demonstrate that the tissue stiffness in osteoarthritic bone is decreased at the bone matrix level. This decreased stiffness affects the ability of bone to sustain weight, and absorb energy from impact and may be due to many factors such as altered mineralization and changes in the collagen of the bone matrix.

The hardness properties of OA trabecular bone at the matrix level have been examined in using micro-indentation techniques and electron probe microanalysis. Lereim *et al.*[35] used the Brinell Hardness Test (with a 5 mm indentation) and reported a 50% reduction of hardness in subchondral plate of the tibial plateau OA bone. A study by Coats *et al.*[36] examined the hardness properties of trabecular structure and similarly found a reduction of hardness in OA trabecular bone. It was interesting to note that the trabecular bone closest to the joint line was "harder" than bone farther from the joint line, demonstrating different responses to mechanical loading in different parts of the joint.

Bone Apparent Level

On the apparent level, on a scale of millimeters to centimeters, changes in OA bone involve alterations to subchondral cortical bone, trabecular bone, and the global mechanical properties of the joint.

Trabecular Bone Architecture

Changes in trabecular bone architecture of osteoarthritic joints are evident in OA[37–39] and can be visualized in Fig. 1. Increased trabecular thickness and decreased trabecular spacing is common in OA bone. One study found increased trabecular thickness in the principal compressive stress regions of the femoral head from human femoral specimens with OA.[37] Ding et al.[38] examined OA bone from human tibial specimens using micro-computed tomography and found that OA trabecular bone was thicker and more "plate-like" than normal, healthy bone. They hypothesized that the increase in trabecular thickness and density but decrease in connectivity in OA trabecular bone suggest a mechanism of altered bone remodeling in early OA. This altered bone remodeling leads to a change of trabeculae from rod-like to plate-like which is opposite to that of normal aging. Similarly results were found by Fazzalari et al. who used trabecular bone samples from severe osteoarthritic specimens taken following total hip replacement surgery.[39] They also found an increase in trabecular number and reduced trabecular spacing in OA.

Aside from examining the changes in trabecular structure using bone cores, it is also interesting to evaluate whether the trabecular structure differs depending on the location of the bone sample (e.g. medial or lateral side of the joint, or its proximity to the joint line), whether there are changes depending on the type of joint (e.g. proximal/distal femur, tibia, vertebra), and whether there are differences depending on the severity of OA. Studies have used MRI to quantify trabecular structure in different regions of the joint to determine whether there are differences in trabecular structure. MR imaging can be used to quantify apparent bone volume fracture, apparent trabecular thickness, apparent trabecular spacing, and apparent trabecular number, using a spatial resolution on the order of the trabecular thickness. One study by Beuf et al.[40] found differences in trabecular structure between the femur and the tibia in osteoarthritic knees using MRI. It was interesting to note that they also found that the differences in trabecular structure between the two anatomic sites became less pronounced in patients with more severe OA. This demonstrates that trabecular structure is constantly changing, and may become less heterogeneous as the disease progresses. Possibly, at the initial stages of OA, the femur and tibia behave differently, but as the disease progresses, the responses become less disparate. Thus, changes in trabecular microarchitecture should be evaluated separately in different regions of the joint and in patients with different disease severity.

Other imaging studies have found that bone microstructure is dependent on location.[41,42] Lindsey *et al.*[41] examined patients with OA of the knee using MRI. They found that as cartilage was lost on the medial side of the joint, there was an increase in bone on the medial side of the joint, and a loss of bone on the lateral side of the joint. These results demonstrated the response of bone to OA varies depending on location within the same joint. The authors suggest that bone responses may be due to joint malalignment. OA can be affected by varus or valgus alignment which distributes the forces during stance toward the medial and lateral sides of the joint, respectively. In the case of varus alignment, the cartilage and bone on the medial side of the joint experience more mechanical stress. Therefore, as the cartilage degenerates on the medial side of the joint, the bone may respond to the increased loading, by getting stronger. There may be an unloading effect on the lateral side of the joint, and the bone may respond by getting weaker. Another longitudinal study[42] found that cartilage degeneration was related to trabecular bone loss closer to the joint line, and trabecular bone gain farther from the joint line. The authors hypothesize that cartilage loss is related to subchondral plate sclerosis (greater absorption of local stresses and decreased load transmission). Thus, osteopenia occurs in the subarticular bone, and there is reactive bone formation farther from the joint line, compensating for the localized bone loss. Therefore, in OA, the trabecular structure has a varied response on the medial/lateral and proximal/distal areas of the joint, demonstrating the importance of location when examining trabecular bone structure in OA.

Subchondral bone is the bone located directly below the cartilage. Subchondral bone sclerosis, a thickening of the bone below the cartilage, is a prominent feature of OA which can result from increased rate of bone apposition and decreased rate of bone resorption. Subchondral bone sclerosis is often evident *in vivo* on both radiographs and on MR imaging scans. Radiography of OA joints in patients has shown that the formation of subchondral sclerosis occurs many months before changes in articular cartilage thickness.[43,44] A radiographic study by Buckland-Wright *et al.*[44] has shown evidence of increased subchondral bone sclerosis in the hand and knee of patients with OA, and well as increased trabecular number in the subchondral trabecular bone.

Apparent Level Mechanical Properties

The mechanical properties of OA bone on an apparent level are altered during the progression of the disease. Normal subchondral bone attenuate loads through the joint more than either the articular cartilage or surrounding soft tissues.[45] In a normal joint, the subchondral bone absorbs up to 50% of the load, and the cartilage absorbs only 1% to 3%.[45,46] In an OA joint, however, the sclerotic subchondral bone is less able to absorb and dissipate the energy of an impulsive load, increasing the force transmitted through the joint. Therefore, the OA knee absorbs only about half as much load as a normal knee.[46] Because the subchondral bone in OA is remodeling actively in response to the increased mechanical stress, much of the newly formed bone does not have sufficient time to mineralize fully. Therefore, from a material standpoint, this bone is less highly mineralized and is less stiff in OA patients than bone from age-matched healthy controls.[33,47]

Studies have evaluated the differences in trabecular apparent modulus a measure of the trabecular bone stiffness in trabecular bone specimens from patients with different severities of OA. A research study examining human trabecular specimens of the femoral condyle with mild OA found a 40% increase in apparent modulus.[48] Another study examining trabecular bone specimens from the femoral head of patients with severe OA also found increased apparent modulus of the bone.[49] Using a mechanical compression testing Li and Aspden[32] found a significantly increased OA bone stiffness compared to normal in specimens from patients having hip arthroplasty, total hip replacement surgery. These studies demonstrate that trabecular bone stiffness is increased in patients with both mild and severe OA.

It is uncertain whether changes in the subchondral bone precede or follow those in the overlying cartilage in OA. These changes are critically important in the initiation of cartilage damage and the progression of cartilage breakdown in OA. One of the first theories on the initiating factors in OA was proposed by Radin and Rose.[50] They hypothesized that the initiating factor in the pathogenesis of OA is an increased stiffness in subchondral bone in OA which adversely affects the bone's ability to absorb energy. A micro-fracture of the trabecular bone initiates the process of bone stiffening. The micro-fracture is followed by increased bone remodeling and localized stiffening of bone. Specifically, the healing of the micro-fractures (evident through callous formation) causes the bone to increase in stiffness. The subchondral bone loses its mechanical ability to withstand loading (due to its decrease in energy absorbing capacity). The changes in mechanical properties of the bone consequently increase the stress in the overlying cartilage and lead to cartilage degeneration. Therefore, Radin and Rose proposed that the onset of OA may be due to microfractures in bone.

Clinical Observations

Since soft tissue such as cartilage or the meniscus cannot be seen on radiographs, features based on bone are used for the classification of OA. Using the Kellgren Lawrence scale, radiologists are able to classify different grades of OA using markers based on bone observations such as joint space width, osteophytes, and subchondral cysts.

Joint Space Narrowing, Osteophytes, and Subchondral Cysts

One of the main characteristics of OA is joint space narrowing (JSN), or the decrease in the space between two joints (e.g. proximal tibia and the distal femur). Figure 2 demonstrates the difference in joint space between a normal and OA subject. JSN is directly related to the amount of cartilage; the less cartilage, the smaller the joint space width. Joint space has been historically evaluated on a radiograph. Radiographic JSN is currently the recommended primary end point in trials assessing new treatments for OA.[51,52] The underlying assumption in the use of radiographic JSN is that longitudinal reduction in the joint space is an accurate measure of a reduction in articular cartilage volume. This is not necessarily true, since radiographic joint space is comprised of addition

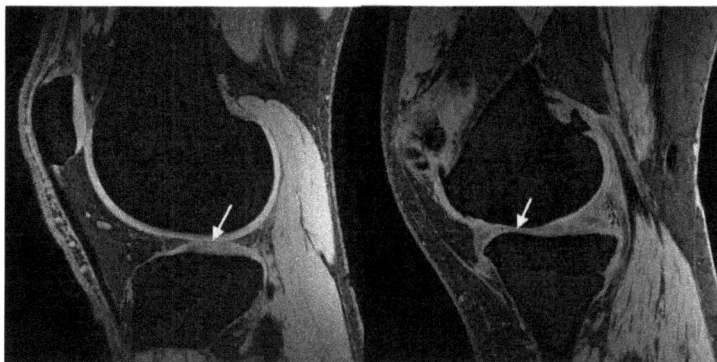

Fig. 2. MRI of a normal (left) and OA (right) knee. Joint Space Narrowing (JSN) is commonly observed in osteoarthritic knees. The white arrows highlight the decrease in joint space, the space between the femur and the tibia, in the OA knee.

structures than articular cartilage. Adams *et al.* found that early radiographic JSN reflects meniscal derangement in the absence of cartilage disease and cautions the evaluation of cartilage loss with radiography.[53] Another study found a strong negative association between medial and lateral tibial cartilage volumes and increasing grade of JSN in patients with knee OA.[54] Therefore, it appears that the reliability of cartilage measurement based solely on radiographic JSN may not be accurate.

Osteophytes, bony growths, which appear at the joint margins are also evident in OA knees[55,56] (Fig. 3). They most often appear at the margins of the joint, originally as outgrowths of cartilage and subsequently undergo endochondral ossification. Central osteophytes are not always easily observed on radiographs because the knee's curved articular surfaces can obscure them, but the tomographic nature of MR images allows osteophytes to be more clearly identified.[57] Studies have determined that radiographically diagnosed osteophytes at the tibio-femoral joint[58] and the patello-femoral joint[59] are associated with MR detected cartilage defects in the same joint. Another study of 193 OA patients determined that central osteophytes are common and are associated with full thickness or near full thickness articular cartilage defect.[56] In fact, osteophytes can form early in the development of OA and can be seen prior to JSN. One study analyzed knee radiography from 90 OA patients and found that bony changes such as subchondral bone sclerosis and osteophytes were evident without joint

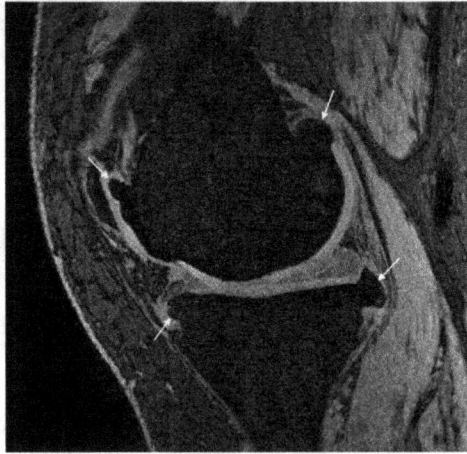

Fig. 3. An MR image of an OA knee. Osteophytes, bony growths, which commonly appear at the joint margins in OA knees are shown with white arrows.

space narrowing in as many as 40% of the OA patients.[43] However, the role of osteophytes, which are central to OA grading systems, is unclear. Although osteophytes may be able to predict pain in OA, they are not related to the severity of pain[60,61] or to OA disease progression.[62] Additionally, the presence of osteophytes and degree of cartilage damage does not correlate. Osteophytes have been observed without any cartilage damage and full thickness cartilage damage without the presence of osteophytes has been shown.[63] However, osteophytes may play a role in knee alignment. One study reported a significant increase in the motion of OA knees with osteophyte removal[64] indicating that osteophytes limit the mobility of OA knees. Another study reported that osteophytes are strongly associated with malalignment on the side of the osteophyte.[62] The authors hypothesized that the association osteophytes have with OA disease progression is partly explained by the association of malalignment with progression. Other evidence supports the concept that osteophytes represent a skeletal adaptation to local mechanical factors that in fact contribute to maintenance of joint function and stability.[55,64,65] Therefore, there remains uncertainty regarding the pathogenic role of osteophytes in OA.

A bone cyst, a fluid-filled cavity within the bone, is another characteristic of OA bone which is often visible on radiographic and MRI scans[66,67] and contains "fibrovascular tissue, linked to active new bone formation."[66,68] According to the intrusion theory, damaged cartilage allows the intrusion of synovial fluid into the bone thus forming a bone cyst which is able to communicate with the joint space.[66,69] Another theory, the bone contrusion theory (mechanical overload theory), suggests that a mechanical overload sufficient enough to cause bone necrosis, bone death, initiates the formation of bone cysts which do not communicate with the joint space.[70–72] Regardless of the primary event, fluid pressure definitely plays a role in the formation of bone cysts in OA.

Knee Alignment

Knee alignment is a key factor that determines the load distribution on the joint. Knee malalignment increases the local stresses in the joint which causes abnormal loading patterns and studies have found that malalignment is a risk factor for the onset of OA.[73–75] Knee alignment is assessed by calculating the angle between the femur and the tibia in the coronal plane. Alignment can be neutral, valgus (knock-kneed), or varus (bow-legged). It is hypothesized that varus malalignment increases the risk for medial OA progression, while valgus malalignment increases the risk for lateral OA progression.[74] This risk factor may be due to the fact that varus alignment increases forces in the medial compartment and valgus alignment increases forces in the lateral compartment. Additionally, there is a high prevalence of bone marrow edema, a lesion within the bone marrow, in knees with malalignment.[74] Sharma *et al.* further investigated how alignment (varus and valgus) affects the progression of OA in 230 subjects with knee OA.[75] The results of this study demonstrate that medial OA progression (during 18 months) occurred in 31% of the patients with varus alignment at baseline, while lateral OA progression occurred in only 22% of the patients with valgus alignment at baseline. After adjustment for age, sex, and BMI, varus alignment at baseline was associated with a four-fold increase in the odds for medial progression, while valgus alignment at baseline was associated with a nearly five-fold increase in the odds for lateral progression. The severity of alignment correlated with the severity of joint space loss. These results demonstrate that malignment is a significant risk factor for OA progression. Varus or valgus alignment may be influenced by genetic factors, developmental factors, or previous injury.

Another study by Cicuttini *et al.*[76] evaluated the effects of knee angle on tibiofemoral cartilage volume over two years. The study obtained a radiograph and 1.5 T MR image of 117 patients with knee at baseline and at two years. The baseline results demonstrated a negative relationship between knee angle and cartilage volume. Therefore, as knee angle increases, cartilage volume decreases. The longitudinal results show that cartilage volume decreased by 5.2% per year. For every 1° increase in baseline varus knee angle, there was an associated decrease in medial femoral cartilage by 17.7 micro-liters. For every 1° increase in baseline valgus knee angle, there was an associated decrease in medial femoral cartilage by 8 micro-liters. This study demonstrates that malalignment at baseline is associated with cartilage loss over two years and similarly suggests that malalignment is associated with OA progression.

The studies by Sharma *et al.*[74] and Cicuttini *et al.*[76] demonstrate that knee alignment is a risk factor for OA progression. Although each study used a different method to measure OA progression (radiography and MRI), their outcome was similar. In normally aligned knees, the medial side is disproportionately loaded; 60%–80% of compressive load is transmitted to the medial side.[76] Therefore, varus malalignment may have a stronger effect on the OA progression than valgus alignment.

Bone Marrow Edema-Like Lesions (BMEL)

Bone marrow edema-like lesions were originally diagnosed with MRI which has provided a powerful diagnostic tool to evaluate changes in the joint tissues within patients with OA. The term "bone marrow edema" (BME) was introduced in 1988 by Wilson[77] who identified regions of increased signal intensity using fluid sensitive magnetic resonance sequences and decreased signal intensity in the $T1$-weighted images. These bone marrow lesions detected with MRI have been also described as focal areas of increased signal in the subchondral marrow in fat-suppressed $T2$-weighted images.[78,79] Figure 4 shows bone marrow edema-like lesions in an OA knee as visualized by MRI. Although termed as "edema," these lesions have shown surprisingly little edema, accumulation of fluid, based

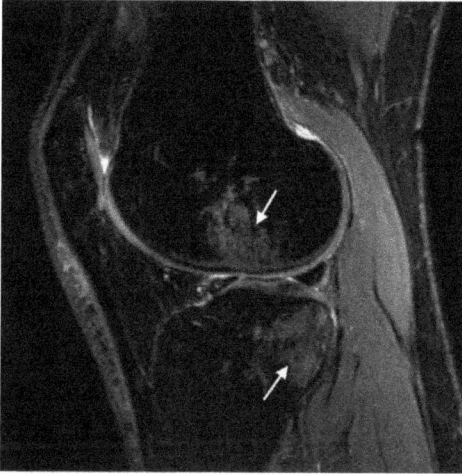

Fig. 4. A fat-suppressed $T2$-weighted FSE MRI of an OA knee in which the bone marrow edema-like lesion (BMEL) appears as a bright signal (white arrows).

on histopathologic examination as previously reported.[78] Instead, this increase in signal has been attributed to a number of other factors, including abnormal trabeculae, bone marrow necrosis, swelling of fat cells, and marrow hemorrhage. Therefore, it has been recently termed as bone marrow edema pattern (BMEP) or bone marrow edema-like lesions (BMEL).

When visualized using MR, BMEL has an ill-defined shape and is therefore difficult to quantify. Most imaging studies used a semi-qualitative evaluation by reporting the presence of high signal[80–82] or by scoring the size of bone bruise volume.[83,84] Quantitative evaluation has been implemented more recently in studies by measuring volume of BMEL manually or semi-automatically using MR images.[85–89] BMEL quantification will allow better classification of these lesions and potentially a better prediction to their prognosis.

BMEL is commonly seen in OA and has been well-documented in studies of patients with mild to severe osteoarthritic knees.[84,90,91] However, the findings on correlation between the presence of BMEL and clinical OA symptoms such as pain and stiffness are not consistent in the literature. BMEL was initially associated with pain in OA since bone marrow is richly innervated with nociceptive, pain-sensing, fibers. Felson *et al.* reported that BMEL on MRI are strongly associated with the presence of pain in knee OA.[83] BMELs were visualized in 272 of 351 (77.5%) persons with painful knees compared with 15 of 50 (30%) persons with no knee pain. The association between BMEL and knee pain in OA was further shown by others.[82,92,93] However it has since been demonstrated that knee effusion and osteophytes are associated with knee OA pain and no other MR findings.[79,84,94]

Regarding the association between BMEL and disease severity, Link *et al.* reported a significant increase of presence of BMEL with increased KL score.[84] Raynauld *et al.* performed a study to evaluate the size changes in BMEL and bone cysts in 107 patients with knee OA over 24 months.[79] The study found an association between cartilage volume loss and the change in BMEL size, independent of any other clinical variable. Additionally, Carrino *et al.* studied the association between BMEL and bone cysts and reported that subchondral cysts develop within regions of subchondral marrow edema-like signal and typically also subjacent to cartilage abnormalities.[95] Felson *et al.* discovered a correlation between BMEL and structure deterioration in knee OA, and between BMEL and frontal plane malalignment.[83] The data in their study showed that much of the relationship of BMEL to radiographic progression was actually explained by their association with malalignment, although there was still a substantial residual association of BMEL with radiographic progression after adjustment of malalignment. The authors concluded that OA disease progression in patients with BMEL may be the consequence of the lesions themselves, or malalignment may produce both the traumatic bone lesions and the wearing away of local cartilage.

BMEL is also commonly observed in acute injuries such as anterior cruciate ligament (ACL) tears,[80,81,85,96,97] where it indicates a so-called bone bruise or impression fracture due to translational injury, where the anterolateral femur impacts the posterolateral tibia (kissing contusions) when the ACL is ruptured. Long-term follow-up studies reported that there was a high prevalence of radiographic OA, pain, and functional limitations in ACL-injured patients 10–20 years after injuries.[98,99] A number of studies have proposed that the cartilage overlying BMEL has sustained irreversible injury during impact, and thus, cartilage degeneration can continue to occur despite the fact that functional stability of the knee is restored following ACL reconstruction.[100,101] Two studies reported that histological samples of the occult bone bruises and overlying cartilage in ACL-injured knees revealed necrosis of osteocytes, degeneration of overlying chondrocytes, and loss of the proteoglycan component in cartilage matrix.[100,102] It is unknown if OA develops due to an irreversible biochemical change caused by the initial ACL injury, an alteration in knee kinematics even after ACL reconstruction, or a combination of both factors. Although the mechanism of OA development in ACL-injured and reconstructed knees remains unclear, there is an interest in investigating clinical significance of BMEL to OA development in such knees because of the observations in the above studies and the association between BMEL and OA progression.

The biochemical composition of bone marrow and BMEL has been studied using proton MR spectroscopy (MRS) techniques. Proton MRS provides a noninvasive method for quantifying biochemical or metabolic changes in tissues. MRS has been used widely in cerebral imaging and other tissues/organs such as prostate, breast, and muscle. However, few studies have investigated MRS in knee bone marrow.[89,103] In the case of bone marrow, the water and lipid contents are of interest.[104–107] Different compartments of lipids can be also investigated using MRS. Of particular interest are indices that provide measures of the unsaturation levels among the triglycerides, which may have potential medical applications.[108,109] Ratios of the methylene or olefinic to methyl resonances are examples of such indices. Figure 5 shows the spectral data in bone marrow with

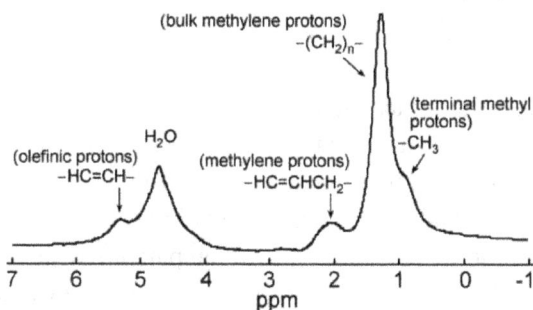

Fig. 5. *In vivo* bone marrow spectral data. Identifiable peaks include olefinic protons ($-CH=CH-$) around 5.35 ppm, water around 4.65 ppm, methylene protons ($-CH=CHCH_2-$) around 2.06 ppm, bulk methylene protons ($-(CH_2)_n-$) around 1.3 ppm, and terminal methyl protons ($-CH_3$) around 0.9 ppm.

identified peaks of olefinic protons ($-CH=CH-$) around 5.35 ppm, water around 4.65 ppm, methylene protons ($-CH=CHCH_2-$) around 2.06 ppm, bulk methylene protons ($-(CH_2)_n-$) around 1.3 ppm, and terminal methyl protons ($-CH_3$) around 0.9 ppm.

The interest in examining lipid compositions within bone marrow of OA is based on the following observations. First, early changes are seen in the adjoining subchondral and trabecular bone in OA as mentioned in previous sections. Second, it is recognized that lipid metabolism plays an important role in bone remodeling.[110] Some investigators have further hypothesized that OA may be a systemic disorder including lipid metabolism.[111] This potential role of lipid metabolism in OA is supported by the association between high body mass index (BMI) and an increased risk of OA,[112,113] not only for knee joints, but also for non-weight-bearing joints such as the hands.[114,115] Plumb et al., have shown that the amount of fat in OA trabecular bone/bone marrow is significantly elevated, and the fat composition is also altered.[116] In addition, adipocytes secrete several highly active molecules including leptin, adiponectin, and resistin. These substances, collectively known as adipocytokines, may function as signaling molecules that influence chondrocyte metabolism in osteoarthritic cartilage.[117–119] Dumond et al., demonstrated that leptin is overexpressed in the human OA knee joint (in both synovial fluid and cartilage tissue) and suggested that leptin contributes to the pathogenesis of OA through stimulation of growth factor synthesis.[117]

Using in vivo 3D MR spectroscopic imaging (MRSI) techniques, bone marrow water and lipid contents were studied in patients with OA ($n = 10$), patients with acute ACL-injuries ($n = 14$) and healthy controls ($n = 8$).[89] Figure 6 presents the typical spectra for a healthy volunteer (Fig. 6a), a patient with OA (Fig. 6b) and a patient with ACL tear (Fig. 6c), respectively. In healthy controls, saturated lipids at 1.3 ppm dominated the signal. All of the patients who had OA or ACL tears showed significantly elevated water at 4.65 ppm in BMEL. Eight out of ten patients with OA, and 13 out of 14 patients with ACL tears showed significantly elevated unsaturated lipids at 5.35 ppm. Significantly elevated water peaks were more focused within BMEL, while significantly elevated unsaturated lipid peaks extended outside the BMEL. Saturated lipids decreased within BMEL. Further quantification of the spectral data showed that the volume of elevated water

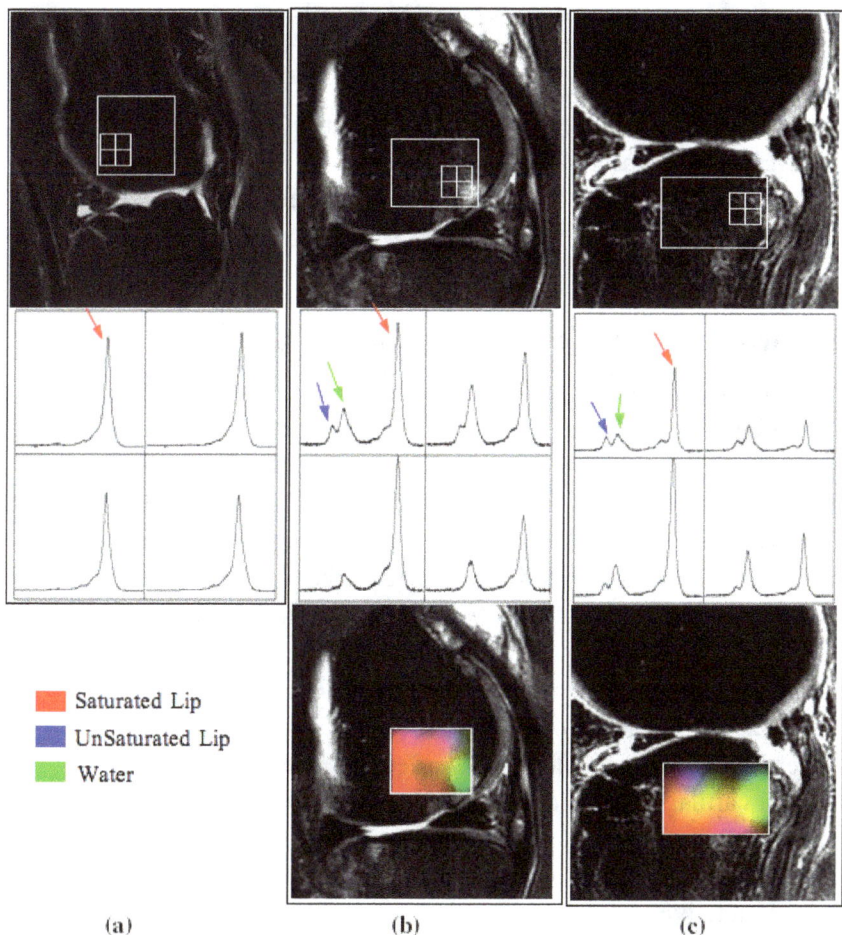

Fig. 6. MR spectral data in bone marrow in a healthy volunteer **(a)**, a patient with OA **(b)**, and a patient with ACL tear **(c)**. In healthy controls, saturated lipid at 1.3 ppm dominated the signal. Significantly elevated unsaturated lipid peaks at 5.35 ppm and water peaks at 4.65 ppm were observed in patients with OA and ACL tear. Significantly elevated water peaks were more focused within BMEL, while significantly elevated unsaturated lipid peaks extended outside the BMEL. Saturated lipids decreased within BMEL.

as derived from MRSI data correlated significantly with the volume of BMEL ($R = 75.5\%$, $P < 0.001$). No correlation was found between the volume of elevated unsaturated lipids and the volume of BMEL. Patients with ACL tears had larger volumes of BMEL, elevated water and elevated unsaturated lipids than patients with OA, but these differences were not significant ($P > 0.05$). These results suggested that there is a significant biochemical changes within the bone marrow of OA and acutely injured knees. These changes are in particular associated with BMEL. However, the origin of the unsaturated lipids remains unclear and further study is warranted on investigating the clinical significance of the changes in bone marrow lipids.

Interaction of Subchondral Bone and Cartilage

The structures in the joint including subchondral bone, trabecular bone, and articular cartilage, collectively withstand mechanical loads that are imposed on the joint. The altered mechanical properties of osteoarthritic bone substantially affect the mechanical loading behavior of the articular cartilage. Since the cartilage may reactively degenerate due to altered loading, it is important to study the interaction between the bone (trabecular and subchondral) and the articular cartilage. One study by Wei *et al.*[120] used finite element models to predict the stress transmission from the trabecular and subchondral bone in the femoral head and neck to the overlying articular cartilage. The results of their study show that the changes in mechanical properties of the subchondral bone affect the stresses experienced by the articular cartilage. Specifically, they found that shear stress on the articular cartilage surface was related to subchondral plate stiffening. However, there was weaker relationship between the shear stress on the cartilage surface and the underlying stiffness of the trabecular bone. These results illustrate the interaction and collective behavior of cartilage and underlying sub-chondral bone in joint loading. Since nutrients from below the subchondral cortical bone may diffuse into the overlying cartilage,[121] the degeneration of bone (especially subchondral) is an important factor in progression of OA. The cartilage overlying the sclerotic subchondral bone degenerates and decreases in volume in OA. Therefore, the cartilage experiences increased mechanical stress. The interplay between the cartilage and bone degenerative changes needs to be further studied to understand whether bone changes, or cartilage changes initiate degeneration in OA. To further understand the pathology of the disease, it would be interesting to evaluate the effects of bone degeneration on other joint tissues, such as the meniscus, that are also involved in OA.

Summary

This chapter is a review of the current understanding of the role of bone in OA. Changes in bone at the matrix level and apparent level are evident in OA. Reduced matrix mechanical properties may be caused by a decrease in bone mineral density (BMD) due to an increase in remodeling activity and due to an alteration in the college structure and network in osteoarthritic joints. At the apparent level, increased trabecular thickness and decreased trabecular spacing as well as the presence of sclerotic bone at the subcondral surface is common in OA bone. The sclerotic subchondral bone is less able to absorb and dissipate the energy of an impulsive load, increasing the force transmitted through the joint. Therefore, the OA knee absorbs only about half as much load as a normal knee. However, it is uncertain whether changes in the subchondral bone precede or follow those in the overlying cartilage in OA. Clinically, because soft tissue such as cartilage or the meniscus cannot be seen on radiographs, features based on bone are used for the classification of OA. Using the Kellgren Lawrence scale, radiologists are able to classify different grades of OA using markers based on bone observations such as joint space width, osteophytes, and subchondral cysts. However additional measures related to bone such as bone marrow edema-like lesions (BMEL) and knee alignment may help improve the clinical diagnosis and grading of OA. MRI has had an enormous impact in understanding the role of bone in OA. MRI has the advantage of being able to non-invasively assess three-dimensional trabecular bone structure without ionizing radiation. Additionally, MRI can depict BMELs which are commonly associated with OA and cannot be assessed in normal radiographs. Numerous studies have used MRI to assess bone changes and bone characteristics in OA.[40–42,54,56–59,61,67,76,79,82,84,92,122] MRI is well-suited for studying the interactions between bone and cartilage in OA because of its superior tissue contrast. The assessment of articular cartilage volume in isolation, is unlikely to be the best available means of determining the severity of OA; use of a combination of measures of multiple joint structures associated with disease (e.g. bone, meniscus, etc.) may help to better assess the severity of knee OA.

References

1. Fernandez-Seara MA, Wehrli SL, Wehrli FW. Diffusion of exchangeable water in cortical bone studied by nuclear magnetic resonance. *Biophys J* 2002;82(1 Pt 1):522–529.

2. Banerjee S, Han ET, Krug R, Newitt DC, Majumdar S. Application of refocused steady-state free-precession methods at 1.5 and 3 T to *in vivo* high-resolution MRI of trabecular bone: simulations and experiments. *J Magn Reson Imaging* 2005;21(6):818–825.

3. Krug R, Han ET, Banerjee S, Majumdar S. Fully balanced steady-state 3D-spin-echo (bSSSE) imaging at 3 Tesla. *Magn Reson Med* 2006;56(5):1033–1040.

4. Techawiboonwong A, Song HK, Magland JF, Saha PK, Wehrli FW. Implications of pulse sequence in structural imaging of trabecular bone. *J Magn Reson Imaging* 2005;22(5):647–655.

5. Hwang SN, Wehrli FW. Experimental evaluation of a surface charge method for computing the induced magnetic field in trabecular bone. *J Magn Reson* 1999;139(1):35–45.

6. Majumdar S, Genant HK, Grampp S, Newitt DC, Truong VH, Lin JC, Mathur A. Correlation of trabecular bone structure with age, bone mineral density, and osteoporotic status: *in vivo* studies in the distal radius using high resolution magnetic resonance imaging. *J Bone Miner Res* 1997;12(1):111–118.

7. Majumdar S, Newitt D, Jergas M, Gies A, Chiu E, Osman D, Keltner J, Keyak J, Genant H. Evaluation of technical factors affecting the quantification of trabecular bone structure using magnetic resonance imaging. *Bone* 1995;17(4):417–430.

8. Hannan MT, Anderson JJ, Zhang Y, Levy D, Felson DT. Bone mineral density and knee osteoarthritis in elderly men and women. The Framingham Study. *Arthritis Rheum* 1993;36(12):1671–1680.

9. Hart DJ, Mootoosamy I, Doyle DV, Spector TD. The relationship between osteoarthritis and osteoporosis in the general population: the Chingford Study. *Ann Rheum Dis* 1994;53(3):158–162.

10. Nevitt MC, Lane NE, Scott JC, Hochberg MC, Pressman AR, Genant HK, Cummings SR. Radiographic osteoarthritis of the hip and bone mineral density. The Study of Osteoporotic Fractures Research Group. *Arthritis Rheum* 1995;38(7): 907–916.

11. Burger H, van Daele PL, Odding E, Valkenburg HA, Hofman A, Grobbee DE, Schutte HE, Birkenhager JC, Pols HA. Association of radiographically evident osteoarthritis with higher bone mineral density and increased bone loss with age. The Rotterdam Study. *Arthritis Rheum* 1996;39(1):81–86.

12. Sowers M, Lachance L, Jamadar D, Hochberg MC, Hollis B, Crutchfield M, Jannausch ML. The associations of bone mineral density and bone turnover markers with osteoarthritis of the hand and knee in pre- and perimenopausal women. *Arthritis Rheum* 1999;42(3):483–489.

13. Bergink AP, Uitterlinden AG, Van Leeuwen JP, Hofman A, Verhaar JA, Pols HA. Bone mineral density and vertebral fracture history are associated with incident and progressive radiographic knee osteoarthritis in elderly men and women: the Rotterdam Study. *Bone* 2005;37(4):446–456.

14. Zhang Y, Hannan MT, Chaisson CE, McAlindon TE, Evans SR, Aliabadi P, Levy D, Felson DT. Bone mineral density and risk of incident and progressive radiographic knee osteoarthritis in women: the Framingham Study. *J Rheumatol* 2000;27(4):1032–1037.

15. Hart DJ, Cronin C, Daniels M, Worthy T, Doyle DV, Spector TD. The relationship of bone density and fracture to incident and progressive radiographic osteoarthritis of the knee: the Chingford Study. *Arthritis Rheum* 2002;46(1):92–99.

16. Hochberg MC, Lethbridge-Cejku M, Tobin JD. Bone mineral density and osteoarthritis: data from the Baltimore Longitudinal Study of Aging. *Osteoarthr Cartil* 2004;12(Suppl A):S45–48.

17. Burr DB. Anatomy and physiology of the mineralized tissues: role in the pathogenesis of osteoarthrosis. *Osteoarthr Cartil* 2004;12(Suppl A):S20–30.

18. Gevers G, Dequeker J. Collagen and non-collagenous protein content (osteocalcin, sialoprotein, proteoglycan) in the iliac crest bone and serum osteocalcin in women with and without hand osteoarthritis. *Coll Relat Res* 1987;7(6):435–442.

19. Mansell JP, Bailey AJ. Abnormal cancellous bone collagen metabolism in osteoarthritis. *J Clin Invest* 1998;101(8):1596–1603.

20. Mansell JP, Tarlton JF, Bailey AJ. Biochemical evidence for altered subchondral bone collagen metabolism in osteoarthritis of the hip. *Br J Rheumatol* 1997;36(1):16–19.

21. Bailey AJ, Mansell JP, Sims TJ, Banse X. Biochemical and mechanical properties of subchondral bone in osteoarthritis. *Biorheology* 2004;41(3–4):349–358.

22. Bailey AJ, Sims TJ, Knott L. Phenotypic expression of osteoblast collagen in osteoarthritic bone: production of type I homotrimer. *Int J Biochem Cell Biol* 2002;34(2):176–182.

23. Seibel MJ, Duncan A, Robins SP. Urinary hydroxy-pyridinium crosslinks provide indices of cartilage and bone involvement in arthritic diseases. *J Rheumatol* 1989;16(7):964–970.

24. Bailey AJ, Mansell JP, Trevor SJ, Xavier B. Biochemical and mechanical properties of subchondral bone in osteoarthritis. In: Stoltz JF, editor. *Mechanobiology: Cartilage and Chondrocyte*, Vol. 3. IOS Press, 2004, pp. 349–358.

25. Hilal G, Martel-Pelletier J, Pelletier JP, Ranger P, Lajeunesse D. Osteoblast-like cells from human subchondral osteoarthritic bone demonstrate an altered phenotype *in vitro*: possible role in subchondral bone sclerosis. *Arthritis Rheum* 1998;41(5):891–899.

26. Bakker AD, Klein-Nulend J, Tanck E, Heyligers IC, Albers GH, Lips P, Burger EH. Different responsiveness to mechanical stress of bone cells from osteoporotic versus osteoarthritic donors. *Osteoporos Int* 2006;17(6):827–833.

27. Westacott CI, Webb GR, Warnock MG, Sims JV, Elson CJ. Alteration of cartilage metabolism by cells from osteoarthritic bone. *Arthritis Rheum* 1997;40(7):1282–1291.

28. Sanchez C, Deberg MA, Bellahcene A, Castronovo V, Msika P, Delcour JP, Crielaard JM, Henrotin YE. Phenotypic characterization of osteoblasts from the sclerotic zones of osteoarthritic subchondral bone. *Arthritis Rheum* 2008;58(2):442–455.

29. Burr DB. The importance of subchondral bone in the progression of osteoarthritis. *J Rheumatol Suppl* 2004;70:77–80.

30. Vener MJ, Thompson RC Jr, Lewis JL, Oegema TR Jr. Subchondral damage after acute transarticular loading: an *in vitro* model of joint injury. *J Orthop Res* 1992;10(6):759–765.

31. Li B, Aspden RM. Material properties of bone from the femoral neck and calcar femorale of patients with osteoporosis or osteoarthritis. *Osteoporos Int* 1997;7(5):450–456.

32. Li B, Aspden RM. Composition and mechanical properties of cancellous bone from the femoral head of patients with osteoporosis or osteoarthritis. *J Bone Miner Res* 1997;12(4):641–651.

33. Li B, Aspden RM. Mechanical and material properties of the subchondral bone plate from the femoral head of patients with osteoarthritis or osteoporosis. *Ann Rheum Dis* 1997;56(4):247–254.

34. Day JS, Ding M, van der Linden JC, Hvid I, Sumner DR, Weinans H. A decreased subchondral trabecular bone tissue elastic modulus is associated with pre-arthritic cartilage damage. *J Orthop Res* 2001;19(5):914–918.

35. Lereim P, Goldie I, Dahlberg E. Hardness of the subchondral bone of the tibial condyles in the normal state and in osteoarthritis and rheumatoid arthritis. *Acta Orthop Scand* 1974;45(4):614–627.

36. Coats AM, Zioupos P, Aspden RM. Material properties of subchondral bone from patients with osteoporosis or osteoarthritis by microindentation testing and electron probe microanalysis. *Calcif Tissue Int* 2003;73(1):66–71.

37. Fazzalari NL, Darracott J, Vernon-Roberts B. Histomorphometric changes in the trabecular structure of a selected stress region in the femur in patients with osteoarthritis and fracture of the femoral neck. *Bone* 1985;6(3):125–133.

38. Ding M, Odgaard A, Hvid I. Changes in the three-dimensional microstructure of human tibial cancellous bone in early osteoarthritis. *J Bone Joint Surg Br* 2003;85(6):906–912.

39. Fazzalari NL, Parkinson IH. Fractal properties of subchondral cancellous bone in severe osteoarthritis of the hip. *J Bone Miner Res* 1997;12(4):632–640.

40. Beuf O, Ghosh S, Newitt DC, Link TM, Steinbach L, Ries M, Lane N, Majumdar S. Magnetic resonance imaging of normal and osteoarthritic trabecular bone structure in the human knee. *Arthritis Rheum* 2002;46(2):385–393.

41. Lindsey CT, Narasimhan A, Adolfo JM, Jin H, Steinbach LS, Link T, Ries M, Majumdar S. Magnetic resonance evaluation of the interrelationship between articular cartilage and trabecular bone of the osteoarthritic knee. *Osteoarthr Cartil* 2004;12(2):86–96.

42. Blumenkrantz G, Lindsey CT, Dunn TC, Jin H, Ries MD, Link TM, Steinbach LS, Majumdar S. A pilot, two-year longitudinal study of the interrelationship between trabecular bone and articular cartilage in the osteoarthritic knee. *Osteoarthr Cartil* 2004;12(12):997–1005.

43. Buckland-Wright JC, MacFarlane DG, Jasani MK, Lynch JA. Quantitative microfocal radiographic assessment of osteoarthritis of the knee from weight bearing tunnel and semiflexed standing views. *J Rheumatol* 1994;21(9):1734–1741.

44. Buckland-Wright C. Subchondral bone changes in hand and knee osteoarthritis detected by radiography. *Osteoarthr Cartil* 2004;12(Suppl A):S10–19.

45. Radin EL, Paul IL, Lowy M. A comparison of the dynamic force transmitting properties of subchondral bone and articular cartilage. *J Bone Joint Surg Am* 1970;52(3):444–456.

46. Hoshino A, Wallace WA. Impact-absorbing properties of the human knee. *J Bone Joint Surg Br* 1987;69(5):807–811.

47. Grynpas MD, Alpert B, Katz I, Lieberman I, Pritzker KP. Subchondral bone in osteoarthritis. *Calcif Tissue Int* 1991;49(1):20–26.

48. Pugh JW, Radin EL, Rose RM. Quantitative studies of human subchondral cancellous bone. Its relationship to the state of its overlying cartilage. *J Bone Joint Surg Am* 1974;56(2):313–321.

49. Brown AN, McKinley TO, Bay BK. Trabecular bone strain changes associated with subchondral bone defects of the tibial plateau. *J Orthop Trauma* 2002;16(9): 638–643.

50. Radin EL, Rose RM. Role of subchondral bone in the initiation and progression of cartilage damage. *Clin Orthop Relat Res* 1986(213):34–40.

51. Altman R, Brandt K, Hochberg M, Moskowitz R, Bellamy N, Bloch DA, Buckwalter J, Dougados M, Ehrlich G, Lequesne M, Lohmander S, Murphy WA, Jr., Rosario-Jansen T, Schwartz B, Trippel S. Design and conduct of clinical trials in patients with osteoarthritis: recommendations from a task force of the Osteoarthritis Research Society. Results from a workshop. *Osteoarthr Cartil* 1996;4(4):217–243.

52. Abadie E, Ethgen D, Avouac B, Bouvenot G, Branco J, Bruyere O, Calvo G, Devogelaer JP, Dreiser RL, Herrero-Beaumont G, Kahan A, Kreutz G, Laslop A, Lemmel EM, Nuki G, Van De Putte L, Vanhaelst L, Reginster JY. Recommendations for the use of new methods to assess the efficacy of disease-modifying drugs in the treatment of osteoarthritis. *Osteoarthr Cartil* 2004;12(4):263–268.

53. Adams JG, McAlindon T, Dimasi M, Carey J, Eustace S. Contribution of meniscal extrusion and cartilage loss to joint space narrowing in osteoarthritis. *Clin Radiol* 1999;54(8):502–506.

54. Cicuttini FM, Wluka AE, Forbes A, Wolfe R. Comparison of tibial cartilage volume and radiologic grade of the tibiofemoral joint. *Arthritis Rheum* 2003;48(3):682–688.

55. van der Kraan PM, van den Berg WB. Osteophytes: relevance and biology. *Osteoarthr Cartil* 2007;15(3):237–244.

56. McCauley TR, Kornaat PR, Jee WH. Central osteophytes in the knee: prevalence and association with cartilage defects on MR imaging. *AJR Am J Roentgenol* 2001;176(2):359–364.

57. Waldschmidt JG, Braunstein EM, Buckwalter KA. Magnetic resonance imaging of osteoarthritis. *Rheum Dis Clin North Am* 1999;25(2):451–465.

58. Boegard T, Rudling O, Petersson IF, Jonsson K. Correlation between radiographically diagnosed osteophytes and magnetic resonance detected cartilage defects in the tibiofemoral joint. *Ann Rheum Dis* 1998;57(7):401–407.

59.   Boegard T, Rudling O, Petersson IF, Jonsson K. Correlation between radiograph-
       ically diagnosed osteophytes and magnetic resonance detected cartilage defects in
       the patellofemoral joint. *Ann Rheum Dis* 1998;57(7):395–400.
60.   Cicuttini FM, Baker J, Hart DJ, Spector TD. Association of pain with radiological
       changes in different compartments and views of the knee joint. *Osteoarthr Cartil*
       1996;4(2):143–147.
61.   Sengupta M, Zhang YQ, Niu JB, Guermazi A, Grigorian M, Gale D, Felson DT,
       Hunter DJ. High signal in knee osteophytes is not associated with knee pain.
       Osteoarthr Cartil 2006;14(5):413–417.
62.   Felson DT, Gale DR, Elon Gale M, Niu J, Hunter DJ, Goggins J, Lavalley
       MP. Osteophytes and progression of knee osteoarthritis. *Rheumatology (Oxford)*
       2005;44(1):100–104.
63.   Alonge TO, Oni OO. An investigation of the frequency of co-existence of
       osteophytes and circumscribed full thickness articular surface defects in the knee
       joint. *Afr J Med Med Sci* 2000;29(2):151–153.
64.   Pottenger LA, Phillips FM, Draganich LF. The effect of marginal osteophytes
       on reduction of varus-valgus instability in osteoarthritic knees. *Arthritis Rheum*
       1990;33(6):853–858.
65.   Messent EA, Ward RJ, Tonkin CJ, Buckland-Wright C. Differences in trabecular
       structure between knees with and without osteoarthritis quantified by macro and
       standard radiography, respectively. *Osteoarthr Cartil* 2006;14(12):1302–1305.
66.   Landells JW. The bone cysts of osteoarthritis. *J Bone Joint Surg Br* 1953;35-
       B(4):643–649.
67.   Pouders C, De Maeseneer M, Van Roy P, Gielen J, Goossens A, Shahabpour M.
       Prevalence and MRI-anatomic correlation of bone cysts in osteoarthritic knees. *AJR
       Am J Roentgenol* 2008;190(1):17–21.
68.   Dequeker J. The inverse relationship between osteoporosis and osteoarthrosis. *Verh
       K Acad Geneeskd Belg* 1987;49(4):273–309.
69.   Schmalzried TP, Akizuki KH, Fedenko AN, Mirra J. The role of access of joint
       fluid to bone in periarticular osteolysis. A report of four cases. *J Bone Joint Surg
       Am* 1997;79(3):447–452.
70.   Woods CG. Subchondral bone cysts. *J Bone Joint Surg Br* 1961;43-B:758–766.
71.   Sabokbar A, Crawford R, Murray DW, Athanasou NA. Macrophage-osteoclast
       differentiation and bone resorption in osteoarthrotic subchondral acetabular cysts.
       Acta Orthop Scand 2000;71(3):255–261.
72.   Durr HD, Martin H, Pellengahr C, Schlemmer M, Maier M, Jansson V. The cause
       of subchondral bone cysts in osteoarthrosis: a finite element analysis. *Acta Orthop
       Scand* 2004;75(5):554–558.
73.   Cerejo R, Dunlop DD, Cahue S, Channin D, Song J, Sharma L. The influence of
       alignment on risk of knee osteoarthritis progression according to baseline stage of
       disease. *Arthritis Rheum* 2002;46(10):2632–2636.
74.   Sharma L. Local factors in osteoarthritis. *Curr Opin Rheumatol* 2001;13(5):
       441–446.
75.   Sharma L, Song J, Felson DT, Cahue S, Shamiyeh E, Dunlop DD. The role of
       knee alignment in disease progression and functional decline in knee osteoarthritis.
       JAMA 2001;286(2):188–195.

76. Cicuttini F, Wluka A, Hankin J, Wang Y. Longitudinal study of the relationship between knee angle and tibiofemoral cartilage volume in subjects with knee osteoarthritis. *Rheumatology (Oxford)* 2004;43(3):321–324.

77. Wilson AJ, Murphy WA, Hardy DC, Totty WG. Transient osteoporosis: transient bone marrow edema? *Radiology* 1988;167(3):757–760.

78. Zanetti M, Bruder E, Romero J, Hodler J. Bone marrow edema pattern in osteoarthritic knees: correlation between MR imaging and histologic findings. *Radiology* 2000;215(3):835–840.

79. Raynauld JP, Martel-Pelletier J, Berthiaume MJ, Abram F, Choquette D, Haraoui B, Beary JF, Cline GA, Meyer JM, Pelletier JP. Correlation between bone lesion changes and cartilage volume loss in patients with osteoarthritis of the knee as assessed by quantitative magnetic resonance imaging over a 24-month period. *Ann Rheum Dis* 2008;67(5):683–688.

80. Bretlau T, Tuxoe J, Larsen L, Jorgensen U, Thomsen HS, Lausten GS. Bone bruise in the acutely injured knee. *Knee Surg Sports Traumatol Arthrosc* 2002;10(2): 96–101.

81. Costa-Paz M, Muscolo DL, Ayerza M, Makino A, Aponte-Tinao L. Magnetic resonance imaging follow-up study of bone bruises associated with anterior cruciate ligament ruptures. *Arthroscopy* 2001;17(5):445–449.

82. Sowers MF, Hayes C, Jamadar D, Capul D, Lachance L, Jannausch M, Welch G. Magnetic resonance-detected subchondral bone marrow and cartilage defect characteristics associated with pain and X-ray-defined knee osteoarthritis. *Osteoarthr Cartil* 2003;11(6):387–393.

83. Felson DT, Chaisson CE, Hill CL, Totterman SM, Gale ME, Skinner KM, Kazis L, Gale DR. The association of bone marrow lesions with pain in knee osteoarthritis. *Ann Intern Med* 2001;134(7):541–549.

84. Link TM, Steinbach LS, Ghosh S, Ries M, Lu Y, Lane N, Majumdar S. Osteoarthritis: MR imaging findings in different stages of disease and correlation with clinical findings. *Radiology* 2003;226(2):373–381.

85. Roemer FW, Bohndorf K. Long-term osseous sequelae after acute trauma of the knee joint evaluated by MRI. *Skeletal Radiol* 2002;31(11):615–623.

86. Schmid MR, Hodler J, Vienne P, Binkert CA, Zanetti M. Bone marrow abnormalities of foot and ankle: STIR versus T1-weighted contrast-enhanced fat-suppressed spin-echo MR imaging. *Radiology* 2002;224(2):463–469.

87. Mayerhoefer ME, Breitenseher M, Hofmann S, Aigner N, Meizer R, Siedentop H, Kramer J. Computer-assisted quantitative analysis of bone marrow edema of the knee: initial experience with a new method. *AJR Am J Roentgenol* 2004;182(6):1399–1403.

88. Davies NH, Niall D, King LJ, Lavelle J, Healy JC. Magnetic resonance imaging of bone bruising in the acutely injured knee–short-term outcome. *Clin Radiol* 2004;59(5):439–445.

89. Li X, Ma BC, Bolbos RI, Stahl R, Lozano J, Zuo J, Lin K, Link TM, Safran M, Majumdar S. Quantitative assessment of bone marrow edema-like lesion and overlying cartilage in knees with osteoarthritis and anterior cruciate ligament tear using MR imaging and spectroscopic imaging at 3 Tesla. *J Magn Reson Imaging* 2008;28(2):453–461.

90.		Felson DT, McLaughlin S, Goggins J, LaValley MP, Gale ME, Totterman S, Li W, Hill C, Gale D. Bone marrow edema and its relation to progression of knee osteoarthritis. *Ann Intern Med* 2003;139(5 Pt 1):330–336.

91.		Kornaat PR, Bloem JL, Ceulemans RY, Riyazi N, Rosendaal FR, Nelissen RG, Carter WO, Hellio Le Graverand MP, Kloppenburg M. Osteoarthritis of the knee: association between clinical features and MR imaging findings. *Radiology* 2006;239(3):811–817.

92.		Hayes CW, Jamadar DA, Welch GW, Jannausch ML, Lachance LL, Capul DC, Sowers MR. Osteoarthritis of the knee: comparison of MR imaging findings with radiographic severity measurements and pain in middle-aged women. *Radiology* 2005;237(3):998–1007.

93.		Torres L, Dunlop DD, Peterfy C, Guermazi A, Prasad P, Hayes KW, Song J, Cahue S, Chang A, Marshall M, Sharma L. The relationship between specific tissue lesions and pain severity in persons with knee osteoarthritis. *Osteoarthr Cartil* 2006;14(10):1033–1040.

94.		Hunter DJ, Zhang YQ, Niu JB, Tu X, Amin S, Clancy M, Guermazi A, Grigorian M, Gale D, Felson DT. The association of meniscal pathologic changes with cartilage loss in symptomatic knee osteoarthritis. *Arthritis Rheum* 2006;54(3):795–801.

95.		Carrino JA, Blum J, Parellada JA, Schweitzer ME, Morrison WB. MRI of bone marrow edema-like signal in the pathogenesis of subchondral cysts. *Osteoarthr Cartil* 2006;14(10):1081–1085.

96.		Hernandez-Molina G, Guermazi A, Niu J, Gale D, Goggins J, Amin S, Felson DT. Central bone marrow lesions in symptomatic knee osteoarthritis and their relationship to anterior cruciate ligament tears and cartilage loss. *Arthritis Rheum* 2008;58(1):130–136.

97.		Bolbos RI, Ma CB, Link TM, Majumdar S, Li X. In vivo T1rho quantitative assessment of knee cartilage after anterior cruciate ligament injury using 3 Tesla magnetic resonance imaging. *Invest Radiol* 2008;43(11):782–788.

98.		Lohmander LS, Ostenberg A, Englund M, Roos H. High prevalence of knee osteoarthritis, pain, and functional limitations in female soccer players twelve years after anterior cruciate ligament injury. *Arthritis Rheum* 2004;50(10):3145–3152.

99.		von Porat A, Roos EM, Roos H. High prevalence of osteoarthritis 14 years after an anterior cruciate ligament tear in male soccer players: a study of radiographic and patient relevant outcomes. *Ann Rheum Dis* 2004;63(3):269–273.

100.		Johnson DL, Urban WP, Jr, Caborn DN, Vanarthos WJ, Carlson CS. Articular cartilage changes seen with magnetic resonance imaging-detected bone bruises associated with acute anterior cruciate ligament rupture. *Am J Sports Med* 1998;26(3):409–414.

101.		Faber KJ, Dill JR, Amendola A, Thain L, Spouge A, Fowler PJ. Occult osteochondral lesions after anterior cruciate ligament rupture. Six-year magnetic resonance imaging follow-up study. *Am J Sports Med* 1999;27(4):489–494.

102.		Fang C, Johnson D, Leslie MP, Carlson CS, Robbins M, Di Cesare PE. Tissue distribution and measurement of cartilage oligomeric matrix protein in patients with magnetic resonance imaging-detected bone bruises after acute anterior cruciate ligament tears. *J Orthop Res* 2001;19(4):634–641.

103. Mulkern RV, Meng J, Oshio K, Williamson DS, Lilly HS, Guttmann CR, Jaramillo D. Spectroscopic imaging of the knee with line scan CPMG sequences. *J Comput Assist Tomogr* 1995;19(2):247–255.

104. Bao S, Guttmann CR, Mugler JP 3rd, Brookeman JR, Panych LP, Kraft RA, Oshio K, Jaramillo D, Jolesz FA, Williamson DS, Mulkern RV. Spin-echo planar spectroscopic imaging for fast lipid characterization in bone marrow. *Magn Reson Imaging* 1999;17(8):1203–1210.

105. Jensen KE. Magnetic resonance imaging and spectroscopy of the bone marrow *in vivo* — with special attention to the possibilities for tissue characterization in patients with leukemia. *Dan Med Bull* 1992;39(5):369–390.

106. Amano Y, Kumazaki T. Proton MR imaging and spectroscopy evaluation of aplastic anemia: three bone marrow patterns. *J Comput Assist Tomogr* 1997;21(2):286–292.

107. Griffith J, Yeung D, Antonio G, Lee F, Hong A, Wong S, Lau E, Leung, PC. Vertebral bone mineral density, marrow perfusion, and fat content in healthy men and men with osteoporosis: dynamic contrast-enhanced MR imaging and MR spectroscopy. *Radiology* 2005;236(3):945–951.

108. Mulkern R, Meng J, Bowers J, Oshio K, Zuo C, Li H, Kraft R, Williamson D, Jaramillo D. *In vivo* bone marrow lipid characterization with line scan Carr-Purcell-Meiboom-Gill proton spectroscopic imaging. *Magn Reson Imaging* 1997;15(7):823–837.

109. Yeung D, Griffith J, Antonio G, Lee F, Woo J, Leung P. Osteoporosis is associated with increased marrow fat content and decreased marrow fat unsaturation: a proton MR spectroscopy study. *J Magn Reson Imaging* 2005;22(2):279–285.

110. Duque G. Bone and fat connection in aging bone. *Curr Opin Rheumatol* 2008;20(4):429–434.

111. Aspden R, Scheven B, Hutchison J. Osteoarthritis as a systemic disorder including stromal cell differentiation and lipid metabolism. *Lancet* 2001;357(9262): 1118–1120.

112. Cicuttini F, Baker J, Spector T. The association of obesity with osteoarthritis of the hand and knee in women: a twin study. *J Rheumatol* 1996;23(7):1221–1226.

113. Oliveria S, Felson D, Cirillo P, Reed J, Walker A. Body weight, body mass index, and incident symptomatic osteoarthritis of the hand, hip, and knee. *Epidemiology* 1999;10(2):161–166.

114. Grotle M, Hagen K, Natvig B, Dahl F, Kvien T. Obesity and osteoarthritis in knee, hip and/or hand: an epidemiological study in the general population with 10 years follow-up. *BMC Musculoskelet Disord* 2008;9:132.

115. Kalichman L, Li L, Kobyliansky E. Prevalence, pattern and determinants of radiographic hand osteoarthritis in Turkmen community-based sample. *Rheumatol Int* 2009;29(10):1143–1149.

116. Plumb M, Aspden R. High levels of fat and (n-6) fatty acids in cancellous bone in osteoarthritis. *Lipids Health Dis* 2004;18:3–12.

117. Dumond H, Presle N, Terlain B, Mainard D, Loeuille D, Netter P, Pottie P. Evidence for a key role of leptin in osteoarthritis. *Arthritis Rheum* 2003;48(11):3118–3129.

118. Presle N, Pottie P, Dumond H, Guillaume C, Lapicque F, Pallu S, Mainard D, Netter P, Terlain B. Differential distribution of adipokines between serum and synovial

fluid in patients with osteoarthritis. Contribution of joint tissues to their articular production. *Osteoarthr Cartil* 2006;14(7):690–695.

119. Lago R, Gomez R, Otero M, Lago F, Gallego R, Dieguez C, Gomez-Reino J, Gualillo O. A new player in cartilage homeostasis: adiponectin induces nitric oxide synthase type II and pro-inflammatory cytokines in chondrocytes. *Osteoarthr Cartil* 2008;16(9):1101–1109.

120. Wei HW, Sun SS, Jao SH, Yeh CR, Cheng CK. The influence of mechanical properties of subchondral plate, femoral head and neck on dynamic stress distribution of the articular cartilage. *Med Eng Phys* 2005;27(4):295–304.

121. Dequeker J, Mokassa L, Aerssens J, Boonen S. Bone density and local growth factors in generalized osteoarthritis. *Microsc Res Tech* 1997;37(4):358–371.

122. Bolbos RI, Zuo J, Banerjee S, Link TM, Ma CB, Li X, Majumdar S. Relationship between trabecular bone structure and articular cartilage morphology and relaxation times in early OA of the knee joint using parallel MRI at 3 T. *Osteoarthr Cartil* 2008;16(10):1150–1159.

Index